METHODS IN MOLECULAR BIOLOGY

Series Editor
John M. Walker
School of Life and Medical Sciences
University of Hertfordshire
Hatfield, Hertfordshire, AL10 9AB, UK

For further volumes:
http://www.springer.com/series/7651

Proteases and Cancer

Methods and Protocols

Edited by

Santiago Cal and Alvaro J. Obaya

Instituto Universitario de Oncología (IUOPA), Universidad de Oviedo, Oviedo, Asturias, Spain

Humana Press

Editors
Santiago Cal
Instituto Universitario de Oncología (IUOPA)
Universidad de Oviedo
Oviedo, Asturias, Spain

Alvaro J. Obaya
Instituto Universitario de Oncología (IUOPA)
Universidad de Oviedo
Oviedo, Asturias, Spain

ISSN 1064-3745 ISSN 1940-6029 (electronic)
Methods in Molecular Biology
ISBN 978-1-4939-7594-5 ISBN 978-1-4939-7595-2 (eBook)
https://doi.org/10.1007/978-1-4939-7595-2

Library of Congress Control Number: 2017963090

Printed on acid-free paper

This Humana Press imprint is published by Springer Nature
The registered company is Springer Science+Business Media, LLC
The registered company address is: 233 Spring Street, New York, NY 10013, U.S.A.

Preface

Proteases are widely involved in homeostatic processes, and hence they are also important players in different biological settings such as development, apoptosis, reproduction, host defense, or blood coagulation, among others. Consequently, alterations in the activity of these proteolytic enzymes are involved in a plethora of pathological diseases. In fact, proteases are crucial factors in the regulation and maintenance of all biological events regarding tissue wealth and organization, from keeping the correct cellular microenvironment to their involvement in important intracellular processes. As an example to which many of the methods of this volume are aimed, protease activity involvement in cancer has been widely studied since these enzymes have been traditionally associated with tumor development, from escaping tight cellular contact in the original tissue to cell nesting in far away and different cellular environments. However, an increasing number of studies also connect proteolytic activities to tumor-protective effects.

This volume of the *Methods in Molecular Biology* series provides to the readers various methods aimed to unravel the role of proteases belonging to different catalytic classes as well as to fully comprehend their importance in different cellular processes associated with cancer. Potential readers include a broad audience of basic and clinical researchers across different fields including molecular and cellular biologists or oncologists, biochemists, chemists, or physicians. This book also contains suitable applications that could be employed for Ph.D. students in different disciplines of health sciences. All these methods have been arranged in 27 chapters which cover from classical biochemical assays to the more intricate models of 3D imaging of proteolytic activity. In this sense, Chapter 1 describes considerations to be taken at the initial steps of analyzing the complete set of all genes encoding proteolytic enzymes, the degradome of any given species. Chapters 2 and 3 describe protocols to identify specific cleavage sites of proteases. The quantification of protease activity on cell surface or in a mitochondrial environment is described in Chapters 4–6. Chapter 7 includes a protocol for the production of functional catalytic domains of MMPs. Chapters 8–11 are focused in the description of several methods of assaying proteolytic activity and validate biological processes through Western blot and zymography or through the use of fluorogenic substrates. CRISPR/Cas9 system is used as an example of targeting cathepsin B expression in Chapter 12. The validation of protease participation in cellular behavior requires the employment of sophisticated techniques mimicking in vivo situations; some of these using 2D and 3D cellular models are described in Chapters 13–16. Angiogenesis and lymphangiogenesis are processes known to rely on proteolytic activity, and methods to their analysis are shown in Chapters 17–20. Carcinogenesis models for studying protease participation in various types of cancer are explained in Chapter 21, and protocols to detect in vivo imaging of their activity in Chapter 22. The next chapters describe methods to induce silencing of protease genes in order to study mechanisms involved in cancer and aging (Chapter 23), to decipher genetic and epigenetic alterations of metallopeptidases (Chapter 24), to alter the ubiquitin-proteasome system (Chapter 25), or to produce highly selective antibody to be employed as protease inhibitors with a potential therapeutic utility (Chapter 26). In addition, strategies to target metalloproteinases are thoroughly reviewed in the last chapter of this volume (Chapter 27).

We would like all of you to enjoy this volume in which we hope you find protocols and ideas for your research in the proteolytic world. We are especially grateful to all contributors, experts in the field and known for their participation in developing the techniques described herein. We also want to thank Dr. John Walker, editor-in-chief of *Methods in Molecular Biology* series, for his support especially during the first months of the elaboration of this volume.

Oviedo, Spain

Santiago Cal
Alvaro J. Obaya

Contents

Contributors

AHMED AL-SAMADI • *Department of Oral and Maxillofacial Diseases, Clinicum, University of Helsinki, Helsinki, Finland*
HANNA ALA-HONGISTO • *Translational Cancer Biology, Research Programs Unit and Medicum, Faculty of Medicine, University of Helsinki, Helsinki, Finland*
ANDREU ALIBÉS • *Program of Predictive and Personalized Medicine of Cancer, Germans Trias i Pujol Research Institute (PMPPC-IGTP), Barcelona, Spain*
SERGIO ALONSO • *Program of Predictive and Personalized Medicine of Cancer, Germans Trias i Pujol Research Institute (PMPPC-IGTP), Barcelona, Spain*
ÁNGEL ÁLVAREZ-EGUILUZ • *Departamento Bioquímica y Biología Molecular, Instituto Universitario de Oncología (IUOPA), Universidad de Oviedo, Oviedo, Spain*
ALICIA G. ARROYO • *Matrix Metalloproteinases in Angiogenesis and Inflammation Laboratory, Centro Nacional de Investigaciones Cardiovasculares Carlos III (CNIC), Madrid, Spain*
PIRJO ÅSTRÖM • *Cancer and Translational Medicine Research Unit, University of Oulu, Oulu, Finland; Medical Research Center, Oulu University Hospital, Oulu, Finland*
JOSEPH S. BEDNASH • *Department of Medicine, Acute Lung Injury Center of Excellence, University of Pittsburgh, UPMC Montefiore, Pittsburgh, PA, USA*
DENIS BELITSKIN • *Translational Cancer Biology, Research Programs Unit and Medicum, Faculty of Medicine, University of Helsinki, Helsinki, Finland*
SANTIAGO CAL • *Departamento de Bioquímica y Biología Molecular, Instituto Universitario de Oncología (IUOPA), Facultad de Medicina, Universidad de Oviedo, Oviedo, Asturias, Spain*
ANAMARIA ARANHA CAMARGO • *Centro de Oncologia Molecular, Hospital Sírio Libanês, São Paulo, Brazil*
DIANA CAMPOS-IGLESIAS • *Departamento de Bioquímica y Biología Molecular, Instituto Universitario de Oncología (IUOPA), Universidad de Oviedo, Oviedo, Spain*
AASTHA CHHABRA • *Peptide and Proteomics Division, Defence Institute of Physiology and Allied Sciences (DIPAS), DRDO, Delhi, India; Department of Biotechnology, Japyee Institute of Information Technology, Noida, UP, India*
CRISTINA CLEMENTE • *Matrix Metalloproteinases in Angiogenesis and Inflammation Laboratory, Centro Nacional de Investigaciones Cardiovasculares Carlos III (CNIC), Madrid, Spain*
ERICO TOSONI COSTA • *Centro de Oncologia Molecular, Hospital Sírio Libanês, São Paulo, Brazil*
ANDER DÍAZ-NAVARRO • *Departamento Bioquímica y Biología Molecular, Instituto Universitario de Oncología (IUOPA), Universidad de Oviedo, Oviedo, Spain*
TANIA DURRÉ • *Laboratory of Tumor and Developmental Biology, GIGA-Cancer, University of Liège, Liège, Belgium*
YAIZA ESPAÑOL • *Departamento de Bioquímica y Biología Molecular, Facultad de Medicina, Instituto Universitario de Oncología (IUOPA), Universidad de Oviedo, Oviedo, Spain*
ÁLVARO F. FERNÁNDEZ • *Center for Autophagy Research, Department of Internal Medicine, University of Texas Southwestern Medical Center, Dallas, TX, USA*

Rubén Fernández-Rodríguez • *GENYO, Centre for Genomics and Oncological Research, Pfizer/Universidad de Granada/Junta de Andalucía, Granada, Spain*

Alicia R. Folgueras • *Departamento de Bioquímica y Biología Molecular, Facultad de Medicina, Instituto Universitario de Oncología (IUOPA), Universidad de Oviedo, Oviedo, Spain*

Tania Fontanil • *Departamento de Bioquímica y Biología Molecular, Instituto Universitario de Oncología (IUOPA), Universidad de Oviedo, Oviedo, Asturias, Spain*

Julia M. Fraile • *Departamento de Bioquímica y Biología Molecular, Instituto Universitario de Oncología (IUOPA), Universidad de Oviedo, Oviedo, Spain*

José M.P. Freije • *Departamento de Bioquímica y Biología Molecular, Instituto Universitario de Oncología (IUOPA), Universidad de Oviedo, Oviedo, Spain*

Sandra Freitas-Rodríguez • *Departamento de Bioquímica y Biología Molecular, Facultad de Medicina, Instituto Universitario de Oncología (IUOPA), Universidad de Oviedo, Oviedo, Spain*

Melissa García-Caballero • *Laboratory of Tumor and Developmental Biology, GIGA-Cancer, University of Liège, Liège, Belgium*

Juana María García-Pedrero • *Servicio de Otorrinolaringología, Hospital Universitario Central de Asturias and Instituto Universitario de Oncología del Principado de Asturias, (IUOPA) and IISPA Oviedo, Spain; Centro de Investigación Biomédica en Red de Cáncer (CIBERONC), Madrid, Spain*

Marta Garzón-Arango • *Servicio de Otorrinolaringología, Hospital Universitario Central de Asturias and Instituto Universitario de Oncología del Principado de Asturias (IUOPA), Oviedo, Spain*

Xin Ge • *Department of Chemical and Environmental Engineering, University of California, Riverside, CA, USA*

Manu Gnanamony • *Department of Pediatrics, University of Illinois College of Medicine at Peoria, Peoria, IL, USA*

Christopher S. Gondi • *Department of Internal Medicine, University of Illinois College of Medicine at Peoria, Peoria, IL, USA; Department of Surgery, University of Illinois College of Medicine at Peoria, Peoria, IL, USA; Department of Pathology, University of Illinois College of Medicine at Peoria, Peoria, IL, USA*

Beatriz González • *Program of Predictive and Personalized Medicine of Cancer, Germans Trias i Pujol Research Institute (PMPPC-IGTP), Barcelona, Spain*

Adam G. Grieve • *Sir William Dunn School of Pathology, University of Oxford, Oxford, UK*

Ritva Heljasvaara • *Oulu Center for Cell-Matrix Research, Biocenter Oulu, Faculty of Biochemistry and Molecular Medicine, University of Oulu, Oulu, Finland; Department of Biomedicine, Centre for Cancer Biomarkers CCBIO, University of Bergen, Bergen, Norway*

Francisco Hermida-Prado • *Servicio de Otorrinolaringología, Hospital Universitario Central de Asturias and Instituto Universitario de Oncología del Principado de Asturias, (IUOPA), Oviedo, Spain*

Konstantina Karamanou • *Biochemistry, Biochemical Analysis & Matrix Pathobiology Research Group, Laboratory of Biochemistry, Department of Chemistry, University of Patras, Patras, Greece*

Keiji Kikuchi • *Division of Cancer Cell Research, Kanagawa Cancer Center Research Institute, Yokohama, Japan*

Juha Klefström • *Translational Cancer Biology, Research Programs Unit and Medicum, Faculty of Medicine, University of Helsinki, Helsinki, Finland*

NAOHIKO KOSHIKAWA • *Division of Cancer Cell Research, Kanagawa Cancer Center Research Institute, Yokohama, Japan; Institute of Medical Science, University of Tokyo, Tokyo, Japan*

HIROKO KOZUKA-HATA • *Institute of Medical Science, University of Tokyo, Tokyo, Japan*

FRÉDÉRIC KRIDELKA • *Department of Obstetrics and Gynecology, CHU Liège, Liège, Belgium*

KI BAEK LEE • *Department of Chemical and Environmental Engineering, University of California, Riverside, CA, USA*

VLADIMIR LEKSA • *Molecular Immunology Unit, Institute for Hygiene and Applied Immunology, Centre for Pathophysiology, Infectiology & Immunology, Medical University of Vienna, Vienna, Austria; Laboratory of Molecular Immunology, Institute of Molecular Biology, Slovak Academy of Sciences, Bratislava, Slovak Republic*

RAMA K. MALLAMPALLI • *Department of Medicine, Acute Lung Injury Center of Excellence, University of Pittsburgh, UPMC Montefiore, Pittsburgh, PA, USA; Department of Cell Biology and Physiology and Bioengineering, University of Pittsburgh, Pittsburgh, PA, USA; Medical Specialty Service Line, Veterans Affairs Pittsburgh Healthcare System, Pittsburgh, PA, USA*

DIMITRA MANOU • *Biochemistry, Biochemical Analysis and Matrix Pathobiology Research Group, Laboratory of Biochemistry, Department of Chemistry, University of Patras, Patras, Greece*

YAMINA MOHAMEDI • *Departamento de Bioquímica y Biología Molecular, Instituto Universitario de Oncología (IUOPA), Universidad de Oviedo, Oviedo, Asturias, Spain*

ANGELA MONCADA-PAZOS • *Sir William Dunn School of Pathology, University of Oxford, Oxford, UK*

HIDEAKI NAGASE • *Kennedy Institute of Rheumatology, Nuffield Department of Orthopaedics, Rheumatology and Musculoskeletal Sciences, University of Oxford, Oxford, UK*

DONG HYUN NAM • *Department of Chemical and Environmental Engineering, University of California, Riverside, CA, USA*

AGNÈS NOËL • *Laboratory of Tumor and Developmental Biology, GIGA-Cancer, University of Liège, Liège, Belgium*

PIA NYBERG • *Biobank Borealis of Northern Finland, Oulu University Hospital, Oulu, Finland; Medical Research Center, Oulu University Hospital and University of Oulu, Oulu, Finland; Institute of Cancer Research and Translational Medicine, University of Oulu, Oulu, Finland*

ALVARO J. OBAYA • *Departamento de Biología Funcional, Instituto Universitario de Oncología (IUOPA), Facultad de Medicina, Universidad de Oviedo, Oviedo, Asturias, Spain*

CHRISTOPHER M. OVERALL • *Department of Oral Biological and Medical Sciences, Faculty of Dentistry, University of British Columbia, Vancouver, BC, Canada; Centre for Blood Research, University of British Columbia, Vancouver, BC, Canada; Department of Biochemistry and Molecular Biology, University of British Columbia, Vancouver, BC, Canada*

MASAAKI OYAMA • *Institute of Medical Science, University of Tokyo, Tokyo, Japan*

ANUPAMA PAL • *Department of Radiation Oncology, University of Michigan, Ann Arbor, MI, USA*

SHISHIR M. PANT • *Translational Cancer Biology, Research Programs Unit and Medicum, Faculty of Medicine, University of Helsinki, Helsinki, Finland*

MANUEL PERUCHO • *Program of Predictive and Personalized Medicine of Cancer, Germans Trias i Pujol Research Institute (PMPPC-IGTP), Barcelona, Spain*

ZOI PIPERIGKOU • *Biochemistry, Biochemical Analysis & Matrix Pathobiology Research Group, Laboratory of Biochemistry, Department of Chemistry, University of Patras, Patras, Greece*

MARÍA CARMEN DEL PLAZA-CALONGE • *GENYO, Centre for Genomics and Oncological Research, Pfizer/Universidad de Granada/Junta de Andalucía, Granada, Spain*

XOSE S. PUENTE • *Departamento Bioquímica y Biología Molecular, Instituto Universitario de Oncología (IUOPA), Universidad de Oviedo, Oviedo, Spain; Centro de Investigación Biomédica en Red de Cáncer (CIBERONC), Madrid, Spain*

PEDRO M. QUIRÓS • *Centro de Investigación Biomédica en Red de Cáncer (CIBERONC), Madrid, Spain; Departamento de Bioquímica y Biología Molecular, Universidad de Oviedo, Oviedo, Spain*

VIBHA RANI • *Department of Biotechnology, Jaypee Institute of Information Technology, Noida, UP, India*

SILVIA REDONDO-GARCÍA • *GENYO, Centre for Genomics and Oncological Research, Pfizer/Universidad de Granada/Junta de Andalucía, Granada, Spain*

ALNAWAZ REHEMTULLA • *Department of Radiation Oncology, University of Michigan, Ann Arbor, MI, USA*

FRANCISCO JAVIER RODRÍGUEZ-BAENA • *GENYO, Centre for Genomics and Oncological Research, Pfizer/Universidad de Granada/Junta de Andalucía, Granada, Spain*

JUAN CARLOS RODRÍGUEZ-MANZANEQUE • *GENYO, Centre for Genomics and Oncological Research, Pfizer/Universidad de Granada/Junta de Andalucía, Granada, Spain*

ÁLVARO SAHÚN-ESPAÑOL • *Matrix Metalloproteinases in Angiogenesis and Inflammation Laboratory, Centro Nacional de Investigaciones Cardiovasculares Carlos III (CNIC), Madrid, Spain*

TUULA SALO • *Department of Oral and Maxillofacial Diseases, Clinicum, University of Helsinki, Helsinki, Finland; Cancer and Translational Medicine Research Unit, University of Oulu, Oulu, Finland; Medical Research Center, Oulu University Hospital, Oulu, Finland*

YARDENA SAMUELS • *Molecular Cell Biology Department, Weizmann Institute of Science, Rehovot, Israel*

SALVATORE SANTAMARIA • *Centre for Haematology, Imperial College London, London, UK*

VICTORIA SANZ-MORENO • *Tumour Plasticity Laboratory, Randall Division of Cell and Molecular Biophysics, King's College London, London, UK*

HERBERT B. SCHILLER • *Molecular Immunology Unit, Institute for Hygiene and Applied Immunology, Centre for Pathophysiology, Infectiology and Immunology, Medical University of Vienna, Vienna, Austria; Comprehensive Pneumology Center, Helmholtz Zentrum München, Member of the German Center for Lung Research (DZL), Munich, Germany*

MOTOHARU SEIKI • *Institute of Medical Science, University of Tokyo, Tokyo, Japan*

NESTOR SOLIS • *Department of Oral Biological and Medical Sciences, Faculty of Dentistry, University of British Columbia, Vancouver, BC, Canada; Centre for Blood Research, University of British Columbia, Vancouver, BC, Canada*

HANNES STOCKINGER • *Molecular Immunology Unit, Institute for Hygiene and Applied Immunology, Centre for Pathophysiology, Infectiology and Immunology, Medical University of Vienna, Vienna, Austria*

SAÚL ÁLVAREZ TEIJEIRO • *Servicio de Otorrinolaringología, Hospital Universitario Central de Asturias and Instituto Universitario de Oncología del Principado de Asturias, (IUOPA), Oviedo, Spain*
TOPI A. TERVONEN • *Translational Cancer Biology, Research Programs Unit and Medicum, Faculty of Medicine, University of Helsinki, Helsinki, Finland*
ACHILLEAS D. THEOCHARIS • *Biochemistry, Biochemical Analysis and Matrix Pathobiology Research Group, Laboratory of Biochemistry, Department of Chemistry, University of Patras, Patras, Greece*
MAUREEN VAN DE VELDE • *Laboratory of Tumor and Developmental Biology, GIGA-Cancer, University of Liège, Liège, Belgium*
GLORIA VELASCO • *Departamento de Bioquímica y Biología Molecular, Facultad de Medicina, Instituto Universitario de Oncología (IUOPA), Universidad de Oviedo, Oviedo, Spain*
MARÍA ÁNGELES VILLARONGA • *Servicio de Otorrinolaringología, Hospital Universitario Central de Asturias and Instituto Universitario de Oncología del Principado de Asturias, Oviedo, Spain*
VIJAY WALIA • *Laboratory of Cell and Developmental Signaling, National Cancer Institute-Frederick, Frederick, MD, USA*

Chapter 1

Dissecting Degradomes: Analysis of Protease-Coding Genes

Ángel Álvarez-Eguiluz, Ander Díaz-Navarro, and Xose S. Puente

Abstract

Proteases constitute up to 3% of all protein-coding genes in a vertebrate genome and participate in numerous physiological and pathological processes. The characterization of the degradome of one organism, the set of all genes encoding proteolytic enzymes, and the comparison to the degradome of other species have proved useful to identify genetic differences that are helpful to elucidate the molecular basis of diverse biological processes, the different susceptibility to disease, and the evolution of the structure and function of proteases. Here we describe the main procedures involved in the characterization of the degradome of an organism for which its genome sequence is available.

Key words Proteases, Genome, Disease, Bioinformatics

1 Introduction

All living organisms rely on their ability to perform complex molecular reactions which ultimately constitute what we define as life. In order to carry out those reactions, either by replicating their genetic material, obtaining energy, or synthesizing their own biomolecules, cells require the use of specific proteins or nucleic acids with enzymatic activity. Proteases constitute a large group of enzymes which can be detected in all kingdoms of life [1]. Due to their ability to irreversibly hydrolyze peptide bonds, proteases can either activate or inactivate specific proteins, constituting important players in numerous biological processes, such as development, homeostasis, apoptosis, reproduction, or host defense, among others [2]. Furthermore, changes in the activity of proteolytic enzymes are frequently involved in numerous pathological processes, with more than 100 human hereditary diseases caused by mutations in protease-coding genes, and others in which proteases activity is altered [3].

Santiago Cal and Alvaro J. Obaya (eds.), *Proteases and Cancer: Methods and Protocols*, Methods in Molecular Biology, vol. 1731, https://doi.org/10.1007/978-1-4939-7595-2_1, © Springer Science+Business Media, LLC 2018

The study of the set of proteases present in an organism, referred to as the degradome [4], constitutes an important task in biomedical research. Many proteolytic enzymes form complex networks (Fig. 1) involved in specific cellular or physiological processes such as apoptosis, blood coagulation, extracellular matrix remodeling, or food digestion. Differences in protease-coding genes can therefore provide clues about molecular processes that have played a role in the evolution of certain species or help in the identification of pharmacological targets. However, and despite the continuous advances in genome sequencing, the complete characterization of the degradome of an organism is still a poorly automated process, in which expert annotation and curation are usually required.

Although all proteases perform the same catalytic reaction, the hydrolysis of a peptide bond, this activity has evolved independently several times leading to the emergence of numerous proteolytic enzymes with different mechanisms capable of performing this type of reaction [1]. According to their catalytic mechanism, proteases are classified in seven different classes. In cysteine, serine, and threonine proteases, the catalytic nucleophile is the sulfhydryl or hydroxyl group of the corresponding side chain. In aspartic, glutamate, and metalloproteases, an activated water molecule acts as a nucleophile to attack the peptide bond of the substrate, whereas in the recently identified class of asparagine proteases, an asparagine residue is able to form a succinimide ring, cleaving its own peptide bond [5]. Within each catalytic class, proteases are classified in different families and clans based on sequence and structure similarity. Some of these families have originated through the divergent evolution of a common ancestor, while in other cases, proteases from different families within the same catalytic class have evolved independently [1]. This makes the identification of protease-coding genes a complex task because no common sequence motif can be used to query a vertebrate genome to search for all protease-coding genes, as might be the case for other type of protein families, such as cytochromes P450 or protein-tyrosine kinases. In those cases, a simple motif search can yield all possible candidates for those particular families in a specific genome. In this chapter, we will discuss the main procedures used for the study of the degradome of an organism, with special emphasis in vertebrate genomes. We will discuss the most common strategies applied, as well as potential limitations and sources of errors in this type of analysis, providing examples of differential genes identified for each case.

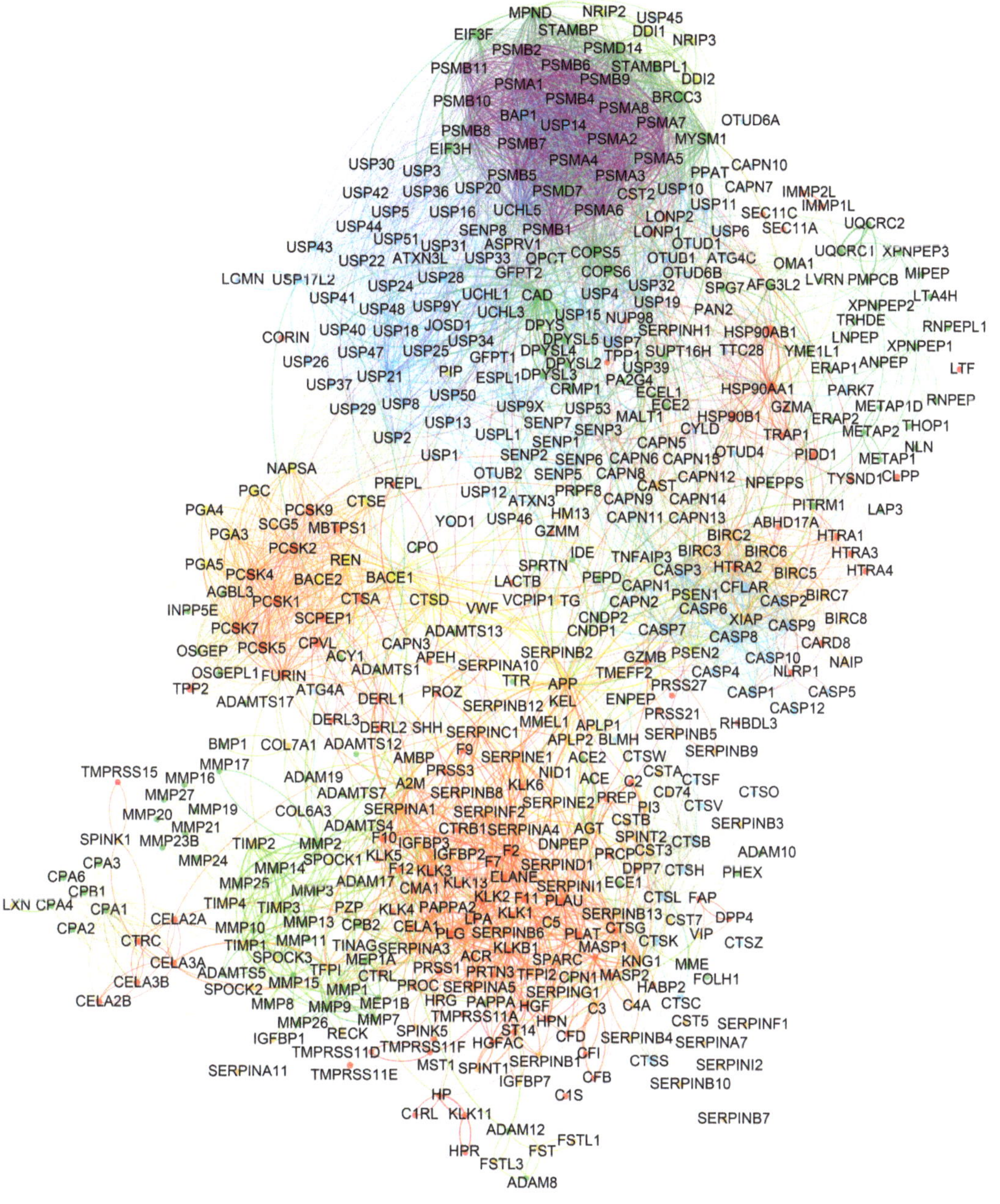

Fig. 1 Human degradome co-occurrence network. Each node represents a protease or protease inhibitor, and connecting lines indicate experimental evidence for the association of those two corresponding proteins. The size of a node is proportional to the number of connections. Stronger connections are represented with thicker edges. Nodes are color coded according to the catalytic class in which the protein appears (yellow, aspartyl proteases; blue, cysteine proteases; green, metalloproteases; red, serine proteases; purple, threonine proteases; and orange, protease inhibitors), and edges have the same color as their source node. Proteins with many pathway associations can be found central to the map. Several clusters of proteases and inhibitors corresponding to specific processes can be detected, including caspases involved in apoptosis on the center right of the figure, proteasome and ubiquitylation on the top, or extracellular matrix remodeling on the left middle bottom

2 Materials

2.1 Databases

Due to the heterogeneity in structure and sequence found in proteolytic enzymes, the first step to characterize the degradome of an organism will rely on the use of specific databases with known proteases and sequences from diverse species. In this regard, the most comprehensive protease database is MEROPS, the peptidase database [6], containing near one million proteases belonging to more than 4500 different species. By contrast, the mammalian degradome database is focused on mammalian proteases, with curated entries for human, chimpanzee, and rodents, as well as with information about major differences between these model organisms and human hereditary diseases caused by mutations in protein-coding genes [3, 7]. Other useful resources include protein family databases such as Pfam or InterPro [8, 9], as well as nucleotide and protein databases such as GenBank or EMBL, where complete or partial sequences from virtually all living organisms exist.

2.2 Sequence Comparison Tools

To study the degradome of a newly sequenced genome, the most common procedure consists in performing sequence comparisons between known proteases in other organisms and the predicted proteins encoded by the target genome. The Basic Local Alignment Search Tool (BLAST) [10] provides enough sensitivity and specificity to detect all orthologous sequences between two evolutionary close organisms. In its TBLASTN configuration, it also allows protein sequence searches against a translated genome, which is useful to identify pseudogenes or search for missing proteases with high sensitivity. BLAST searches can be complemented by the analysis of Hidden Markov Models (HMM) corresponding to protease families, by using programs like HMMER [11].

3 Methods

3.1 Building Degradomes

It is very likely that a set of proteases for the target species has already been annotated in the MEROPS database, which can provide a good starting point to build its degradome (Fig. 2).

Depending on the number of available protease sequences, this information can be used to assess the completeness of the genome to be analyzed and the quality of the assembly. The inability to identify a previously known protease in a newly generated genome reflects that the obtained genome assembly might be incomplete to fully characterize all coding genes. Furthermore, the absence of some exons, or the presence of exons from the same gene in different order and different contigs or chromosomal regions, might

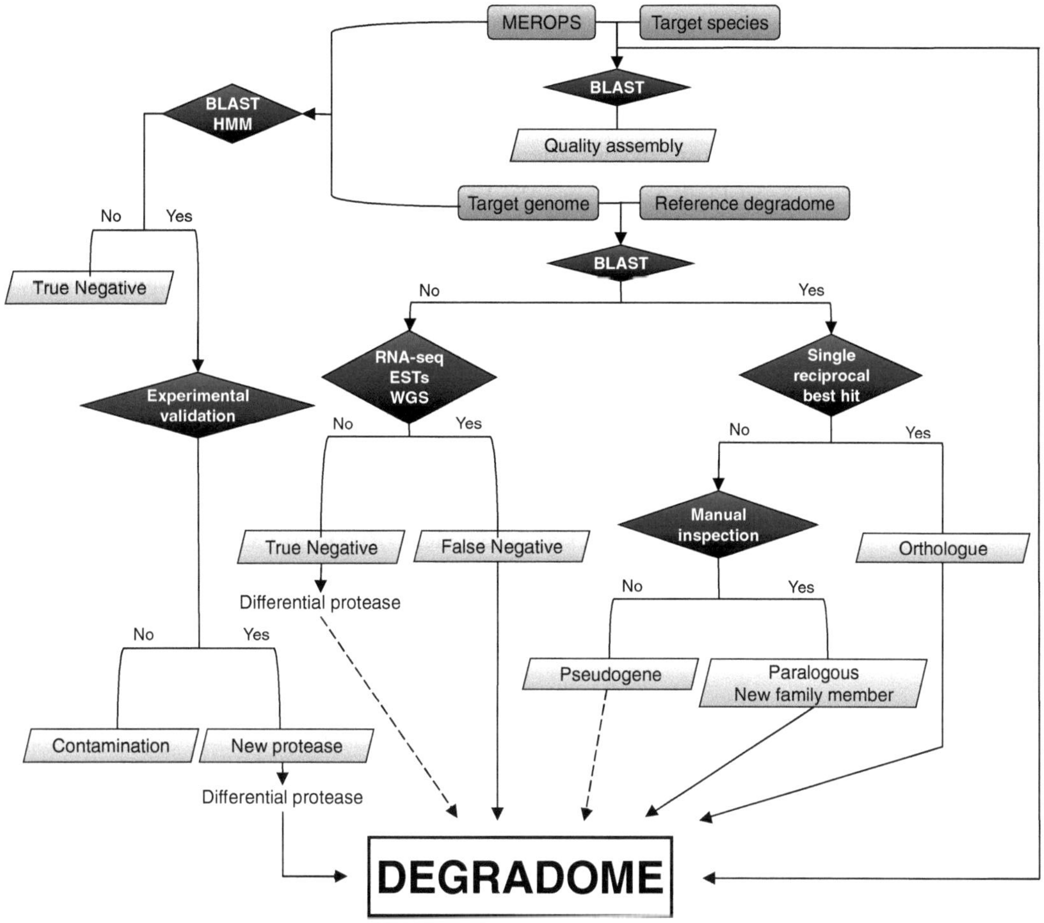

Fig. 2 Flowchart with the main steps involved in the construction of a degradome. The process starts with the search of proteases from the target species in the MEROPS database. Next, BLAST searches are carried out between a reference degradome and the target genome, allowing the detection of most protease-coding genes in the target species. Then, an iterative process using BLAST, TBLASTN, or HMM searches would be included to identify additional family members or new protease families, as well as manual inspection to identify potential false-positive or false-negative hits

also indicate a poor quality assembly. This information about the quality and accuracy of a new generated genome assembly is of outmost importance when trying to interpret differences in the protease repertoire between this species and others, as genome incompleteness, and not true biological changes, might account for some of the differences observed when comparing degradomes.

3.2 Protein Sequence Comparison

Once previously known proteases have been annotated, a second step in the construction of a degradome consists in the comparison with proteases from other related organisms. This step is usually sufficient to classify most proteases present in a particular species, because, despite the existence of more than 260 different families of proteases [6], most organisms from the same class (i.e., mammals) usually contain proteases belonging to the same catalytic families [7, 12, 13]. Therefore, sequence comparison constitutes the most powerful strategy to annotate protease-coding genes from a newly generated genome. Nevertheless, the approaches and potential pitfalls in this strategy largely depend on the type of event that has been acting through evolution. In this regard, we can consider the evolution of protease-coding genes in five different scenarios:

1. In the most simple and frequent scenario, a protease gene has been conserved, and a clear orthologue can be detected within closely related species.
2. A protease is lost due to the accumulation of truncating mutations or to a gene deletion event.
3. A protease or group of proteases is expanded due to gene duplication events.
4. A protease is retained or acquired and is not present in the degradome of the organisms used for comparison.
5. A protease losses its proteolytic activity due to changes in specific catalytic sites.

Although gene evolution can include more possible scenarios, these are the most common ones encountered when building degradomes from vertebrate species, and the type of pitfalls arising when dealing with each type of scenario is different and worth describing herein.

3.3 Identifying One-to-One Orthologues

In the most simple and frequent scenario, a protease gene has been conserved through evolution, so orthologues can be detected within closely related species. For vertebrate organisms, this represents the most common case. Therefore, a direct comparison of proteases from a well-annotated organism such as human, using the BLAST algorithm against the protein sequences predicted from the genome of the query organism, can yield most one-to-one orthologues shared by both species. This approach is both simple to perform and powerful to detect most protease-coding genes in a vertebrate genome (*see* **Note 1**). However, this approach can result in false negatives (failure to identify bona fide orthologues) or false positives (label as protease something that it is not). There are several reasons why a true protease might fail to be detected using this simple approach (*see* **Notes 2** and **3**).

Nevertheless, the most common reason for obtaining false negatives is the quality of the genome assembly. This could cause either the absence of a complete gene, or some of its exons, leading to the classification of the corresponding protease as absent from this organism, or truncated. By this reason, it is important to perform quality control measurements with already known protease-coding genes or at least known protein-coding genes, in order to estimate the completeness of the genome assembly. Furthermore, the existence of additional genomic information, such as RNA-seq data, Expressed Sequence Tags (ESTs), or whole-genome sequence (WGS) from other individuals, provides additional lines of evidence that can be extremely useful when trying to determine whether a gene has been lost or is absent due to limitations of the assembly quality (*see* **Note 4**).

On the other hand, a search for protease orthologues can also result in the appearance of false positives, which is discussed together with the loss of protease genes in Subheading 3.4.

3.4 Loss of Protease-Coding Genes

The birth and death of genes in an organism constitute a qualitative change which sometimes allows us to deduce physiological functions that might have been altered due to this change, such as the loss of a particular proteolytic activity. For instance, loss of the enamel-specific protease MMP20 in avian species can be attributed to the loss of teeth in birds [14], while loss of gastric proteases in platypus is accompanied by the lack of functional stomach in this mammal [12]. Therefore, careful examination of missing proteases can provide important clues to our understanding of evolutionary traits in our species of interest. The two main mechanisms by which a gene can be inactivated includes complete or partial deletion and the accumulation of truncating mutations affecting the coding sequence. Although these alterations are easily identifiable through bioinformatics analysis, manual inspection is highly recommended in order to avoid false positives or negatives. Thus, as mentioned in Subheading 3.1, low-quality assemblies can result in the lack of certain genes or exons from the assembly, giving rise to false negatives. Similarly, sequencing errors can lead to the presence of insertion/deletions or substitutions that might appear as truncating mutations (*see* **Note 5**).

However, the identification of pseudogenes, or the distinction from false positives, is not a trivial process. Gene prediction algorithms might erroneously classify a pseudogene as a protein-coding gene either by reporting a putative transcript in which the mutated/lost exon is skipped or by selecting an alternative splicing site that generates a long open reading frame that otherwise would be disrupted by the presence of a premature stop codon or frameshift mutation in the genome. Therefore, caution must be taken with proteases in which the predicted sequence is shorter by lack of one exon or part of it when compared to the orthologous gene in closer species, as they might constitute potential pseudogenes. In any case, functional validation, either by using RNA-seq to confirm that a truncating variant is expressed, or that a predicted shorter transcript is real, or through experimental validation, is necessary to determine that a protease gene has been pseudogenized in a particular species.

3.5 Gene Duplication and Family Expansion

Similar to gene deletions, the creation of novel members of a family through gene duplication events could help explain some of the processes that have acted during the evolution of this species, shaping its genome. For instance, the number of proteases in mice and rats is 14% and 11% higher than in humans, respectively [7, 13]. Most of these differences are due to the expansion of specific protease families during rodent evolution. They include placental and testin subfamilies of cathepsins, independent expansion of glandular kallikreins in mice and rats, or the expansion of a small cluster of mast cell chymases and granzymes composed of just four genes in humans which have undergone numerous cycles of duplication in rodents, resulting in 17 and 24 genes in mice and rats, respectively [13]. These data show that reproduction and host defense constitute physiological processes on which selection has been acting on during rodent evolution, shaping their genome and degradome composition.

Gene duplication events lead to the generation of paralogous genes. When using protease sequences from one organism (species A) to characterize the degradome of our organism of interest (species B), gene duplication events are detected by the presence of two genes in B with high sequence identity, that when compared back to species A, both genes have the same gene in A as their best hit. In most cases, gene duplication events occur in tandem, and, therefore, two almost identical copies of a gene appear within the same locus. Although this fact could in principle facilitate the identification of duplicated protease-coding genes, in practice the detection and annotation of duplicated genes are challenging. Thus, in the case of very recently duplicated genes, both paralogous genes are almost 100% identical, and this usually leads to both sequences being artificially collapsed into one during the assembly process. Therefore, the ability to detect recently duplicated genes from genome assembly data is relatively low, and our sensitivity increases as more time has passed since the duplication event took place.

An additional factor that must be taken into account for the identification and annotation of duplicated proteases is the fact that most duplication events occur in genomic regions where clusters of protease-coding genes already exist. Usually, together with genes, these regions also contain numerous pseudogenes, as evidence of previous unsuccessful duplications. These complex regions can be error prone during the assembly process, resulting either in the collapse of two genes into one or even the generation of chimeric genes with exons and introns from a gene and a pseudogene. This can cause the formation of unique structures that raise the interest of the researcher but usually do not stand further experimental validation (*see* **Note 6**).

3.6 Proteases Not in the Species of Reference

As mentioned before, the use of a reference degradome from a well-annotated organism can be extremely useful to classify the degradome of another species. However, this approach might reduce the ability to detect proteases which are not present in the reference organism. Therefore, when all orthologous genes have been annotated for a particular protease family, the next step would include an iterative process using BLAST or HMM searches and parsing results to classify all hits as either protease-coding genes or pseudogenes. By performing this iterative step, it is possible to identify additional family members which, despite not being orthologues, share enough sequence similarity to be detected using BLAST or HMM models. An example of this approach is the identification of the aspartyl protease nothepsin in the platypus genome [15]. This protease is involved in processing vitellogenin or other egg-yolk proteins and, although present in all vertebrates and invertebrates which lie eggs, has being pseudogenized in marsupials and eutherians. Nevertheless, by performing sequence similarity searches using human proteases, and analyzing residual results, it is possible to identify additional members that provide information about the biology of monotremas.

Once a protease family is completed, the same iterative process is performed with subsequent families. The overall result of this process would be a list of all proteases encoded by the genome of interest. However, depending on the type of organism, it might contain proteases from families not present in the organism that has been used as reference (human in this case). Therefore, a comparison using BLAST or HMM models for additional protease families is now performed. Due to the fact that some protease families are very specific to certain organisms, including virus, bacteriophages, bacteria, or fungi, most comparisons will yield a negative result. In the case of a positive result, it is strongly required to determine the molecular mechanism by which this protease has been acquired in this organism to prevent inclusion of false positives (*see* **Note 7**).

3.7 Functional Genes Losing Proteolytic Activity

About 20% of all human genes evolutionary derived from protease-coding genes lack proteolytic activity and are referred to as non-protease homologues. Orthologues in other organisms usually share this lack of proteolytic activity. However, there are some examples, such as caspase 12, in which this gene encodes a functional protease in rodents and chimpanzee, while in some human populations is a non-protease homologue conferring higher risk of sepsis, while in other human populations is a pseudogene due to the presence of a premature stop codon [16, 17]. Therefore, once sequences corresponding to proteolytic genes have been compiled, an analysis of residues involved in catalytic activity might help to identify genes that might have lost their proteolytic activity in our species of interest. The use of programs to identify protein families such as Pfam or InterPro, as well as multiple sequence alignments, can facilitate this process.

3.8 Data Integration

Finally, in order to identify changes in individual genes that might be responsible for specific evolutionary traits in one species, literature is reviewed to determine the function of differential proteases identified in this analysis. The existence of diseases or phenotypes associated with changes in a gene in humans or other species or the effect of knocking out a gene in a model organism can provide evidence for its participation in specific traits observed in the target species. Depending on the evolutionary distance between compared species, the ability to unequivocally associate a gene change to a particular trait or phenotype can be challenging. Closer species will have few or even no changes in their degradomes, allowing a more in-depth study of the potential consequences of these changes. By contrast, as further apart two species are, more differential proteases and more phenotypic changes between them will be detected, making the genotype-phenotype association more difficult to interpret.

4 Notes

1. A common source of noise in the identification of proteases by performing BLAST searches between a known protease and the genome of the target organism is the presence of pseudogenes, either processed or unprocessed, for that protease in the target genome. Pseudogenes can make more difficult the identification of true orthologues, requiring additional steps to annotate a particular protease. A common procedure to establish the most likely orthologous sequence will involve the analysis of shared synteny by looking at flanking genes to the protease gene of interest. Although chromosomal rearrangements might have split an ancestral block in different blocks, synteny is usually conserved between organisms that diverged up to hundreds of millions of years ago, providing a good reference point to determine which of the multiple sequence hits might be the most likely orthologue. The classification of the rest of sequence

hits in either gene duplications or pseudogenes is discussed in Subheadings 3.4 and 3.5.

2. One reason to obtain false negatives is that our protein-protein comparison was relying on the protein sequences predicted from our genome, and those predictions failed to identify one of the protease-coding genes in the genome. If that is the case, an alternative approach is to perform a sequence alignment between the human protein and the DNA sequence of our genome using an algorithm such as TBLASTN. If there is a gene encoding an orthologous protease, this procedure will allow us to identify exons corresponding to this gene. With this information, it is possible to reconstruct the protein sequence corresponding to the missing protease.
3. In other cases, the inability to detect a protease when performing a sequence comparison against a human protease might be due to both species being too distantly related or one of those genes evolving under positive selection. In the case of using human proteins as queries and failing to get the corresponding orthologue, it can be helpful to use as query the orthologue from a more evolutionary closer organism, as the number of changes between those species will be lower than with a more distantly related organism. For genes evolving under positive selection, the number of non-synonymous substitutions at non-synonymous sites will be higher than the number of synonymous substitutions at synonymous sites. However, by using a protein sequence from an evolutionary closer organism, it would be possible to identify that protease, as the expected number of variant sites is small.
4. RNA-seq data, or even WGS data from the same individual or additional individuals, is nowadays easy to generate and provides an independent set of sequences in which to confirm or discard findings obtained from the analysis of a genome assembly. In general, these massive approaches provide a fast and cost-effective alternative to validate findings obtained by analyzing a single assembly. Thus, searching for proteases which are missing from the assembly, by using RNA-seq or WGS data, can lead to the detection of reads corresponding to the orthologous protease, suggesting that a gap in the assembly, and not a gene deletion, is the most likely cause for its absence in the analyzed genome.
5. To distinguish between true truncating mutations and sequencing errors, availability of additional sequence data (either RNA-seq or WGS) can provide an independent line of evidence to distinguish between true deletions or mutations and lack of coverage or sequencing errors in the genome assembly.

6. Experimental validation of genes or variants within highly repetitive regions can be challenging when using PCR. Primers will likely anneal to different genes/pseudogenes preventing a clear result. Although cumbersome, the use of BACs or fosmids can overcome some of the intrinsic difficulties which are faced when validating results from regions showing a high percentage of identity.
7. The identification of a protease from a family not present in other evolutionary closer organisms might indicate that either this protease has been retained during evolution and lost in the remaining species, that is the result of horizontal gene transfer (HGT), or that it has appeared due to contamination of the sample with parasites or molecular biology reagents. For instance, blood-borne parasites constitute a source of contamination that can lead to the identification of false HGT events. Thus, if the DNA sample for sequencing was obtained from blood from an individual which was infected by a blood-borne parasite such as a virus, a bacteria, or a protozoan, DNA from that parasite will be also extracted and sequenced. This might result in the presence of genes from that parasite in the final genome assembly, leading to the identification of potential HGT events. Although HGT cannot be discarded, the presence of numerous genes from the same parasite in a genome assembly of its host is most likely due to sample contamination with the parasite than to HGT. Nevertheless, experimental validation would be required to determine whether HGT or sample contamination is responsible for the presence of otherwise alien proteases in the genome of our species of interest.

References

1. Rawlings ND, Barrett AJ (1993) Evolutionary families of peptidases. Biochem J 290:205–218
2. Lopez-Otin C, Bond JS (2008) Proteases: multifunctional enzymes in life and disease. J Biol Chem 283(45):30433–30437. https://doi.org/10.1074/jbc.R800035200
3. Perez-Silva JG, Espanol Y, Velasco G et al (2016) The Degradome database: expanding roles of mammalian proteases in life and disease. Nucleic Acids Res 44(D1):D351–D355. https://doi.org/10.1093/nar/gkv1201
4. Lopez-Otin C, Overall CM (2002) Protease degradomics: a new challenge for proteomics. Nat Rev Mol Cell Biol 3(7):509–519. https://doi.org/10.1038/nrm858
5. Rawlings ND, Barrett AJ, Bateman A (2011) Asparagine peptide lyases: a seventh catalytic type of proteolytic enzymes. J Biol Chem 286(44):38321–38328. https://doi.org/10.1074/jbc.M111.260026
6. Rawlings ND, Barrett AJ, Finn R (2016) Twenty years of the MEROPS database of proteolytic enzymes, their substrates and inhibitors. Nucleic Acids Res 44(D1):D343–D350. https://doi.org/10.1093/nar/gkv1118
7. Puente XS, Sanchez LM, Overall CM et al (2003) Human and mouse proteases: a comparative genomic approach. Nat Rev Genet 4(7):544–558. https://doi.org/10.1038/nrg1111
8. Finn RD, Coggill P, Eberhardt RY et al (2016) The Pfam protein families database: towards a more sustainable future. Nucleic Acids Res 44(D1):D279–D285. https://doi.org/10.1093/nar/gkv1344
9. Finn RD, Attwood TK, Babbitt PC et al (2017) InterPro in 2017-beyond protein

family and domain annotations. Nucleic Acids Res 45(D1):D190–D199. https://doi.org/10.1093/nar/gkw1107

10. Altschul SF, Gish W, Miller W et al (1990) Basic local alignment search tool. J Mol Biol 215(3):403–410. https://doi.org/10.1016/S0022-2836(05)80360-2
11. Mistry J, Finn RD, Eddy SR et al (2013) Challenges in homology search: HMMER3 and convergent evolution of coiled-coil regions. Nucleic Acids Res 41(12):e121. https://doi.org/10.1093/nar/gkt263
12. Ordonez GR, Hillier LW, Warren WC et al (2008) Loss of genes implicated in gastric function during platypus evolution. Genome Biol 9(5):R81. https://doi.org/10.1186/gb-2008-9-5-r81
13. Puente XS, Lopez-Otin C (2004) A genomic analysis of rat proteases and protease inhibitors. Genome Res 14(4):609–622. https://doi.org/10.1101/gr.1946304
14. Quesada V, Velasco G, Puente XS et al (2010) Comparative genomic analysis of the zebra finch degradome provides new insights into evolution of proteases in birds and mammals. BMC Genomics 11:220. https://doi.org/10.1186/1471-2164-11-220
15. Warren WC, Hillier LW, Marshall Graves JA et al (2008) Genome analysis of the platypus reveals unique signatures of evolution. Nature 453(7192):175–183. https://doi.org/10.1038/nature06936
16. Puente XS, Gutierrez-Fernandez A, Ordonez GR et al (2005) Comparative genomic analysis of human and chimpanzee proteases. Genomics 86(6):638–647. https://doi.org/10.1016/j.ygeno.2005.07.009
17. Saleh M, Vaillancourt JP, Graham RK et al (2004) Differential modulation of endotoxin responsiveness by human caspase-12 polymorphisms. Nature 429(6987):75–79. https://doi.org/10.1038/nature02451

Chapter 2

Identification of Protease Cleavage Sites and Substrates in Cancer by Carboxy-TAILS (C-TAILS)

Nestor Solis and Christopher M. Overall

Abstract

Determination of drug targets and development of novel therapeutics for the treatment of different cancers are actively ongoing areas of research. Proteases being the second largest group of enzymes in humans present themselves as attractive targets for blocking and activation to treat malignancies. However, determination of the protease cleavage substrates is often missed by utilizing conventional modern proteomic approaches. The relatively low abundance of proteolytically processed, and mostly semi-tryptic, peptides compared to tryptic peptides generated in shotgun proteomics compounded with their poorer identification rates makes the identification of such critical peptides challenging and so are mostly overlooked. Our laboratory introduced Terminal Amine Isotopic Labeling of Substrates (TAILS) to identify N-terminal peptides from cleavage events. In this chapter we present a protocol from our complementary method carboxy-TAILS (C-TAILS) to identify C-terminal peptides in metabolically labeled cancer cell lines.

Key words Proteolysis, Proteolytic regulation, Metabolic labeling, Protease substrate

1 Introduction

Proteins have been classically characterized as the molecular effectors of the cell—the products of genes that catalyze all necessary reactions for life or provide structural components that the cell utilizes for form and function. As cancer is not a single disease, but rather a summation of dysregulated events in the cell, it is unsurprising to see that proteins have modified spatiotemporal expression and aberrant posttranslational modifications in comparison to healthy tissue counterpart cells [1]. Protein phosphorylation in cancer has been well studied with critical pathways identified by dysregulated phosphorylation/dephosphorylation levels such as the MAPK pathway [2]. Glycosylation has also emerged as an important posttranslational modification on the cancer cell surface with examples of increased sialylation on terminal sugars of complex polysaccharide chains attached to proteins on cellular surfaces which modify their interaction with the extracellular matrix and

Santiago Cal and Alvaro J. Obaya (eds.), *Proteases and Cancer: Methods and Protocols*, Methods in Molecular Biology, vol. 1731, https://doi.org/10.1007/978-1-4939-7595-2_2, © Springer Science+Business Media, LLC 2018

can aid cancer cells in invasion [3, 4]. However, the most overlooked yet most abundant posttranslational modification is proteolytic processing. There are over 500 proteases in humans, making them the second largest group of enzymes in humans, and they control a plethora of biological aspects required for life [5]. Proteases and peptidases act as a concerted network—the protease web [6]—which is tightly controlled to result in highly tuned modulators responsible for key processes, notably, coagulation, apoptosis, and complement activation as the classically studied pathways. However, proteolytic processing is a key regulator of cytokine and other bioactive mediator functions involved in tissue homeostasis and its dysregulation in cancer. This is still an active area of research with a high potential for development of therapeutics. It is important to note that 5–10% of all drugs against different human diseases target the protease class of enzymes [7].

The method of choice for systematically identifying and quantifying proteins is mass spectrometry-based proteomics [8]. Methods for extracting, tryptically digesting, and utilizing increasingly powerful mass spectrometers and bioinformatic tools have made it possible to profile entire proteomes with unprecedented accuracy, confidence, and speed [9]. When comparing tumors and cell lines to normal or wild-type counterparts using bottom-up approaches, whole proteomes are extracted and digested with trypsin into peptides—which are far more amenable to liquid chromatography tandem mass spectrometry-based (LS-MS/MS) analyses due to their chromatographic properties, ionization characteristics, and beneficial fragmentation patterns due to these peptides ending in arginine or lysine [10]. Yet, these workflows which are becoming routine for biochemistry labs across the world do not allow for the identification of cleavage sites in substrates due to these species being (1) less abundant compared to internally generated tryptic peptides and (2) having semi-tryptic cleavage sites which are frequently missed by bioinformatic search tools [11]. As such, when attempting to decipher the role of particular endo- or exopeptidases, the location of cleavage will be lost in an expansive sea of tryptic peptides that do not inform of proteolytic regulation. Consequently, these cleaved peptides as hallmarks of substrate cleavages must be enriched.

We have presented a method for determining cleavage sites N-terminally, termed Terminal Amine Isotopic Labeling of Substrates (TAILS) [12, 13]. Here we show a complementary protocol for determining cleavage sites C-terminally using a negative selection method—carboxy-TAILS (C-TAILS) (Fig. 1) [14]. Identification of the cleavage site by both methods provides validation of proteolytic processing and can be validated biochemically. Proteomes are extracted and blocked at their cysteines to prevent aggregate formation. Primary amines (lysines and N termini) are blocked via a dimethylation reaction or acetylation reaction [15], to prevent the cross-reactivity at the subsequent carboxylic acid

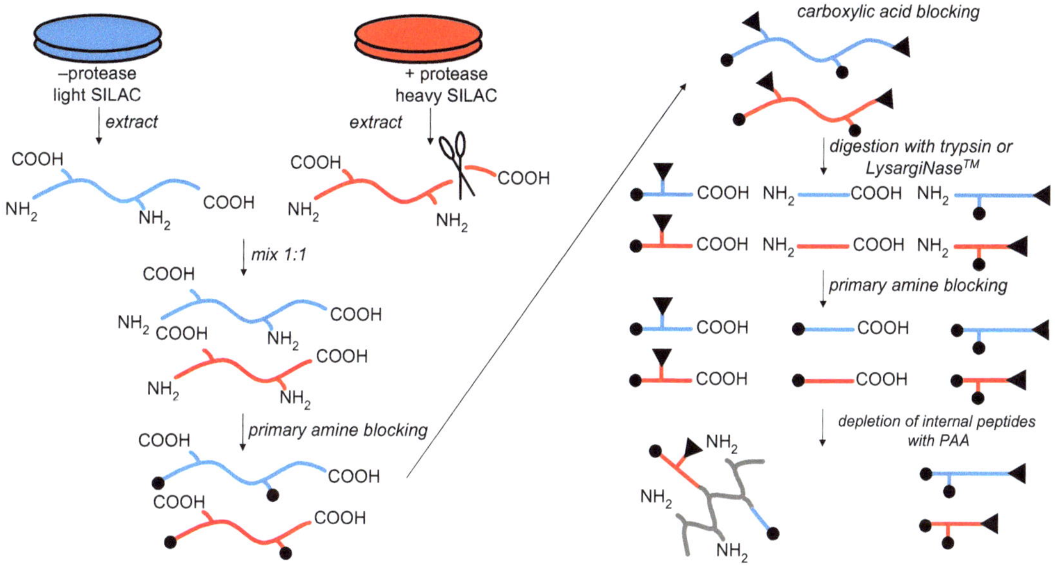

Fig. 1 Carboxy-TAILS (C-TAILS). Cancer cell lines are grown in light or heavy SILAC conditions. Here blue represents the light labeled cell line lacking the protease of interest, while in red is the cell line with the activity of said protease. Proteomes are extracted, reduced, and alkylated (not shown for simplicity) and then mixed at equal amounts which enables robust quantification. Primary amines are blocked using reductive dimethylation, and carboxylic acids are then blocked using EDAC/s-NHS chemistry. Proteins are then digested into peptides generating new primary amines and carboxylic acids. Newly formed primary amines are blocked using reductive dimethylation. Peptides with freely available carboxylic acids are depleted using a polyallylamine (PAA) polymer using EDAC chemistry, and unreacted peptides are recovered by ultrafiltration for LC-MS/MS analysis

labeling step. Carboxylic acids when activated react with primary amines, which, if coming from peptides and proteins, can lead to the formation of aggregates that are not amenable for analysis. Following cleanup, the amine-labeled proteins are activated with EDAC and s-NHS to react their carboxylic acids (glutamate, aspartate, and C termini) with a tag—in this method ethanolamine. There are novel developments in tags that can increase C-terminal peptide identification, and the reader is welcome to explore those avenues [16].

The presence of a tag at the C terminus of the protein allows for negative selection of the protein's natural C-terminal peptide and neo-C-terminal peptide generated after protease cleavage and as a marker to qualify which peptides are bona fide C-terminal peptides. Proteomes are precipitated and digested with trypsin. We also presented LysargiNase™ as a protease suitable for proteomic analysis due to its ability to cleave specifically N-terminally to arginines and lysines, thus providing complementary coverage to trypsin and enhancing C-terminal peptide identification, while retaining beneficial properties for these peptides for LC-MS/MS which otherwise would have been lost with trypsin [17].

Trypsin or LysargiNase™ digestion into peptides forms new primary amines and carboxylic acids. Peptide amines are blocked for the same reasons as at the protein level, and this also allows for the introduction of an isotopic or isobaric tag if performing sample comparisons by relative quantification. Alternately, SILAC labeling can be performed for quantitative analyses. Hence, the peptide mixture is composed of amine-blocked peptides that either (a) have a C-terminal tag introduced at the protein level which correspond to the true ends of proteins or (b) peptides with no C-terminal tag and are internal tryptic or LysargiNase™ peptides that we aim to deplete. A polyallylamine polymer can then react with the latter class of peptides using the same EDAC/s-NHS chemistry leaving behind the initially C-terminally tagged peptides. These C-terminally tagged peptides are isolated from the polymer using a spin filter device with a large molecular weight cutoff and can be analyzed by LC-MS/MS and later identified by database search engines.

2 Materials

2.1 Metabolic Labeling and Cell Culture Reagents

1. Arginine- and lysine-free DMEM or RPMI (dependent on cell type).
2. Dialyzed fetal bovine serum (FBS).
3. Cell culture supplements as required (antibiotics, nonessential amino acids, etc.).
4. Cell culture grade amino acids: "light" L-leucine (Leu0) and "heavy" $^{13}C_6$ L-leucine (Leu6).
5. Phosphate-buffered saline buffer (PBS): 137 mM NaCl, 2.7 mM KCl, 10 mM Na_2HPO_4, and 1.8 mM KH_2PO_4 in water.
6. 10× EDTA solution: 100 mM ethylenediaminetetraacetic acid in water.
7. Cell lysis buffer (e.g., RIPA buffer).
8. Protease inhibitor cocktail.

2.2 Proteome Preparation Reagents

1. Protein quantification kit.
2. DTT solution: 1 M dithiothreitol in water.
3. IAA solution: 500 mM iodoacetamide in water.
4. Methanol.
5. Chloroform.
6. Chemically resistant conical tubes (15 mL volume).
7. GuCl solution: 6 M guanidinium chloride in water.
8. NaOH solution 1: 1 M sodium hydroxide in water.
9. NaOH solution 2: 0.1 M sodium hydroxide in water.

10. HEPES buffer 1: 1 M 4-(2-hydroxyethyl)-1-piperazineethanesulfonic acid in water, pH 7.5.
11. HEPES buffer 2: 200 mM 4-(2-hydroxyethyl)-1-piperazineethanesulfonic acid in water, pH 7.5.

2.3 Amine and Carboxylic Acid Derivatizing Reagents

1. Formaldehyde solution: 2 M CH_2O in water.
2. Sodium cyanoborohydride solution: 1 M $NaBH_3CN$ in water.
3. Formic acid (1%).
4. MES buffer 1: 400 mM 2-(*N*-morpholino)ethanesulfonic acid in water, pH 5.0.
5. MES buffer 2: 1 M 2-(*N*-morpholino)ethanesulfonic acid in water, pH 5.0.
6. Ethanolamine hydrochloride solution: 1 M C_2H_7NO (ethanolamine salt) in water.
7. EDAC solution: 800 mM 1-ethyl-3-(3-dimethylaminopropyl) carbodiimide in DMSO.
8. s-NHS solution: 500 mM sulfo-N-hydroxysuccinimide in DMSO.
9. Dimethyl sulfoxide (DMSO).

2.4 Digestion Enzymes

1. Sequencing-grade trypsin.
2. Calcium chloride solution: 1 M $CaCl_2$ in water.
3. LysargiNase™ (sequencing grade) (http://www.sbu.csic.es/research-groups/proteolysis-lab/lysarginase/#price-and-availability).

2.5 Polymer Depletion and Peptide Purification Reagents

1. PAA polymer solution: 30 mM polyallylamine polymer in water.
2. Spin-filter ultrafiltration device with 30,000 Da molecular weight cutoff.

2.6 Data Acquisition and Analysis Platforms

1. Liquid chromatography (C_{18}) tandem mass spectrometry system capable of performing high-throughput peptide identification analysis, e.g., Q-TOF platforms, Orbitrap systems, etc.
2. Database search engine and software package—we recommend the freely available MaxQuant software [18].

3 Methods

The method shown here describes a two-way comparison (often wild-type and protease knockout) but can be expanded to more channels utilizing appropriate isotopic or isobaric labeling techniques, for example, treatment with protease inhibitors. We recommend firstly attempting this protocol with no metabolic or isobaric labeling—using only inexpensive dimethylation reagents—to ensure the technique is optimal for the experimental settings of the researcher before embarking on the costlier SILAC or isobaric tagging reagents. Furthermore, due to the nature of this protocol, we advise using metabolic labeling as it enables easier processing and increased robustness for quantification.

3.1 Metabolic Labeling of Cancer Cell Lines

1. Prepare cell growth medium with required media component (RPMI, DMEM, etc.) depleted of arginine and lysine. Supplement media with isotopically labeled light L-leucine (Leu0) for condition 1 (henceforth termed "wild type") and with isotopically heavy $^{13}C_6$ L-leucine (Leu6) for condition 2 (henceforth termed "knockout"). Supplement media with heat-inactivated 10% dialyzed FBS and other additives as required (e.g., antibiotics).
2. Grow wild-type and knockout cells in their respective media to conditions desired. Cells are to be grown in fresh media for every doubling for at least five doublings to ensure complete incorporation of amino acids.
3. Ensure that cells have been completely metabolically labeled. An aliquot of cells can be extracted at five doublings and digested for LC-MS analysis. Database searching should reveal the percentage of peptides that converted to the heavy form. Labeling must be in excess of 98% for accurate quantification.
4. Once labeling is confirmed to be complete for the heavy amino acid-containing cell line, appropriate chemical or biological treatment can be performed. In this method, wild-type and protease knockout cancer cells will be compared.
5. For a T75 dish, wash cells with phosphate-buffered saline (PBS) three times (10 mL) and lyse with RIPA buffer (700 μL) containing 10 mM EDTA (1:10 dilution of EDTA solution) and protease inhibitor cocktail. Scrape cells off the cell culture flask and do not use trypsin for lifting the cells as it will interfere with downstream analysis (*see* **Note 1**).
6. Lyse cells on ice and use a tip-probe sonicator to burst cells and shear DNA which interferes with downstream analysis.
7. Take an aliquot of each wild-type and knockout lysates and perform a protein quantification procedure of choice (typically BCA assay) and mix lysates at 1:1 ratio in order to have 1.5–2.0 mg of protein in 1 mL volume to begin chemical labeling (*see* **Note 2**).

3.2 Proteome Preparation and Purification for 1 mL Volume

1. Cysteines must be blocked to prevent formation of protein aggregates due to disulfide bonding. Prepare 100 μL fresh stock of DTT solution and add 10 μL to the lysate and incubate at 37 °C for 1 h to reduce proteins. Final concentration of DTT is 10 mM.

2. Prepare 100 μL fresh stock of IAA solution and add 20 μL to the lysate and incubate at 25 °C for 30 min in the dark. Final concentration of IAA is 20 mM.
3. Quench by adding DTT solution again as in Subheading 3.2, **step 1**.
4. Protein lysates must be precipitated prior to the next step as it is sensitive to the presence of primary amines. The investigator is welcome to use any protein precipitation method of his/her choice. Here we quickly describe the usage of Wessel and Flugge's chloroform/methanol method for 1 mL volumes [19]:
   (a) Transfer lysate to 15-mL-sized chemically resistant conical tubes (~1 mL).
   (b) Add 3 mL water.
   (c) Add 4 mL ice-cold methanol. Vortex vigorously.
   (d) Add 1 mL chloroform. Vortex vigorously.
   (e) Centrifuge in a swing-bucket rotor at 3000 × *g* for 5 min to separate into three phases.
   (f) Carefully pipette into waste the top layer.
   (g) The interphase which consists of purified protein is then transferred carefully to a microfuge tube (*see* **Note 3**).
   (h) Add 1000 μL methanol, vortex vigorously, and centrifuge at 9000 × *g* for 2 min at 4 °C.
   (i) Remove the supernatant into waste and repeat the methanol washing two more times to ensure removal of contaminants.
5. Following protein precipitation, the pellet is resuspended in 500 μL of GuCl solution. If protein does not fully resuspend, add NaOH solution 1 in 100 μL aliquots or alternatively briefly tip-probe sonicate to ensure solubilization. Add 200 μL of HEPES buffer 1 and make up to 1 mL with water.

3.3 Protein-Level Dimethylation

Protein-level labeling is as in TAILS and is required for C-TAILS as carboxylic acids on proteins cannot be labeled in one step due to the lack of reactivity of these groups. The most effective way of reacting carboxylic acids in aqueous conditions is by condensation reactions of the carboxylic acid with primary amines. As such, protein amines must be made unavailable such that they do not react with the carboxylic acids in their direct proximity. Primary amines on proteins are reacted with formaldehyde in a fast, effective, and inexpensive reaction, and as such this step requires having no primary amines in the buffers (e.g., Tris is not permitted) and small primary amine molecules available from the lysate (e.g., freely available amino acids and nucleic acids).

1. Prepare 100 μL of the following solutions fresh: sodium cyanoborohydride solution and formaldehyde solution.
2. Add 22 μL formaldehyde solution and immediately after add 22 μL of sodium cyanoborohydride solution, mix, and incubate at 37 °C for 3 h. Final concentration of formaldehyde is 80 mM. Final concentration of sodium cyanoborohydride is 40 mM.
3. Acidify with 1% formic acid to a final concentration of 0.1% and incubate at room temperature for 1 h. Excess reagents will react to form bubbles.
4. Perform protein precipitation of choice or as in Subheading 3.2, **step 4**.

3.4 Protein-Level Amidation

Primary amines on proteins being blocked now permit the tagging of the C terminus which permits inference of the biologically occurring end of the protein by mass spectrometry in later stages. The chemistry employed is an amidation reaction utilizing a small primary amine molecule to attach to the C-terminal end of proteins and peptides which prevent these species being captured by the polymer employed at a latter stage. This is performed using 1-ethyl-3-(3-dimethylaminopropyl)carbodiimide (EDAC) and sulfo-N-hydroxysuccinimide (s-NHS). EDAC activates carboxylic acids to make them more reactive and is stabilized by s-NHS to form an amine-reactive intermediate which is available for reaction with the primary amine used for tagging. Unfortunately, EDAC is unstable in aqueous solution, thus requiring multiple addition steps to push the reaction in the forward direction.

1. Resuspend the protein pellet in 200 μL of GuCl solution and ensure it is solubilized. Avoid adding basic solutions and tip-probe sonicate as required.
2. Add 200 μL of MES buffer 1. Ensure that final pH is still 5.0.
3. Prepare 150 μL of EDAC solution, s-NHS solution, and ethanolamine solution (*see* **Note 4**).
4. Add 25 μL s-NHS solution and 25 μL EDAC solution to the protein solution, and incubate at 25 °C for 30 min. Final concentration of s-NHS is 50 mM. Final concentration of EDAC is 80 mM.
5. Add 25 μL ethanolamine solution. Final concentration of ethanolamine is 200 mM.
6. Vortex vigorously and spin down (*see* **Note 5**). Incubate for 1 h at 25 °C.
7. Add equivalent amounts as in Subheading 3.4 **step 4**, and incubate for an additional hour at 25 °C.

8. Repeat as in Subheading 3.4 **step 7** and incubate overnight at 25 °C.
9. Perform a protein precipitation of choice or as in Subheading 3.2, **step 4**.

3.5 Proteome Digestion

As with all bottom-up proteomic approaches, proteins are digested, albeit they have been tagged prior to this step. Peptides generated will either have the C-terminal tag—our peptides of interest—or will be unmodified. A complementary strategy of trypsin is our recently introduced protease, LysargiNase™, which makes for increased coverage and better ionization properties of C-terminal peptides [17]. Digestion with either enzyme generates new primary amines and new carboxylic acids. As at the protein level, these primary amines need to be blocked to prevent cross-reactions. Internal tryptic or LysargiNase™ peptides bearing a freely available carboxylic acid are later removed by an amine-containing polymer.

1. Resuspend protein pellet in 50–100 μL of GuCl solution and tip-probe sonicate. Dilute to a final volume of 1000 μL with HEPES buffer 2.
2. Add 10 μL of calcium chloride solution. Final concentration of 10 mM $CaCl_2$.
3. Split the sample into two separate tubes, one for trypsin and the other for LysargiNase™.
4. Add trypsin in a protease-to-substrate ratio of 1:100 (w/w), while LysargiNase™ is added in a protease-to-substrate ratio of 1:25 (w/w).
5. Incubate at 37 °C overnight. LysargiNase™ is a thermostable enzyme and can be incubated up to 54 °C for faster digestion or to aid denaturation of digestion-recalcitrant proteins.
6. Add half the protease amount from Subheading 3.5, **step 4** and digest further for 2 h.

3.6 Peptide-Level Dimethylation

This step is required to not only prevent cross-linking at the next step but also is the step where isobaric and isotopic labeling happens if not performing metabolic labeling. In this method the samples have been metabolically labeled which allowed for their mixing at the very beginning of the process. However, in many cases direct metabolic labeling might not be applicable, and while application of techniques such as super-SILAC is relevant [20], chemical tagging might be appropriate where multiplexing is desired. As such, each channel must be dealt separately from the beginning until this stage which incurs variability between channels and less quantitative accuracy. However, if chemical labeling is to be performed, do so here using isotopically coded dimethylation tags, isobaric tagging via iTRAQ or TMT, etc.

1. Prepare 100 μL of the following solutions fresh: sodium cyanoborohydride solution and formaldehyde solution.
2. Add 22 μL formaldehyde solution and immediately after add 22 μL of sodium cyanoborohydride solution, mix, and incubate at 37 °C for 3 h. Final concentration of formaldehyde is 80 mM. Final concentration of sodium cyanoborohydride is 40 mM.
3. Acidify with 1% formic acid to a final concentration of 0.1% and incubate at room temperature for 1 h. Excess reagents will react to form bubbles.
4. Perform C_{18} purification and lyophilize peptides.

3.7 Polymer Depletion

The PAA polymer needs to be washed or dialyzed prior to use to remove low molecular weight adducts. This is described in Subheading 3.7, **step 1** and can be performed in parallel with Subheading 3.7, **steps 2–4**.

1. Aliquot 400 μL PAA polymer solution:
   (a) Prewash 30 kDa cutoff spin filter device with NaOH solution 2 by adding 400 μL and spinning for 5 min at 5000 × *g*. Repeat twice more with water.
   (b) Add the PAA polymer solution to the spin filter device, and centrifuge for 10 min at 12,000 × *g*.
   (c) Add 300 μL water, mix PAA polymer solution in the device, and centrifuge as in Subheading 3.7, **step 1a**. Perform this twice.
   (d) Retrieve PAA polymer solution by adding 100 μL MES buffer 2 then pipetting out of the device or inverting the membrane device and gently spinning into a fresh tube. Keep this tube for Subheading 3.7, **step 5**.
2. Prepare 150 μL of EDAC solution and 150 μL s-NHS solution.
3. Resolubilize lyophilized peptides with 200 μL MES buffer 1 (*see* **Note 6**).
4. Add 25 μL s-NHS solution and 25 μL EDAC solution and then incubate for 30 min at 25 °C. Ensure pH is 5.0. Final concentration of s-NHS is 50 mM. Final concentration of EDAC is 80 mM.
5. Add the PAA polymer solution from Subheading 3.7, **step 1** to the peptide solution. Ensure pH is 5.0, mix well by vortexing, spin down, and incubate for 1 h at 25 °C.
6. Add equivalent amounts as in Subheading 3.7, **step 4**, and incubate for an additional hour at 25 °C.
7. Repeat Subheading 3.7, **step 6**, and incubate overnight at 25 °C.

8. Prepare a new centrifugal filter device, and prepare it as outlined in Subheading 3.7, **step 1a** and **1b**.
9. Add the PAA/peptide solution to the centrifugal membrane, and centrifuge for 10 min at 12,000 × *g* at room temperature.
10. Collect filtrate and add 300 μL of water to the membrane, mix the contents, and centrifuge as said on Subheading 3.7, **step 9**.
11. Collect and combine filtrates.
12. All collected filtrate is acidified to 0.1% formic acid and purified by C_{18} prior to LC-MS/MS. Lyophilize eluent peptides.

3.8 LC-MS/MS and Bioinformatics

Data-dependent acquisition methods can be performed to identify C-terminal peptides. While the mass spectrometric methods will not be discussed here, it is important to note that as these mixtures are highly simplified compared to shotgun samples, thus, fractionation and extremely high sequencing speeds are not obligatory. TAILS and C-TAILS rely frequently on single-peptide identifications to identify a protein, and as such focusing on generating high-quality MS/MS spectra is key to confidently profile the true ends of proteins.

1. Resuspend peptides in buffer A from the LC-MS/MS system employed.
2. Acquire data using data-dependent acquisition favoring quality of spectra over quantity of spectra. It is important to note here that the presence of longer peptides due to lysine blocking may warrant the utilization of different fragmentation methods. While collision-induced dissociation (CID) favors typical tryptic peptides, other methods such as electron-transfer dissociation (ETD) may provide additional complementary information benefiting from higher charge state peptides [21].
3. Perform database searching using algorithm of choice. Utilization of MaxQuant with the Andromeda algorithm provides a simple platform for managing peptide modifications on the C terminus and quantitative measurements [22].
4. In the case of using SILAC with heavy and light amino acids, the quantitative labels in MaxQuant can be selected as Leu0 for the light channel and Leu6 (+6.020129 Da) and for the heavy channel.

   Carbamidomethylation of cysteine (+57.021464 Da) and dimethylation of lysine and N termini (+28.031300 Da) are fixed modifications. To check if labeling of carboxylic acids is complete, search using amidation of aspartate, glutamate, and C termini as variable modifications using the appropriate mass residue of the tag employed. For ethanolamine the mass increase is +43.042199 Da (monoisotopic mass of ethanolamine = 61.0152763 Da). Once checked, C-TAILS data can then utilize amidation of aspartate, glutamate as fixed modifications, while modification at the C terminus is variable.

Choice of digestion enzyme is either trypsin ([K/R]|) or LysargiNase™ (|[K/R]) using semi-cleavage at the C terminus. Utilization of *a*-ions improves scoring with LysargiNase™ digests [17]. These identifications will often be predominated with *b*-type and *a*-type ion ladders.

Mass accuracy parameters are determined by the instrument used. We recommend using a protein FDR of 5% as many proteins will be identified by a single peptide and as such require lenient cutoffs for later validation.

5. Peptides identified fall into three categories:
   (a) Heavy (protease KO): light (wild type) = 1:1. Background proteolysis events which do not concern the protease of interest.
   (b) Heavy (protease KO): light (wild type) < 2:1. The peptide is in less abundance in KO cells, which implies activity of the protease of interest in the wild type. These constitute biologically interesting substrates and spectra need to be checked manually for correct assignation as well as presence of the tag at the C terminus.
   (c) Heavy (protease KO): light (wild type) > 2:1. There is a higher amount of processing of this substrate in knockout cells which suggests that the protease of interest inhibited or cleaved a secondary protease or set of proteases which performed the cleavage observed. These constitute biologically interesting substrates and spectra need to be checked manually for correct assignation as well as presence of the tag at the C terminus.

4 Notes

1. Efficient removal of serum albumin greatly increases the recovery of proteins and peptides from the cell and reduces complexity.
2. Avoid using volumes larger than 1 mL. It makes precipitation of larger volumes more cumbersome and prone to losses.
3. Critical: breaking the protein pellet makes transferring significantly more challenging and can result in large losses of yields. The pellet can be transferred by picking it up with a pipette tip or small spatula and placing it inside a microfuge tube containing 100 μL of chloroform.
4. Ethanolamine can be substituted by the primary amine of choice of the investigator.
5. It is critical to observe if protein precipitates, which, if so, requires less amounts of protein to obtain a lower effective concentration.
6. Save 10% of the sample for LC-MS/MS checking prior to depletion (*see* Subheading 3.8, **step 1**).

Acknowledgments

N.S. is funded by the Michael Smith Foundation for Health Research of Canada (Grant ID:16642) and by the National Health and Medical Research Council of Australia (APP1126842). C.M.O holds a Canada Research Chair in Protease Proteomics and Systems Biology.

References

1. Krueger KE, Srivastava S (2006) Posttranslational protein modifications: current implications for cancer detection, prevention, and therapeutics. Mol Cell Proteomics 5(10):1799–1810. https://doi.org/10.1074/mcp.R600009-MCP200
2. Burotto M, Chiou VL, Lee JM et al (2014) The MAPK pathway across different malignancies: a new perspective. Cancer 120(22):3446–3456. https://doi.org/10.1002/cncr.28864
3. Dennis JW, Laferte S, Waghorne C et al (1987) Beta 1-6 branching of Asn-linked oligosaccharides is directly associated with metastasis. Science 236(4801):582–585
4. Ma X, Dong W, Su Z et al (2016) Functional roles of sialylation in breast cancer progression through miR-26a/26b targeting ST8SIA4. Cell Death Dis 7(12):e2561. https://doi.org/10.1038/cddis.2016.427
5. Puente XS, Sanchez LM, Overall CM et al (2003) Human and mouse proteases: a comparative genomic approach. Nat Rev Genet 4(7):544–558. https://doi.org/10.1038/nrg1111
6. Fortelny N, Cox JH, Kappelhoff R et al (2014) Network analyses reveal pervasive functional regulation between proteases in the human protease web. PLoS Biol 12(5):e1001869. https://doi.org/10.1371/journal.pbio.1001869
7. Overall CM, Blobel CP (2007) In search of partners: linking extracellular proteases to substrates. Nat Rev Mol Cell Biol 8(3):245–257. https://doi.org/10.1038/nrm2120
8. Aebersold R, Mann M (2003) Mass spectrometry-based proteomics. Nature 422(6928):198–207. https://doi.org/10.1038/nature01511
9. Hebert AS, Richards AL, Bailey DJ et al (2014) The one hour yeast proteome. Mol Cell Proteomics 13(1):339–347. https://doi.org/10.1074/mcp.M113.034769
10. Steen H, Mann M (2004) The ABC's (and XYZ's) of peptide sequencing. Nat Rev Mol Cell Biol 5(9):699–711. https://doi.org/10.1038/nrm1468
11. Solis N, Overall CM (2016) Mass spectrometry-based methodologies for studying proteolytic networks and the degradome. In: Bradshaw RA, Stahl PD (eds) Encyclopedia of cell biology, vol 1. Elsevier, Waltham MA, pp 568–581
12. Kleifeld O, Doucet A, auf dem Keller U et al (2010) Isotopic labeling of terminal amines in complex samples identifies protein N-termini and protease cleavage products. Nat Biotechnol 28(3):281–288. https://doi.org/10.1038/nbt.1611
13. Kleifeld O, Doucet A, Prudova A et al (2011) Identifying and quantifying proteolytic events and the natural N terminome by terminal amine isotopic labeling of substrates. Nat Protoc 6(10):1578–1611. https://doi.org/10.1038/nprot.2011.382
14. Schilling O, Barre O, Huesgen PF et al (2010) Proteome-wide analysis of protein carboxy termini: C terminomics. Nat Methods 7(7):508–511. https://doi.org/10.1038/nmeth.1467
15. Zhang Y, He Q, Ye J et al (2015) Systematic optimization of C-terminal amine-based isotope labeling of substrates approach for deep screening of C-Terminome. Anal Chem 87(20):10354–10361. https://doi.org/10.1021/acs.analchem.5b02451
16. Somasundaram P, Koudelka T, Linke D et al (2016) C-terminal charge-reversal Derivatization and parallel use of multiple proteases facilitates identification of protein C-termini by C-Terminomics. J Proteome Res 15(4):1369–1378. https://doi.org/10.1021/acs.jproteome.6b00146
17. Huesgen PF, Lange PF, Rogers LD et al (2015) LysargiNase mirrors trypsin for protein C-terminal and methylation-site identification. Nat Methods 12(1):55–58. https://doi.org/10.1038/nmeth.3177
18. Cox J, Mann M (2008) MaxQuant enables high peptide identification rates, individualized p.p.b.-range mass accuracies and proteome-wide protein quantification. Nat Biotechnol 26(12):1367–1372. https://doi.org/10.1038/nbt.1511
19. Wessel D, Flugge UI (1984) A method for the quantitative recovery of protein in dilute solution in the presence of detergents and lipids. Anal Biochem 138(1):141–143

20. Geiger T, Cox J, Ostasiewicz P et al (2010) Super-SILAC mix for quantitative proteomics of human tumor tissue. Nat Methods 7(5):383–385. https://doi.org/10.1038/nmeth.1446
21. Good DM, Wirtala M, McAlister GC et al (2007) Performance characteristics of electron transfer dissociation mass spectrometry. Mol Cell Proteomics 6(11):1942–1951. https://doi.org/10.1074/mcp.M700073-MCP200
22. Tyanova S, Temu T, Cox J (2016) The MaxQuant computational platform for mass spectrometry-based shotgun proteomics. Nat Protoc 11(12):2301–2319. https://doi.org/10.1038/nprot.2016.136

Chapter 3

Identification of Proteolytic Cleavage Sites of EphA2 by Membrane Type 1 Matrix Metalloproteinase on the Surface of Cancer Cells

Keiji Kikuchi, Hiroko Kozuka-Hata, Masaaki Oyama, Motoharu Seiki, and Naohiko Koshikawa

Abstract

Proteolytic cleavage of membrane proteins can alter their functions depending on the cleavage sites. We recently demonstrated that membrane type 1 matrix metalloproteinase (MT1-MMP) converts the tumor suppressor EphA2 into an oncogenic signal transducer through EphA2 cleavage. The cleaved EphA2 fragment that remains at the cell surface may be a better target for cancer therapy than intact EphA2. To analyze the cleavage site(s) of EphA2, we purified the fragments from tumor cells expressing MT1-MMP and Myc- and 6× His-tagged EphA2 by two-step affinity purification. The purified fragment was digested with trypsin to generate proteolytic peptides, and the amino acid sequences of these peptides were determined by nano-LC-mass spectrometry to identify the MT1-MMP-mediated cleavage site(s) of EphA2.

Key words MT1-MMP, EphA2, Proteolytic cleavage, Myc tag, His tag, Affinity purification, Nano-LC-mass spectrometry

1 Introduction

Membrane type 1 matrix metalloproteinase (MT1-MMP) has potent proinvasive and growth-promoting activities due to proteolytic modification of extracellular matrix (ECM) components and membrane molecules such as the α subunit of integrin, CD44, CD63, transglutaminase, and heparin-binding epidermal growth factor (EGF)-like growth factor (HB-EGF) [1]. In addition to these targets, we and another group found that MT1-MMP cleaves the tyrosine kinase receptor EphA2 [2, 3]. Although EphA2 is a key factor in the suppression or enhancement of ErbB-receptor-mediated signals, whose opposing functions are switched by the availability of EphA2 ligands [4, 5], proteolytic regulation of EphA2 by MT1-MMP is a likely mechanism to convert the tumor

Santiago Cal and Alvaro J. Obaya (eds.), *Proteases and Cancer: Methods and Protocols*, Methods in Molecular Biology, vol. 1731, https://doi.org/10.1007/978-1-4939-7595-2_3, © Springer Science+Business Media, LLC 2018

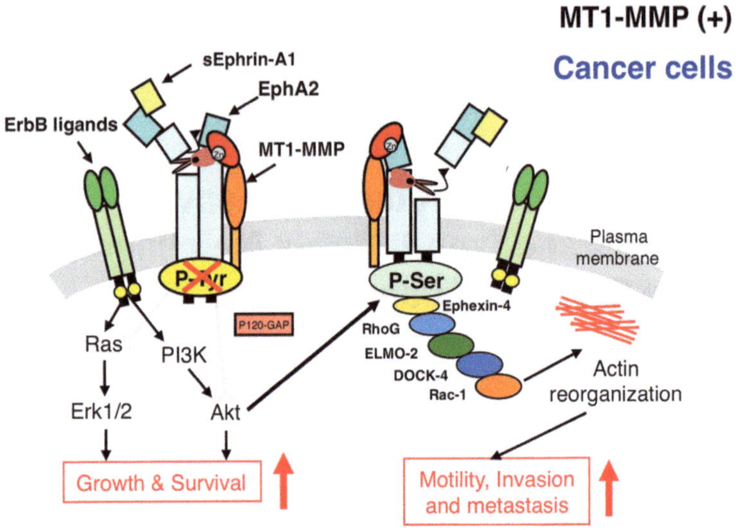

Fig. 1 Schematic representation of membrane type 1 MT1-MMP-mediated proteolytic conversion of EphA2 functions in cancer cells. In cancer cells expressing both EphA2 and MT1-MMP, MT1-MMP cleaves and converts EphA2 into a ligand-insensitive form. MT1-MMP thus acts as a trigger for ligand-independent EphA2 signals, which cooperate with ErbB-receptor-mediated signals to promote tumor growth, invasion, and metastasis. Obtained from [3], with permission from the publisher

suppressor EphA2 into an oncogenic signal transducer (Fig. 1; reproduced from Koshikawa et al., 2015, with permission from Cancer Research) [3]. Thus, the cleaved EphA2 fragment and a corresponding specific antibody may be a better target and tool, respectively, for cancer therapy and diagnosis.

To characterize the MT1-MMP-cleaved EphA2, the fragment(s) were purified from the colorectal carcinoma cell line HCT116 expressing MT1-MMP with or without C-terminally Myc−/6× His-tagged EphA2. Western blotting with anti-EphA2 cytoplasmic domain polyclonal antibody (pAb) showed the intact EphA2 protein (130 kDa) and two cleaved fragments (55 and 60 kDa) in whole cell lysates (Fig. 2a, whole lysate +). The EphA2 fragments were purified and characterized as follows. First, the cell lysates were subjected to immunoprecipitation (IP) with anti-Myc monoclonal antibody (mAb). The eluate was subjected to sodium dodecyl sulfate polyacrylamide gel electrophoresis (SDS-PAGE) and Western blotting using an anti-EphA2 cytoplasmic domain pAb (Fig. 2A, B). The fraction purified by IP with an anti-Myc mAb contained abundant contaminant proteins, including immunoglobulin heavy chain and others, which hampers sequencing (Fig. 2B, Myc IP +). To further purify the fraction obtained by IP with anti-Myc mAb, the sample was subjected to purification using nickel-nitrilotriacetic acid (Ni-NTA) beads, which resulted in

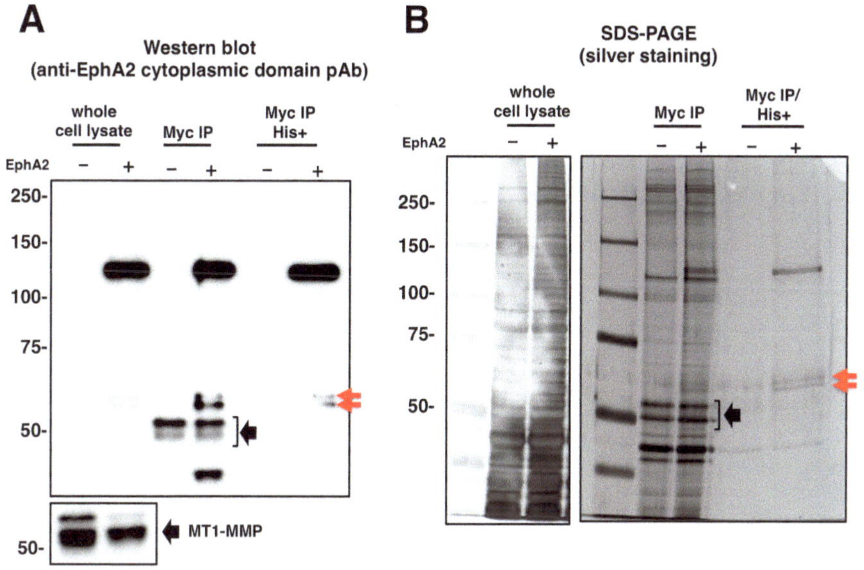

Fig. 2 Sequential purification of EphA2 fragments after MT1-MMP cleavage. The C-terminally dual-tagged EphA2 was transfected into the colon carcinoma cell line HCT116. Whole cell lysates extracted from HCT116 cells expressing the Myc and 6× His EphA2 with or without MT1-MMP were subjected to Western blotting and SDS-PAGE (**A** and **B**). Immunoprecipitation of EphA2 fragments with anti-Myc monoclonal antibody showed contamination with abundant immunoglobulin proteins as indicated by a black arrow (Myc IP, **A** and **B**). Further purification of the fragments was performed by Ni-NTA affinity beads using His tags. Highly purified intact EphA2 and its fragments of 60 and 55 kDa (red arrows) were obtained (**A** and **B**) and used for mass spectrometry analysis

highly purified EphA2 fragments of 60 and 55 kDa as detected in SDS-PAGE (Fig. 2A, B).

To determine the fragments' cleavage sites, each polypeptide band was cut out from a Coomassie brilliant blue (CBB)-stained gel and was subjected to nano-liquid chromatography (LC)-mass spectrometry (MS)/MS analysis (Fig. 3). Sequencing by MS indicated that MT1-MMP cleaves EphA2 between ^{431}S and ^{432}V and between ^{434}I and ^{435}N (Fig. 4), in agreement with previous results using the fibrosarcoma cell line HT1080 [3].

2 Materials

2.1 Cell, Culture, and Transfection

1. Human colon carcinoma cell line HCT116.
2. The complete DMEM medium: high-glucose (4.5 g/L) DMEM, 10% fetal bovine serum (FBS), 10 mM HEPES-NaOH pH 7.2, 15 mM $NaHCO_3$, 2 mM glutamate.
3. Plasmids pLent6-MT1-MMP and pcDNA3.1-Myc−/6× His-tagged EphA2.
4. Lipofectamine 2000.
5. Opti-MEM I Reduced-Serum Medium.

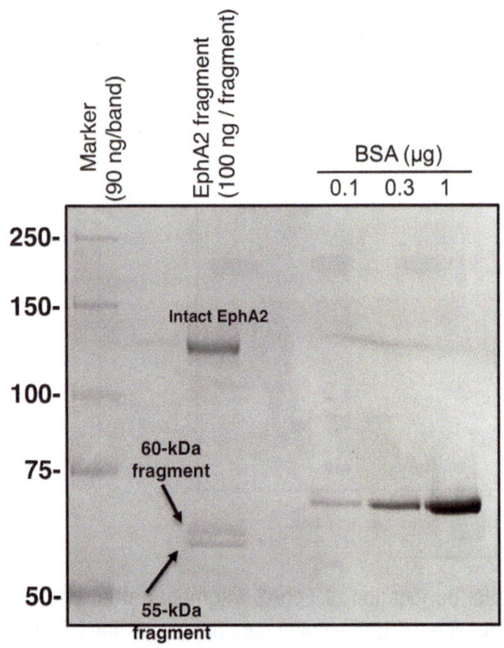

Fig. 3 Evaluation of purity and amount of cleaved EphA2 fragments for mass spectrometry analysis. Arrows show approximately 100 ng of each membrane type 1 matrix proteinase-cleaved EphA2 fragment. Bovine serum albumin (BSA) was used to evaluate the amount of protein (100, 300, and 1000 ng/lane). The molecular weight marker contained 90 ng of each polypeptide

```
1   KEVVLLDFAA AGGELGWLTH PYGKGWDLMQ NIMNDMPIYM YSVCNVMSGD
51  QDNWLRTNWV YRGEAERIFI ELKFTVRDCN SFPGGASSCK ETFNLYYAES
101 DLDYGTNFQK RLFTKIDTIA PDEITVSSDF EARHVKLNVE ERSVGPLTRK
151 GFYLAFQDIG ACVALLSVRV YYKKCPELLQ GLAHFPETIA GSDAPSLATV
201 AGTCVDHAVV PPGGEEPRMH CAVDGEWLVP IGQCLCQAGY EKVEDACQAC
251 SPGFFKFEAS ESPCLECPEH TLPSPEGATS CECEEGFFRA PQDPASMPCT
301 RPPSAPHYLT AVGMGAKVEL RWTPPQDSGG REDIVYSVTC EQCWPESGEC
351 GPCEASVRYS EPPHGLTRTS VTVSDLEPHM NYTFTVEARN GVSGLVTSRS
401 FRTASVSINQ TEPPKVRLEG RSTTSLSVSW SIPPPQQSRV WKYEVTYRKK
451 GDSNSYNVRR TEGFSVTLDD LAPDTTYLVQ VQALTQEGQG AGSKVHEFQT
501 LSPEGSGNLA VIGGVAVGVV LLLVLAGVGF FIHRRRKNQR ARQSPEDVYF
551 SKSEQLKPLK TYVDPHTYED PNQAVLKFTT EIHPSCVTRQ KVIGAGEFGE
601 VYKGMLKTSS GKKEVPVAIK TLKAGYTEKQ RVDFLGEAGI MGQFSHHNII
651 RLEGVISKYK PMMIITEYME NGALDKFLRE KDGEFSVLQL VGMLRGIAAG
701 MKYLANMNYV HRDLAARNIL VNSNLVCKVS DFGLSRVLED DPEATYTTSG
751 GKIPIRWTAP EAISYRKFTS ASDVWSFGIV MWEVMTYGER PYWELSNHEV
801 MKAINDGFRL PTPMDCPSAI YQLMMQCWQQ ERARRPKFAD IVSILDKLIR
851 APDSLKTLAD FDPRVSIRLP STSGSEGVPF RTVSEWLESI KMQQYTEHFM
901 AAGYTAIEKV VQMTNDDIKR IGVRLPGHQK RIAYSLLGLK DQVNTVGIPI
951 SRGPFEQKLI SEEDLNMHTG HHHHHH
```

Ephrin-Binding domain

Cleavage sites

Trans-membrane domain

Fig. 4 Amino acid sequence of EphA2 showing the identified membrane type 1 matrix proteinase (MT1-MMP) cleavage sites. Cleavage sites (red arrows) resulting in the 60- and 55-kDa EphA2 fragments are shown in the amino acid sequence of human EphA2 (^{1}K–^{950}I + Myc and 6x His tag). The ephrin-binding and transmembrane domains are underlined and shown in blue and green, respectively

2.2 Extraction of Cellular Proteins and Immunoprecipitation of Tagged Protein

1. Anti-Myc mAb (clone 4A6).
2. Protein G-conjugated magnetic beads.
3. Ni-NTA agarose.
4. Precast 7.5% polyacrylamide gel.
5. Lysis buffer: 20 mM HEPES-NaOH, pH 7.2, 142.5 mM KCl, 5 mM $MgCl_2$, 1 mM EDTA, 0.2% (v/v) NP-40, protease inhibitor cocktail.
6. Binding buffer: 10 mM Tris–HCl, pH 7.5, 6 M guanidinium-HCl, 0.2% (v/v) NP-40, 10 mM imidazole.
7. Washing buffer: 50 mM sodium phosphate pH 7.5, 300 mM NaCl, 0.2% (v/v) NP-40, 40 mM imidazole.
8. Elution buffer: 50 mM sodium phosphate pH 7.5, 300 mM NaCl, 0.2% (v/v) NP-40, 250 mM imidazole.
9. 4× SDS sample buffer: 25 mM Tris–HCl, pH 6.8, 40% (v/v) glycerol, 9.2% (w/v) sodium dodecyl sulfate, 20% (v/v) 2-mercaptoethanol, 0.04% (w/v) bromophenol blue.
10. SDS running buffer: 25 mM Tris, 192 mM glycine, 0.1% (w/v) sodium dodecyl sulfate.
11. CBB staining solution: 0.25% (w/v) CBB R-250, 45% (v/v) ethanol, 10% (v/v) acetic acid.
12. CBB destaining solution I: 20% (v/v) ethanol, 8% (v/v) acetic acid.
13. CBB destaining solution II: 5% ethanol, 7.5% (v/v) acetic acid.

2.3 In-Gel Protein Digestion for MS

1. Gel reducing solution: 10 mM DTT, 100 mM NH_4HCO_3.
2. Gel alkylating solution: 55 mM iodoacetamide (IAA), 100 mM NH_4HCO_3.
3. Trypsin solution: 40 mM Tris–HCl, pH 8.8, 1 pmol/μL trypsin.
4. Dilution buffer: 50 mM Tris–HCl, pH 8.8.
5. Gel extraction solution: 50% (v/v) CH_3CN, 5% (v/v) formic acid.

3 Methods

3.1 Expression of EphA2 with Myc/6× His Tags in HCT116 Cells

1. Grow the cells at 37 °C in complete DMEM medium in a humidified atmosphere of 5% CO_2 and 95% air.
2. Twenty-four hour before transfection, seed the cells in twelve 10-cm culture dishes at approximately 25% confluence.

3. Mix 48 μg each of expression vectors for Myc−/6× His-tagged EphA2 and MT1-MMP in 6 mL of Opti-MEM I into a 50-mL plastic tube.
4. Mix 240 μL Lipofectamine 2000 in 6 mL of Opti-MEM I in a 50-mL tube and let it stand for 5 min.
5. Gently mix the DNA and Lipofectamine 2000 solutions and incubate at 25 °C for 20 min.
6. Replace the medium in the 12 culture dishes with pre-warmed Opti-MEM I (4 mL/dish).
7. Add 1.02 mL of DNA-Lipofectamine 2000 mix to each dish and mix gently by rocking.
8. Incubate the cells for 5 h in a CO_2 incubator.
9. Aspirate off the medium and add 10 mL of pre-warmed complete DMEM medium to each dish.
10. Culture the cells for 48 h in a CO_2 incubator.

3.2 Immunoprecipitation of Myc−/His-Tagged EphA2 and Its Proteolytic Fragments

1. Wash the cells with PBS three times and add fresh PBS (1 mL/dish).
2. Scrape off the cells and transfer the cell suspension to a 1.5-mL Eppendorf tube.
3. Collect the cells by centrifugation (180 × *g*, 2 min, room temperature) and remove the supernatant (*see* **Note 1**).
4. Resuspend the cells in 1 mL/dish of ice-cold lysis buffer.
5. Pass the cell suspension through a 23-gauge needle syringe ten times and chill on ice for 10 min.
6. Centrifuge at 11,500 × *g*, 4 °C for 10 min and transfer the supernatant (cleared cell lysate) to new 1.5-mL Eppendorf tubes.
7. Add anti-Myc mAb (2 μg/tube) and let it stand for 30 min on ice.
8. Add protein G-conjugated magnetic beads (20 μL/tube) and continuously rotate at 4 °C overnight.
9. Remove the lysate using a magnetic separator.
10. Wash the beads three times with lysis buffer.
11. Transfer the protein G-magnetic beads to a new 1.5-mL Eppendorf tube.
12. Add Ni-NTA binding buffer (up to 800 μL) and continuously mix for 10 min on a rotator.
13. Collect the supernatant (eluate) into a new 1.5-mL Eppendorf tube (Tube A).
14. Resuspend the beads with Ni-NTA binding buffer (400 μL) again and mix for 10 min on a rotator.

15. Remove the supernatant (eluate) from the magnetic beads using a magnetic separator and transfer to Tube A (total volume, 1.2 mL).
16. Add Ni-NTA agarose beads (15 μL/tube) and continuously mix on a rotator at 4 °C for 2 h.
17. Spin down the Ni-NTA beads and wash the beads three times with 1 mL Ni-NTA wash buffer.
18. Resuspend the beads with Ni-NTA elution buffer (30 μL) and let it stand for 5 min at room temperature.
19. Remove the supernatant from the beads by centrifugation at 200 × *g* for 5 min and transfer to a new 1.5-mL Eppendorf tube (Tube B).
20. Repeat **steps 18** and **19**.
21. Collect the supernatant (eluate) in Tube B and store the eluate (60 μL) at −20 °C until SDS-PAGE analysis.

3.3 Isolation of EphA2 Fragments on SDS-PAGE for MS Analysis

1. Mix the eluate (60 μL) with 4× SDS loading buffer (20 μL) and boil the sample for 5 min (*see* **Note 2**).
2. Load the samples (20 μL/lane, 4 lanes) on a 7.5% precast polyacrylamide gel and perform the electrophoresis at 25 mA/gel until the dye front reaches the bottom of the gel (*see* **Note 3**).
3. After electrophoresis, remove the gel using a clean spatula and place the gel on a disposable plastic tray with distilled water.
4. Discard the water and incubate the gel in CBB staining solution with shaking for 30 min at room temperature.
5. Discard the CBB staining solution and incubate the gel in CBB destaining solution I for 30 min at room temperature.
6. Discard the CBB destaining solution I and replace it with CBB destaining solution II. Change the destaining solution II several times until the protein bands appear.
7. Wash the gel with distilled water several times.
8. Cut the protein bands corresponding to EphA2 fragments using a disposable scalpel and place each in a new Eppendorf tube.
9. The excised band can be stored at −80 °C.

3.4 In-Gel Protein Digestion

1. Crush the gel slices to small pieces by passing them through the tip inside a 0.5-mL Eppendorf tube during centrifugation at 9100 × *g*.
2. Add destaining buffer (200 μL/tube) and incubate for 3–10 min at 40 °C.
3. Spin down the gel and discard the supernatant.
4. Repeat **steps 2** and **3** twice.

5. Add gel reducing solution (200 μL/tube) and incubate for 60 min at 56 °C.
6. Cool down the tube to room temperature and then remove the supernatant by centrifugation at 9100 × *g* for 5 min.
7. Add gel alkylating solution (200 μL/tube) and incubate for 45 min at room temperature in the dark.
8. Spin down the gel and wash the sediment with distilled water (400 μL/tube) twice.
9. Add 100% CH_3CN (200 μL/tube) and incubate for 10 min with gentle tapping.
10. The gel pieces will become whitish and form an aggregate.
11. Remove the CH_3CN by centrifugation at 9100 × *g* for 5 min.
12. Dry the gel pieces by vacuum centrifugation.
13. Add trypsin solution (10 μL/tube) and put on ice for 15 min.
14. Add dilution buffer (20 μL/tube) and incubate at 37 °C overnight.
15. Add gel extraction solution (50 μL/tube) and incubate for 10 min with gentle tapping at room temperature.
16. Collect the eluate in a new Eppendorf tube (collection tube A).
17. Repeat **steps 15** and **16**.
18. Add 100% CH_3CN (50 μL/tube) and incubate for 10 min with gentle tapping at room temperature.
19. Collect the supernatant in the collection tube A.
20. Reduce the extract volume to 5–20 μL in the collection tube using vacuum centrifugation.
21. The eluted peptides are ready for nano-LC-MS analysis and can be stored at −80 °C.

4 Notes

1. The cell pellet can be stored at −80 °C after quick freezing in dry ice or liquid nitrogen.
2. It is recommended to wear gloves and a face mask throughout the SDS-PAGE and in-gel protein digestion to avoid contamination of the samples. A slab gel tank, chips, and SDS-PAGE reagents exclusively for use in MS analysis is recommended.
3. Before purification by SDS-PAGE, sample protein concentration must be checked by comparing the band density of a sample aliquot with those of 0.1, 0.3, and 1.0 μg of a standard protein such as bovine serum albumin.

References

1. Itoh Y (2015) Membrane-type matrix metalloproteinases: their functions and regulations. Matrix Biol 44–46:207–223. https://doi.org/10.1016/j.matbio.2015.03.004
2. Sugiyama N, Gucciardo E, Tatti O et al (2013) EphA2 cleavage by MT1-MMP triggers single cancer cell invasion via homotypic cell repulsion. J Cell Biol 201(3):467–484. https://doi.org/10.1083/jcb.201205176
3. Koshikawa N, Hoshino D, Taniguchi H et al (2015) Proteolysis of EphA2 converts it from a tumor suppressor to an oncoprotein. Cancer Res 75(16):3327–3339. https://doi.org/10.1158/0008-5472.CAN-14-2798
4. Miao H, Wang B (2012) EphA receptor signaling--complexity and emerging themes. Semin Cell Dev Biol 23(1):16–25. https://doi.org/10.1016/j.semcdb.2011.10.013
5. Lisabeth EM, Falivelli G, Pasquale EB (2013) Eph receptor signaling and ephrins. Cold Spring Harb Perspect Biol 5(9). https://doi.org/10.1101/cshperspect.a009159

Chapter 4

Biotin-Chasing Assay to Evaluate uPAR Stability and Cleavage on the Surface of Cells

Vladimir Leksa, Herbert B. Schiller, and Hannes Stockinger

Abstract

The plasminogen activation system, i.e., the fibrinolytic system, is one of the major plasma proteolytic pathways. The proteolytic conversion of the zymogen plasminogen to the active serine protease plasmin is on the cell surface catalyzed by the serine protease urokinase-type plasminogen activator (urokinase, uPA). Upon binding to the urokinase receptor (uPAR, CD87), single-chain pro-uPA is processed to double-chain uPA which in turn specifically converts cell-bound plasminogen to plasmin. Plasmin is harnessed in many physiological processes, e.g., blood clots' resolution, or proteolytic activation of growth factors. Plasmin is essential also for migratory cells, for instance, activated immune cells; however, malignant cells hijack plasmin for invasion as well. The activation of plasminogen to plasmin is thus at the physiological level tightly controlled. One of the negative regulators of plasminogen activation has been identified in the cation-independent mannose 6-phosphate/insulin-like growth factor 2 receptor (M6P/IGF2R, CIMPR, CD222). M6P/IGF2R is a multifunctional receptor involved in protein sorting, internalization, and degradation, being considered a tumor suppressor. M6P/IGF2R binds both plasminogen and uPAR and facilitates in this way the proteolytic cleavage of uPAR resulting in the loss of the uPA binding on the cell surface. Hence, this molecular device contributes to the negative feedback loop in regulation of pericellular plasminogen activation and cell invasion.

In this chapter, we describe the experimental approach, i.e., biotin-chasing assay, to evaluate uPAR stability and cleavage on the surface of cells.

Key words Pericellular proteolysis, Plasminogen, Urokinase, Cell migration, Fibrinolysis

Abbreviations

M6P/IGF2R	Mannose 6-phosphate/insulin-like growth factor 2 receptor
mAb	Monoclonal antibody
Plg	Plasminogen
RNAi	RNA interference
shRNA	Short hairpin RNA
uPA	Urokinase-type plasminogen activator
uPAR	Urokinase-type plasminogen activator receptor

Santiago Cal and Alvaro J. Obaya (eds.), *Proteases and Cancer: Methods and Protocols*, Methods in Molecular Biology, vol. 1731, https://doi.org/10.1007/978-1-4939-7595-2_4, © Springer Science+Business Media, LLC 2018

1 Introduction

Proteolytic enzymes—proteases—represent about 2% of all human gene products [1], yet basically all proteins might become a substrate for proteases eventually. Accordingly, proteolysis plays indispensable roles in all biological processes. Components of four major proteolytic cascades, i.e., the coagulation, fibrinolytic, complement, and kinin systems, synchronize their activities to maintain homeostasis. In particular, the fibrinolytic, i.e., plasminogen activation system, is well known for its role in dissolution of fibrin clots [2]. However, the plasminogen activation system is in addition harnessed in a plethora of other physiological processes: it mediates proteolytic activation of growth factors, e.g., TGFβ [3–5], it is central for cell penetration through tissue barriers [6], and it contributes to the removal of protein aggregates, e.g., beta-amyloid deposits in the brain [7]. Hence, it must be tightly controlled. Indeed, a variety of human pathologies are associated with impaired plasminogen activation, e.g., malignant cells' dissemination, deficiencies in immune responses, neurodegeneration, and dysregulated homeostasis [8].

Plasminogen (Plg) is a zymogen secreted by hepatocytes [8]. Its concentration in plasma is high (2 μM). The proteolytic conversion of Plg to plasmin might be catalyzed by (1) tissue-type plasminogen activator (tPA), primarily responsible for Plg activation on the extracellular matrix upon fibrin degradation [9]; (2) the serine protease urokinase-type plasminogen activator (urokinase, uPA), the central enzyme in cell-mediated Plg activation [10]; and (3) bacterial components, such as streptokinase, which in this way increases the virulency of bacteria [11, 12]. uPA is secreted by migrating cells as the inactive zymogen pro-uPA. The single-chain pro-uPA is proteolytically processed to the double-chain uPA upon binding to the urokinase receptor (uPAR, CD87). This conversion is mediated by a variety of proteases including kallikrein, Factor XIIa and plasmin itself. The active uPA in turn specifically converts cell-bound Plg to plasmin [6].

uPAR is a GPI-anchored protein consisting of three homologous domains (D1, D2, and D3) partitioning preferentially in so-called lipid rafts, entities enriched in glycosphingolipids and cholesterol [13]. uPAR is upregulated on migrating cells, e.g., activated leukocytes, endothelial cells, and also invasive malignant cells. The binding site for uPA is encompassed within the N-terminal domain 1 (D1) of uPAR [14]. A proteolytic cleavage of uPAR between D1 and D2 results in the downregulation of uPA binding on the cell surface and thus represents a negative feedback mechanism in cell migration. The cleavage might be mediated by various proteases including plasmin and uPA [15]. Several other molecular devices control Plg activation: uPA and plasmin are inhibited by plasminogen activator inhibitors (e.g., PAI-1) and plasmin inhibitors (e.g., α2-antiplasmin) that are present in plasma [16]. In addition, Plg activation is restricted on the cell surface via terminal-lysine-containing Plg receptors, which usually recognize lysine-binding sites located in kringle domains of Plg. Many heterogeneous Plg receptors have been characterized up to now, and the vast majority of them potentiate plasmin generation [17]. In contrast, we have identified a negative regulator of Plg activation in the cation-independent mannose 6-phosphate/insulin-like growth factor 2 receptor (M6P/IGF2R, CIMPR, CD222).

M6P/IGF2R is a multifunctional type I receptor involved in protein sorting, internalization, and degradation, present largely in the Golgi apparatus and endosomes and on the cell surface. M6P/IGF2R has a crucial role in biogenesis of lysosomes—through recognition of mannose 6-phosphate (M6P), it transports lysosomal enzymes and extracellular ligands [18]. It also internalizes insulin-like growth factor 2 (IGF2), a potent mitogen [19]. Finally, the loss of M6P/IGF2R has been described in many human malignancies; hence, it is considered a tumor suppressor [20]. We have found that M6P/IGF2R binds Plg via its amino-terminal region [21]. The crystal structure of this region, resolved by Olson and colleagues, has unraveled the shape of the Plg-binding site [22]. We have found further that M6P/IGF2R downregulates pericellular Plg activation via Plg internalization [23]. In addition, we have shown that soluble M6P/IGF2R blocks Plg activation by preventing Plg from binding to uPA [24]. Finally, we observed that M6P/IGF2R facilitates the proteolytic truncation of uPAR leading to the loss of uPA binding through D1 and subsequently to blunted Plg activation and cell invasion [25].

The latter observation was surprising since M6P/IGF2R had been proposed to be involved in the internalization of uPAR [26] rather than its cleavage. Nevertheless, we have found no reduction in the uPAR internalization upon M6P/IGF2R knockdown [25]. On the other hand, in the M6P/IGF2R-silenced cells, we detected a significant increase of uPAR stability. In particular, we measured the stability of cell surface uPAR by means of the biotin-chasing assay. First, cells of the human kidney carcinoma cell line TCL-598 were biotinylated on ice. Then, to chase the uPAR stability, the surface-biotinylated cells were incubated for various time intervals at 37 °C. Afterward, the cells were lysed, and biotinylated proteins were precipitated with streptavidin-coupled beads. Finally, the precipitated full-length form of uPAR was analyzed by SDS-PAGE followed by immunoblotting. The bands corresponding to full-length uPAR were normalized to loading control bands and statistically evaluated. The half-life of full-length uPAR was significantly prolonged in M6P/IGF2R-silenced cells when compared to

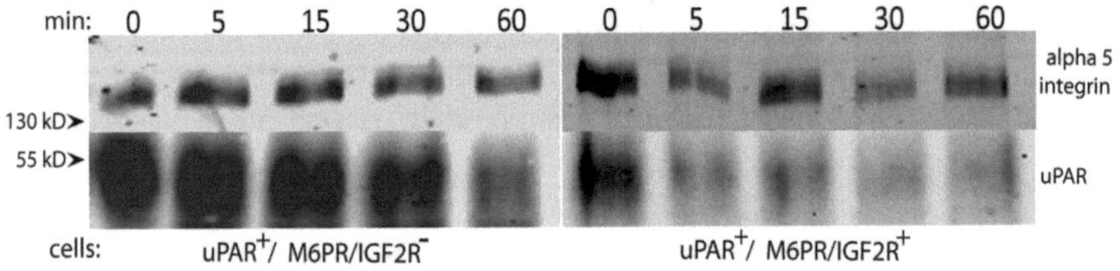

Fig. 1 uPAR cleavage is affected by M6P/IGF2R. Surface-biotinylated M6P/IGF2R-negative mouse fibroblasts transduced either with human uPAR or with both human uPAR and human M6P/IGF2R were incubated in culture medium supplemented with human uPA (10 nM) for the indicated times at 37 °C. After incubation, the cells were lysed, and biotinylated full-length uPAR was analyzed by SDS-PAGE and immunoblotting. Alpha 5 integrin was used as a control

control cells (2 h vs. 30 min). This difference was due to the proteolytic activity of uPA since the uPA inhibitor amiloride prevented the cleavage of uPAR in both silenced and control cells (figure 8 in ref. 25).

We have obtained similar results with mouse fibroblasts derived from M6P/IGF2R knockout mice transduced with human uPAR either alone or together with human M6P/IGF2R. Since mouse fibroblasts did not produce human uPA, we performed the biotin-chasing assay in the presence of human uPA. Both biotinylated uPAR$^+$ and uPAR$^+$/M6P/IGF2R$^+$ fibroblasts expressed predominantly the full-length variant of cell surface uPAR which was rapidly cleaved, especially when M6P/IGF2R was co-expressed. Namely, upon expression of M6P/IGF2R, the half-life of uPAR was shortened from 1 h to 30 min (*see* [25] and Fig. 1).

Hence, by chasing the cell surface-biotinylated uPAR, we concluded that M6P/IGF2R reduced the stability of uPAR. Since M6P/IGF2R can bind both Plg and uPAR [4], the local accumulation of uPA and Plg on the uPAR-M6P/IGF2R complex might lead to the proteolytic removal of the uPA-binding site (Fig. 2). This molecular device thus represents a negative feedback loop in pericellular proteolysis and cell migration.

2 Materials

2.1 Cell Surface Biotinylation and Biotin Chasing

1. Cells: TCL-598—human kidney carcinoma (invasive tumor cell line that secretes pro-uPA), M6P/IGF2R-negative mouse fibroblasts—immortalized fibroblasts from the M6P/IGF2R knockout mouse [27].
2. Medium RPMI 1640: Roswell Park Memorial Institute standard medium containing penicillin, streptomycin, and L-glutamine.
3. Trypsin.
4. EDTA.

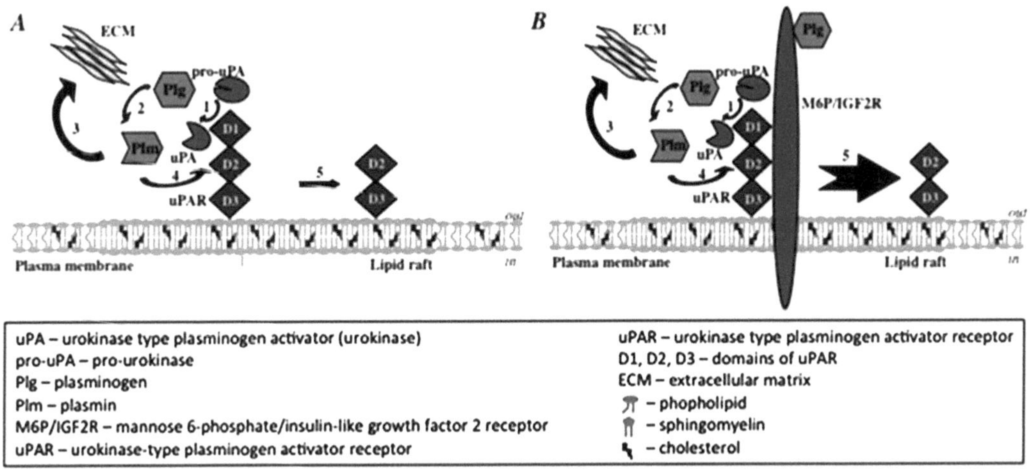

Fig. 2 Scheme showing the pericellular plasminogen/uPAR proteolytic system. (**a**) The GPI-anchored uPAR is localized preferentially within lipid rafts enriched in sphingomyelins and cholesterol. uPAR binds pro-uPA, which is proteolytically converted to the active uPA (1). On the cell surface, uPA activates the zymogen Plg to the active serine protease Plm (2). Plasmin plays a central role in cell migration via degrading extracellular matrix proteins, ECM (3). Plasmin can provide a positive feedback loop via the activation of pro-uPA to uPA (4). In addition, both plasmin and uPA provide also a negative feedback regulatory loop through cleaving uPAR (5). (**b**) M6P/IGF2R is a type I receptor playing crucial role in intracellular protein transport and internalization of extracellular ligands. M6P/IGF2R binds both Plg and uPAR and thus contributes to the cleavage of uPAR

5. FCS: fetal calf serum.
6. PBS—phosphate-buffered saline (1×): 0.137 M NaCl, 2.7 mM KCl, 4.3 mM Na_2HPO_4, 1.4 mM KH_2 PO_4, pH 7.4.
7. $CaCl_2$.
8. $MgCl_2$.
9. Sulfo-NHS-SS-Biotin.
10. Glycine.
11. Urokinase—uPA.
12. uPA inhibitor amiloride.

2.2 Precipitation and Western Blotting

1. Lysis buffer: 20 mM Tris–HCl, 150 mM NaCl, pH 7.5.
2. Detergents: NP40, Triton X-100, SDS (sodium dodecyl sulfate), deoxycholic acid.
3. Protease inhibitors: aprotinin, leupeptin, pepstatin, PMSF (phenylmethylsulfonyl fluoride).
4. RIPA buffer: lysis buffer containing 1% Triton X-100, 0.1% SDS, 0.5.% deoxycholic acid.
5. Streptavidin beads.
6. Tris/SDS separation gel buffer: 1 M Tris–HCl, 0.27% SDS, pH 8.8.

7. Tris/SDS stacking gel buffer: 1 M Tris–HCl, 0.8% SDS, pH 6.8.
8. Isopropanol.
9. SDS-PAGE running buffer (10×): 0.25 M Tris, 1.92 M Glycine, 1% SDS in aqueous solution.
10. SDS-PAGE sample loading buffer—Laemmli buffer (4×): 0.5 M Tris–HCl, 40% glycerol, bromphenol blue, 8% SDS, pH 6.8, and −/+ 5% EtSH for non/reducing conditions [28].
11. Western blotting buffer: 25 mM Tris, 0.2 M glycine, 15% methanol.
12. Washing buffer—TBST—TBS-Tween: 50 mM Tris–HCl, 140 mM NaCl and 0.05% Tween20, pH 7.5.
13. 10% ammonium persulfate (APS).
14. AA solution: 30% acrylamide, 0.8% N,N′-methylenebisacrylamide.
15. Tetramethylethylenediamine (TEMED).
16. Nonfat dry milk.
17. Albumin fraction V (BSA).
18. Polyvinylidene fluoride microporous (PVDF) membrane.
19. Methanol.
20. Whatman paper.
21. Antibodies and conjugates: mAb H2 to uPAR, mAb AB1928 to alpha5 integrin, anti-mouse and anti-rabbit fluorescently labeled secondary conjugates.

3 Methods

3.1 Cell Surface Biotinylation and Biotin Chasing

1. Culture both the adherent human kidney epithelial tumor cell line TCL-598 and the M6P/IGF2R-negative mouse fibroblasts routinely in complete RPMI-1640 and 10% heat-inactivated FCS. Grow the cells at 37 °C and 5% CO_2 in a humidified atmosphere and passage them each third day using trypsin-EDTA solution for adherent cells.
2. Remove medium when the cells are subconfluent in culture flasks (T75), wash the cells two times with PBS (10 mL per flask), and then harvest them with 5 mM EDTA solution in PBS (5 mL) directly in culture flasks for 5 min at 37 °C (*see* **Note 1**).
3. Collect the cells into 50 mL conical centrifuge tubes, dilute them with ice cold PBS (+ $CaCl_2$ 0.1 mM, $MgCl_2$ 1 mM) to 50 mL, and centrifuge at 300 × *g* for 5 min.

4. Remove the medium supernatants and dilute the cells to 50 mL with ice cold PBS washed and centrifuge at 300 × *g* for 5 min (*see* **Note 2**).
5. After the final washing step, count the cells and resuspend the cells in ice cold PBS with 0.5 mg/mL sulfo-NHS-SS-Biotin (1×10^7 cells/mL). Let the cells biotinylate for 30 min on ice on regular vortexing.
6. Stop the biotinylation by a 10-min incubation with 100 μM glycine in PBS on ice.
7. Wash the cells three times with RPMI (10% FCS).
8. Incubate the cells in complete RPMI (10% FCS) at 37 °C. In case of mouse fibroblasts, in the presence of human uPA (10 nM), optionally, add the uPA-specific inhibitor amiloride (10 μM) (*see* **Note 3**).

3.2 Precipitation and Western Blotting

1. Stop the incubation after different time points at 37 °C and centrifuge the cells (300 × *g*, 5 min).
2. Lyse the cells in RIPA buffer (1×10^7 cells/mL) for 30 min on ice.
3. After cell lysis, centrifuge the crude lysate shortly to remove cell debris (1 min) and transfer the supernatant (clean lysate) into new tubes.
4. Precipitate the cell surface-biotinylated proteins with streptavidin beads for 2 h at 4 °C. For this, add the beads to the clean lysate (50 μL of bead solution per 1 mL lysate) and perform the incubation on a shaker.
5. Wash the beads—i.e., centrifuge the beads (300 × *g*, 3 min)—remove the supernatant carefully (without touching the beads), and resuspend the bead pellet in ice cold PBS. Repeat this step four times with ice cold PBS.
6. After the final washing step, remove the supernatant quantitatively (*see* **Note 4**).
7. Elute precipitated proteins from the beads with the SDS-PAGE sample loading buffer (200 μL per 50 μL beads).
8. Prepare the separation gel (10%) and the stacking gel.
9. Boil the samples of **step** 7.
10. Load the samples onto the gel.
11. Run the electrophoresis at constant voltage of 120 V in SDS-PAGE running buffer till the dye front reaches the end of the separation gel.
12. Soak a PVDF membrane 1 min in methanol.
13. Preincubate the PVDF membrane and Whatman papers in Western blotting buffer.

14. Prepare a Western blotting sandwich to transfer the samples from the gel to the membrane at 15 V for 1 h in a semidry system in Western blotting buffer.
15. Block the membrane in 5% nonfat dry milk in TBST for 20 min on a shaker at RT and wash it with TBST.
16. Incubate the membrane with the specific Ab, prepared in 0.5% nonfat dry milk in TBST or in 1% BSA in TBST for 1 h at RT or overnight at 4 °C (*see* **Note 5**).
17. Wash the membrane three times with TBST for 5 min on the shaker.
18. Incubate the membrane with the appropriate fluorescently labeled secondary conjugate prepared in 0.5% nonfat dry milk in TBST or in 0.5% BSA in TBST for 1 h at RT.
19. Wash the membrane three times for 15 min with TBST.
20. Detect and quantify the bands on the immunoblot by analyzing the integrated intensity on the Odyssey infrared imaging system (LI-COR Biosciences).

4 Notes

1. The concentration of EDTA should be tested for each adherent cell line since 5 mM EDTA might be toxic for some cells.
2. It is necessary to resuspend the cellular pellets at first in 5 mL ice cold PBS (+0.1 mM $CaCl_2$, 1 mM $MgCl_2$) before dilution.
3. If necessary, other protease inhibitors might be added as well.
4. Use long and thin tips, the ones for loading the SDS-PAGE samples, which do not allow the beads to be taken in.
5. Alternatively, 5% BSA in TBST might be used.

References

1. Rawlings ND, Barrett AJ (1993) Evolutionary families of peptidases. Biochem J 290(Pt 1): 205–218
2. Rijken DC, Lijnen HR (2009) New insights into the molecular mechanisms of the fibrinolytic system. J Thromb Haemost 7(1):4–13. https://doi.org/10.1111/j.1538-7836.2008.03220.x
3. Lyons RM, Gentry LE, Purchio AF et al (1990) Mechanism of activation of latent recombinant transforming growth factor beta 1 by plasmin. J Cell Biol 110(4):1361–1367
4. Godar S, Horejsi V, Weidle UH et al (1999) M6P/IGFII-receptor complexes urokinase receptor and plasminogen for activation of transforming growth factor-beta1. Eur J Immunol 29(3):1004–1013
5. Leksa V, Godar S, Schiller HB et al (2005) TGF-{beta}-induced apoptosis in endothelial cells mediated by M6P/IGFII-R and mini-plasminogen. J Cell Sci 118(Pt 19):4577–4586
6. Bugge TH (2008) Physiological functions of plasminogen activation: effects of gene deficiencies in human and mice. The cancer degradome: proteases and cancer biology. Springer, New York
7. Dotti CG, Galvan C, Ledesma MD (2004) Plasmin deficiency in Alzheimer's disease

brains: causal or casual? Neurodegener Dis 1(4–5):205–212. https://doi.org/10.1159/000080987
8. Dano K, Behrendt N, Hoyer-Hansen G et al (2005) Plasminogen activation and cancer. Thromb Haemost 93(4):676–681
9. Zorio E, Gilabert-Estelles J, Espana F et al (2008) Fibrinolysis: the key to new pathogenetic mechanisms. Curr Med Chem 15(9):923–929
10. Dass K, Ahmad A, Azmi AS et al (2008) Evolving role of uPA/uPAR system in human cancers. Cancer Treat Rev 34(2):122–136
11. Young KC, Shi GY, DH W et al (1998) Plasminogen activation by streptokinase via a unique mechanism. J Biol Chem 273(5):3110–3116
12. McArthur JD, Cook SM, Venturini C et al (2012) The role of streptokinase as a virulence determinant of streptococcus pyogenes--potential for therapeutic targeting. Curr Drug Targets 13(3):297–307
13. Degryse B (2011) The urokinase receptor system as strategic therapeutic target: challenges for the 21st century. Curr Pharm Des 17(19):1872–1873. doi: BSP/CPD/E-Pub/000498 [pii]
14. Blasi F, Carmeliet P (2002) uPAR: a versatile signalling orchestrator. Nat Rev Mol Cell Biol 3(12):932–943
15. Ragno P (2006) The urokinase receptor: a ligand or a receptor? Story of a sociable molecule. Cell Mol Life Sci 63(9):1028–1037
16. Binder BR, Mihaly J, Prager GW (2007) uPAR-uPA-PAI-1 interactions and signaling: a vascular biologist's view. Thromb Haemost 97(3):336–342
17. Miles LA, Hawley SB, Baik N et al (2005) Plasminogen receptors: the sine qua non of cell surface plasminogen activation. Front Biosci 10:1754–1762
18. Ghosh P, Dahms NM, Kornfeld S (2003) Mannose 6-phosphate receptors: new twists in the tale. Nat Rev Mol Cell Biol 4(3):202–212
19. Macdonald RG, Byrd JC (2003) The insulin-like growth factor II/mannose 6-phosphate receptor: implications for IGF action in breast cancer. Breast Dis 17:61–72
20. Scott CD, Firth SM (2004) The role of the M6P/IGF-II receptor in cancer: tumor suppression or garbage disposal? Horm Metab Res 36(5):261–271
21. Leksa V, Godar S, Cebecauer M et al (2002) The N terminus of mannose 6-phosphate/insulin-like growth factor 2 receptor in regulation of fibrinolysis and cell migration. J Biol Chem 277(43):40575–40582
22. Olson LJ, Yammani RD, Dahms NM et al (2004) Structure of uPAR, plasminogen, and sugar-binding sites of the 300 kDa mannose 6-phosphate receptor. EMBO J 23(10):2019–2028
23. Leksa V, Pfisterer K, Ondrovicova G et al (2012) Dissecting mannose 6-phosphate-insulin-like growth factor 2 receptor complexes that control activation and uptake of plasminogen in cells. J Biol Chem 287(27):22450–22462. https://doi.org/10.1074/jbc.M112.339663
24. Leksa V, Loewe R, Binder B et al (2011) Soluble M6P/IGF2R released by TACE controls angiogenesis via blocking plasminogen activation. Circ Res 108(6):676–685. https://doi.org/10.1161/CIRCRESAHA.110.234732
25. Schiller HB, Szekeres A, Binder BR et al (2009) Mannose 6-phosphate/insulin-like growth factor 2 receptor limits cell invasion by controlling alphaVbeta3 integrin expression and proteolytic processing of urokinase-type plasminogen activator receptor. Mol Biol Cell 20(3):745–756. doi:10.1091/mbc.E08-06-0569
26. Nykjaer A, Christensen EI, Vorum H et al (1998) Mannose 6-phosphate/insulin-like growth factor-II receptor targets the urokinase receptor to lysosomes via a novel binding interaction. J Cell Biol 141(3):815–828
27. Wang ZQ, Fung MR, Barlow DP et al (1994) Regulation of embryonic growth and lysosomal targeting by the imprinted Igf2/Mpr gene. Nature 372(6505):464–467
28. Laemmli UK (1970) Cleavage of structural proteins during the assembly of the head of bacteriophage T4. Nature 227(5259):680–685

Chapter 5

Determination of Aconitase Activity: A Substrate of the Mitochondrial Lon Protease

Pedro M. Quirós

Abstract

Mitochondrial aconitase is a reversible enzyme that catalyzes the conversion of citrate to isocitrate in the tricarboxylic acid cycle. Mitochondrial aconitase is very sensitive to oxidative inactivation and can aggregate and accumulate in the mitochondrial matrix causing mitochondrial dysfunction. Lon protease, one of the major quality control proteases in mitochondria, degrades oxidized aconitase maintaining mitochondrial homeostasis. This chapter describes a step-by-step protocol for a simple and reliable measurement of mitochondrial aconitase, as well as citrate synthase activity, using isolated mitochondria from cells. The protocol is simple and fast, and it is optimized for a 96-well plate using a microplate reader.

Key words Mitochondria, Mitochondrial protease, Lon protease, Cancer, Aconitase, Citrate synthase, Enzyme activity

1 Introduction

LONP1, or Lon protease, is a highly conserve serine protease that plays essential roles regulating mitochondrial function [1]. LONP1 degrades oxidized, misfolded, and damaged proteins in the mitochondrial matrix, contributing to maintain mitochondrial homeostasis [1, 2]. Beside its function as quality control protease, Lon has also been involved in the specific degradation of several mitochondrial proteins, including mitochondrial aconitase (ACO2), succinate dehydrogenase subunit 5 (SDH5), glutaminase C, cytochrome c oxidase isoform COX4–1, steroidogenic acute regulatory protein (StAR), haeme oxygenase-1 (HO-1), 5-aminolevulinic acid synthase (ALAS1), cystathionine β-synthase (CBS), pyruvate dehydrogenase kinase 4 (PDK4), and the mitochondrial transcription factor A (TFAM), among others [3–11]. In addition to TFAM degradation, Lon also binds to mtDNA, participating in mtDNA maintenance and mitochondrial gene expression [11, 12].

Santiago Cal and Alvaro J. Obaya (eds.), *Proteases and Cancer: Methods and Protocols*, Methods in Molecular Biology, vol. 1731, https://doi.org/10.1007/978-1-4939-7595-2_5,

The key role of Lon maintaining mitochondrial function has been extensively studied in multiple organisms and cell lines. Downregulation or inhibition of Lon triggers a vast of mitochondrial and cellular defects, inhibits cellular proliferation, and promotes accelerate aging in yeast and embryonic lethality in mice [13–15]. Conversely, upregulation of Lon protects against several stress conditions and increases healthspan and lifespan in a fungi model [16, 17]. In humans, mutations in LONP1 gene cause CODAS syndrome, a rare and multisystemic developmental disorder characterized by cerebral, ocular, dental, auricular, and skeletal anomalies [18, 19].

Lon is one of the most studied and characterized mitochondrial proteases associated with the tumorigenic process [20, 21]. Several reports have consistently described that its upregulation promotes tumorigenesis and protects tumor cells against stress, increasing their malignance [15, 20, 22]. Contrary, and similarly to normal cells, Lon downregulation impairs cell proliferation and decreases the tumorigenesis of cancer cells [15, 23–27], and, more importantly, mice heterozygous for Lon deletion show a decreased tumor susceptibility [15]. The implications of Lon in the tumorigenic process can be explained by any of its multiple roles in mitochondria. In this regard, several examples have linked specific functions of Lon with an increase in cell survival of cancer cells, including adaptation to hypoxia [4], metabolic reprogramming [15], or resistance to senescence and apoptosis [15, 28]. However, due to its multitasking activity, other functions of Lon may also contribute to the increase in tumorigenesis, as increase in mitochondrial proteostasis, alterations in any of its multiple substrates, or changes in the levels and expression of mtDNA.

Among all multiple substrates of Lon, one of the best characterized is the mitochondrial aconitase, an enzyme that catalyzes a reversible isomerization of citrate to isocitrate in the tricarboxylic acid cycle. Aconitase is very sensitive to oxidation, which inactivates the enzyme and triggers its aggregation and accumulation, compromising mitochondrial function and cellular viability [3]. It is demonstrated that Lon preferentially degrades aconitase after oxidative modification [3] and that inhibition of Lon increases the levels of aconitase, whereas its overexpression decreases its levels and activity [15, 25] (Fig. 1).

This protocol describes the determination of aconitase activity, which can provide an indirect measurement of Lon activity in vivo. The protocol is optimized for a 96-well plate and provides a detailed explanation on how to isolate mitochondria and calculate aconitase activity. Also, it is described the determination of citrate synthase activity, a mitochondrial enzyme that is used to normalize to mitochondrial content.

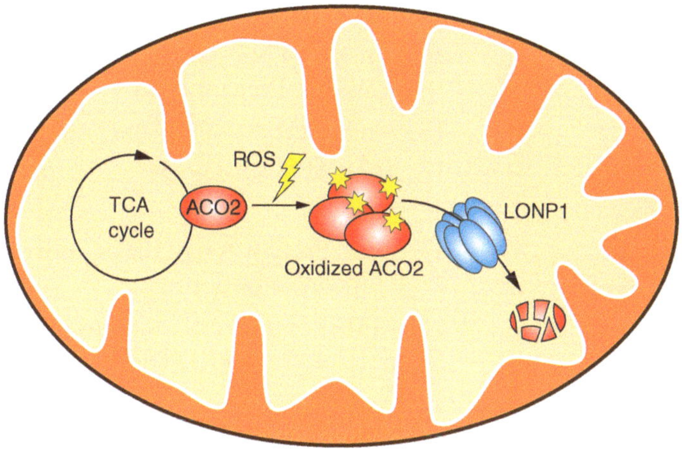

Fig. 1 Mitochondrial Lon protease (LONP1) degrades the tricarboxylic acid (TCA) cycle enzyme aconitase (ACO2). Schematic model representing the proteolytic processing of oxidized ACO2 by LONP1 in the mitochondrial matrix

2 Materials

2.1 Equipment

1. Cell culture dishes treated (100 mm).
2. Glass/Teflon Potter-Elvehjem homogenizer.
3. 15 mL centrifuge tubes (conical bottom).
4. 1.5 mL microcentrifuge tubes.
5. Refrigerated centrifuge and microcentrifuge.
6. Microplate spectrophotometer.

2.2 Reagents and Stock Solutions

1. Double-distilled or Milli-Q-purified water. Use this in all recipes and protocol steps.
2. Cell line of interest.
3. Dulbecco's phosphate-buffered saline (DPBS) without Ca^{2+} and Mg^{2+}. Stored at room temperature (RT).
4. 1 M Tris–HCl, pH 7.4. Store at RT.
5. 0.5 M EDTA pH 8. Store at RT.
6. 1 M sucrose. Aliquot and store at −20 °C.
7. 10 mM potassium phosphate buffer pH 7.4. Store at RT.
8. 0.6 M sodium citrate pH 7.4. Store at RT.
9. Triton X-100. Store at RT.
10. 60 mM $MnCl_2$. Store at RT.
11. 20 mM NADP. Aliquot and store at −20 °C.
12. 200 U/mL isocitrate dehydrogenase ($NADP^+$ dependent). Store at −20 or −80 °C.

13. 1 M Tris–HCl pH 8. Store at RT.
14. 1 mM DTNB (5,5-dithio-bis-(2-nitrobenzoic acid); Ellman's reagent). Prepare fresh.
15. 8 mM acetyl-CoA (7 mg/mL). Aliquot and store at −20 °C.
16. 10 mM oxaloacetate (1.32 mg/mL). Aliquot and store at −20 °C.
17. BCA Protein Assay Kit or other method/kit to quantify protein concentration.
18. Mitochondrial isolation buffer (buffer A): 10 mM of Tris–HCl pH 7.4, 1 mM EDTA, 0.32 M Sucrose. Store at 4 °C.
19. Aconitase activity buffer: 50 mM Tris–HCl, pH 7.4, 6 mM sodium citrate, 0.2% Triton X-100, 0.6 mM $MnCl_2$, 0.2 mM NADP, and 2 U/mL of Isocitrate dehydrogenase. Prepare fresh.
20. Citrate activity buffer: 75 mM Tris–HCl, pH 8.0, 0.1 mM DTNB, 0.1% Triton X-100, and 0.4 mM acetyl-CoA. Prepare fresh.

3 Methods

3.1 Isolation of Mitochondrial-Enriched Fractions from Cells

1. Harvest exponentially growing cells by trypsinization. Use one 100 mm plate of 80–90% confluent cells (around 8×10^6 cells) (*see* **Note 1**).
2. Transfer the cells to a 15 mL tube, and wash the cells twice with cold DPBS by centrifuging at 500 × *g* for 5 min at 4 °C.
3. Resuspend the pellet in 1 mL of buffer A and keep on ice. Buffer A is an isotonic media that protects mitochondria from swelling.
4. Homogenize with a 2 mL glass/Teflon pestle on ice with 15 slow up-down strokes at 600 rpm (*see* **Note 2**).
5. Transfer the homogenized cell to a 1.5 mL tube.
6. Centrifuge 1500 × *g* for 5 min at 4 °C to pellet unbroken cells, debris, and nuclei.
7. Collect the supernatant in a new 1.5 mL tube.
8. *Optional*: resuspend the pellet in 500 μL of buffer A and repeat **steps 4–8**.
9. Centrifuge the supernatants at 12,000 × *g* for 10 min at 4 °C.
10. Carefully discard the supernatant.
11. Pellet contains the mitochondrial-enriched fraction. Pellets can be stored a −80 °C up to 3 months.

3.2 Prepare Samples for Enzymatic Assays

1. Resuspend fresh or frozen mitochondrial pellets in 50–100 μL of 10 mM of potassium phosphate buffer pH 7.4.
2. Subject mitochondrial solution to three cycles of freezing-thawing in liquid nitrogen to disrupt the mitochondrial membranes.

3.3 Protein Assay

1. Measure the protein concentration using a standard protein quantification method as BCA protein assay.

3.4 Aconitase Activity

1. Aconitase activity is determined spectrophotometrically by following the linear increase in absorbance due to the generation of NADPH.
2. Set up the 96-well plate reader at 340 nm and create a template selecting samples and blank in triplicates.
3. Add 99 μL of aconitase activity buffer to all wells.
4. Add 1 μL of isolated mitochondria, of approximately 10 μg/μL, to the sample wells and 1 μL of water to the blank wells.
5. Register the absorbance continually at 340 nm during 5 min at 25 °C to generate a kinetic curve for each sample (*see* **Note 3**).
6. Calculate the slope of the curves using only the linear part of the curve (slope = absorbance/min).

3.5 Citrate Synthase Activity

1. Citrate synthase activity is determined spectrophotometrically by following the linear increase in absorbance produced by the generation of TNB (*see* **Note 4**).
2. Set up the 96-well plate reader at 412 nm and create a template selecting samples and blank in triplicates.
3. Add 27 μL of citrate synthase activity buffer to all wells.
4. Add 1–3 μL of isolated mitochondria, of approximately 10 μg/μL, to the sample wells.
5. Complete adding water to all wells (samples and blank) to get a final volume of 95 μL.
6. Incubate 2 min at 30 °C.
7. Add 5 μL of oxaloacetate (10 mM of stock) to all wells.
8. Register the absorbance continually at 412 nm during 5 min at 30 °C to generate a kinetic curve (*see* **Note 3**).
9. Calculate the slope of the curve using only the linear part of the curve (slope = absorbance/min).

3.6 Calculations

1. Specific activities (μmol of substrate generated per min per mg of protein) of aconitase and citrate synthase are calculated using the Lambert-Beer equation: Absorbance = $\varepsilon \cdot b \cdot c$.
   ε = molar extinction coefficient; b = path length (*see* **Note 5**); c = sample protein concentration.

2. For aconitase activity, ε (NADPH) = 6.22 mM^{-1} cm^{-1}, and for citrate synthase activity, ε (TNB) = 13.8 mM^{-1} cm^{-1}.
3. An enzymatic unit is one μmol of substrate/min, so the specific activity is also represented as U/mg.
4. Therefore, specific activity is calculated as follows:

   $Slope_{final} = Slope_{sample} - Slope_{blank}$

   $Slope_{final}$ (Absorbance/min) = ε · b · c/min

   c = $slope_{final}$/ε · b = μmol min^{-1} mL^{-1} = U mL^{-1}

   Activity = enzymatic unit (U mL^{-1})/protein concentration (mg mL^{-1}) = U mg^{-1}
5. Aconitase activity is normalized to citrate synthase activity (*see* **Note 6**).

   Relative aconitase activity = aconitase activity/citrate synthase activity.

4 Notes

1. In the case of primary cells or fibroblasts, it is recommended to use 150 mm cell culture dishes.
2. Precool the glass/Teflon homogenizer on ice before starting the homogenization. It is recommended to use a motor-driven glass/Teflon pestle to achieve a good homogenization; however, manually, homogenization can also work by doing more strokes (around 30).
3. If an increase in absorbance is not detected, incubate and register absorbance for more time (10–15 min). If the signal is very low, or no differences are observed with blank samples, repeat the reaction using more mitochondrial sample.
4. DTNB (or Ellman's reagent) is a chemical used to quantify the number or concentration of thiol groups in a sample. Thiol groups, such as those generated by citrate synthase from acetyl-CoA and oxaloacetate, react with DTNB in a rapid and stoichiometric reaction, cleaving the disulfide bond and generating 2-nitro-5-thiobenzoate acid (TNB). TNB has a yellow color and can be determined spectrophotometrically by measuring absorbance at 412 nm.
5. Classically, in horizontal spectrophotometry, as happened using cuvette spectrophotometers, path length has been standardized to 1 cm. However, in vertical spectrophotometry, as happened when using microplate readers, the path length depends on the volume of the solution and height of the plate. The path length can be calculated by comparing the absorbance of that solution in a cuvette with the absorbance in the

microplate well. Other option is to use an approximation of 0.29 cm, which is valid for a 96-well plate and 100 μL of an aqueous solution. However, many modern plate readers have implemented a K-factor correction for the path length that depends on the plate and volume of reaction and can be set up in the software instrument.

6. Citrate synthase is considered a stable mitochondrial enzyme whose activity is not subjected to changes in pathological conditions. Therefore, normalization to citrate synthase activity can prevent differences in mitochondrial content or in the mitochondrial yield during the isolation procedure when comparing different lines and conditions.

References

1. Quiros PM, Langer T, Lopez-Otin C (2015) New roles for mitochondrial proteases in health, ageing and disease. Nat Rev Mol Cell Biol 16(6):345–359. https://doi.org/10.1038/nrm3984
2. Pinti M, Gibellini L, Liu Y et al (2015) Mitochondrial Lon protease at the crossroads of oxidative stress, ageing and cancer. Cell Mol Life Sci 72(24):4807–4824. https://doi.org/10.1007/s00018-015-2039-3
3. Bota DA, Davies KJ (2002) Lon protease preferentially degrades oxidized mitochondrial aconitase by an ATP-stimulated mechanism. Nat Cell Biol 4(9):674 680. https://doi.org/10.1038/ncb836
4. Fukuda R, Zhang H, Kim JW et al (2007) HIF-1 regulates cytochrome oxidase subunits to optimize efficiency of respiration in hypoxic cells. Cell 129(1):111–122. https://doi.org/10.1016/j.cell.2007.01.047
5. Granot Z, Kobiler O, Melamed-Book N et al (2007) Turnover of mitochondrial steroidogenic acute regulatory (StAR) protein by Lon protease: the unexpected effect of proteasome inhibitors. Mol Endocrinol 21(9): 2164–2177. https://doi.org/10.1210/me.2005-0458
6. Matsushima Y, Goto Y, Kaguni LS (2010) Mitochondrial Lon protease regulates mitochondrial DNA copy number and transcription by selective degradation of mitochondrial transcription factor A (TFAM). Proc Natl Acad Sci U S A 107(43):18410–18415. https://doi.org/10.1073/pnas.1008924107
7. Tian Q, Li T, Hou W et al (2011) Lon peptidase 1 (LONP1)-dependent breakdown of mitochondrial 5-aminolevulinic acid synthase protein by heme in human liver cells. J Biol Chem 286(30):26424–26430. https://doi.org/10.1074/jbc.M110.215772
8. Kita K, Suzuki T, Ochi T (2012) Diphenylarsinic acid promotes degradation of glutaminase C by mitochondrial Lon protease. J Biol Chem 287(22):18163–18172. https://doi.org/10.1074/jbc.M112.362699
9. Teng H, Wu B, Zhao K et al (2013) Oxygen-sensitive mitochondrial accumulation of cystathionine beta-synthase mediated by Lon protease. Proc Natl Acad Sci U S A 110(31):12679–12684. https://doi.org/10.1073/pnas.1308487110
10. Bezawork-Geleta A, Saiyed T, Dougan DA et al (2014) Mitochondrial matrix proteostasis is linked to hereditary paraganglioma: LON-mediated turnover of the human flavinylation factor SDH5 is regulated by its interaction with SDHA. FASEB J 28(4):1794–1804. https://doi.org/10.1096/fj.13-242420
11. Lu B, Lee J, Nie X et al (2013) Phosphorylation of human TFAM in mitochondria impairs DNA binding and promotes degradation by the AAA+ Lon protease. Mol Cell 49(1):121–132. https://doi.org/10.1016/j.molcel.2012.10.023
12. Lu B, Liu T, Crosby JA et al (2003) The ATP-dependent Lon protease of Mus musculus is a DNA-binding protein that is functionally conserved between yeast and mammals. Gene 306:45–55. https://doi.org/10.1016/S0378-1119(03)00403-7
13. Erjavec N, Bayot A, Gareil M et al (2013) Deletion of the mitochondrial Pim1/Lon protease in yeast results in accelerated aging and impairment of the proteasome. Free Radic Biol Med 56:9–16. https://doi.org/10.1016/j.freeradbiomed.2012.11.019

14. Bota DA, Ngo JK, Davies KJ (2005) Downregulation of the human Lon protease impairs mitochondrial structure and function and causes cell death. Free Radic Biol Med 38(5):665–677. https://doi.org/10.1016/j.freeradbiomed.2004.11.017
15. Quiros PM, Espanol Y, Acin-Perez R et al (2014) ATP-dependent Lon protease controls tumor bioenergetics by reprogramming mitochondrial activity. Cell Rep 8(2):542–556. https://doi.org/10.1016/j.celrep.2014.06.018
16. Luce K, Osiewacz HD (2009) Increasing organismal healthspan by enhancing mitochondrial protein quality control. Nat Cell Biol 11(7):852–858. https://doi.org/10.1038/ncb1893
17. Ngo JK, Pomatto LC, Davies KJ (2013) Upregulation of the mitochondrial Lon protease allows adaptation to acute oxidative stress but dysregulation is associated with chronic stress, disease, and aging. Redox Biol 1(1):258–264. https://doi.org/10.1016/j.redox.2013.01.015
18. Strauss KA, Jinks RN, Puffenberger EG et al (2015) CODAS syndrome is associated with mutations of LONP1, encoding mitochondrial AAA(+) Lon protease. Am J Hum Genet 96(1):121–135. https://doi.org/10.1016/j.ajhg.2014.12.003
19. Dikoglu E, Alfaiz A, Gorna M et al (2015) Mutations in LONP1, a mitochondrial matrix protease, cause CODAS syndrome. Am J Med Genet A 167(7):1501–1509. https://doi.org/10.1002/ajmg.a.37029
20. Quirós PM, Bárcena C, López-Otín C (2014) Lon protease: a key enzyme controlling mitochondrial bioenergetics in cancer. Mol Cell Oncol 1(4):e968505. https://doi.org/10.4161/23723548.2014.968505
21. Bota DA, Davies KJ (2016) Mitochondrial Lon protease in human disease and aging: including an etiologic classification of Lon-related diseases and disorders. Free Radic Biol Med 100:188–198. https://doi.org/10.1016/j.freeradbiomed.2016.06.031
22. Cheng CW, Kuo CY, Fan CC et al (2013) Overexpression of Lon contributes to survival and aggressive phenotype of cancer cells through mitochondrial complex I-mediated generation of reactive oxygen species. Cell Death Dis 4:e681. https://doi.org/10.1038/cddis.2013.204
23. Gibellini L, Pinti M, Boraldi F et al (2014) Silencing of mitochondrial Lon protease deeply impairs mitochondrial proteome and function in colon cancer cells. FASEB J 28(12):5122–5135. https://doi.org/10.1096/fj.14-255869
24. Bernstein SH, Venkatesh S, Li M et al (2012) The mitochondrial ATP-dependent Lon protease: a novel target in lymphoma death mediated by the synthetic triterpenoid CDDO and its derivatives. Blood 119(14):3321–3329. https://doi.org/10.1182/blood-2011-02-340075
25. Gibellini L, Pinti M, Bartolomeo R et al (2015) Inhibition of Lon protease by triterpenoids alters mitochondria and is associated to cell death in human cancer cells. Oncotarget 6(28):25466–25483. https://doi.org/10.18632/oncotarget.4510
26. Liu Y, Lan L, Huang K et al (2014) Inhibition of Lon blocks cell proliferation, enhances chemosensitivity by promoting apoptosis and decreases cellular bioenergetics of bladder cancer: potential roles of Lon as a prognostic marker and therapeutic target in baldder cancer. Oncotarget 5(22):11209–11224. https://doi.org/10.18632/oncotarget.2026
27. Nie X, Li M, Lu B et al (2013) Down-regulating overexpressed human Lon in cervical cancer suppresses cell proliferation and bioenergetics. PLoS One 8(11):e81084. https://doi.org/10.1371/journal.pone.0081084
28. Kao TY, Chiu YC, Fang WC et al (2015) Mitochondrial Lon regulates apoptosis through the association with Hsp60-mtHsp70 complex. Cell Death Dis 6:e1642. https://doi.org/10.1038/cddis.2015.9

Chapter 6

A Simple Cell-Based Assay for the Detection of Surface Protein Shedding by Rhomboid Proteases

Angela Moncada-Pazos and Adam Graham Grieve

Abstract

Rhomboids are intramembrane serine proteases that cleave their substrates within or immediately adjacent to their transmembrane domains, a process known as regulated intramembrane proteolysis. In eukaryotes, two main types of rhomboid proteases can be distinguished based on their subcellular localization: mitochondrial rhomboids and secretase-type rhomboids that target the secretory pathway. The latter class can cleave and release the extracellular domain of all epidermal growth factor-like proteins in *Drosophila* and can liberate epidermal growth factor (EGF) in mammals, in a process known as ectodomain shedding. These released EGFs can then activate the EGF receptor (EGFR). EGFR signaling is crucial for mammalian development and is often deregulated in human cancer. Here we describe a cell-based protocol for detecting the ability of rhomboid proteases to release EGFR ligands into the medium. First, cells are transfected with the corresponding protease- and substrate-expressing vectors; second, cells condition the medium and accumulate shed protein. After this, protein lysates from cells and media are prepared and Western blotting is performed to detect the EGFR ligands that have been released into the medium.

Key words Rhomboid, Serine protease, Regulated intramembrane proteolysis, EGFR ligands

1 Introduction

In 2001 Urban and colleagues [1] were the first to identify that *Drosophila* rhomboid-1 was a novel protease—the first known intramembrane serine protease. Since then, rhomboid proteases have been identified in all forms of life, including archaea, bacteria, and eukaryotes, being one of the most conserved and widespread membrane protein groups [2]. All rhomboids perform hydrolysis using a catalytic dyad of a serine and a histidine [3], within a polytopic six-transmembrane domain core (although in most eukaryotic rhomboids there is an additional seventh transmembrane domain) [4]. This enzymatic mechanism is fundamentally different from classical serine proteases and is the result of

Santiago Cal and Alvaro J. Obaya (eds.), *Proteases and Cancer: Methods and Protocols*, Methods in Molecular Biology, vol. 1731, https://doi.org/10.1007/978-1-4939-7595-2_6, © Springer Science+Business Media, LLC 2018

independent and convergent evolution [2, 5]. The biochemical particularities of these enzymes have demanded the development of specific approaches and methods that have flourished in the last few years, substantially increasing our knowledge of rhomboid function [6].

Among metazoans, rhomboids have been mostly studied in *Drosophila* and mammals. Focussing on secretase rhomboids, five different rhomboids are known in the fruit fly (rho1, rho2, rho3, rho4, rho6) and four in mammals (RHBDL1-4) [7]. The *Drosophila* rhomboids have a well-established role in the cleavage of ligands of the EGFR: Spitz, Gurken, and Keren. Like most of the mammalian EGFR ligands, these growth factors are synthesised as membrane precursors that need to be liberated from the membrane to facilitate activation of the EGFR [1, 8]. In the case of mammalian rhomboids, the identification of substrates has proven more difficult and slower than in *Drosophila*. The first rhomboid substrate reported in mammals was thrombomodulin, an anticoagulant protein cleaved at the cell surface by RHBDL2 [9]. An important question is whether, as in flies, EGFR ligands in mammals are released by rhomboid proteases. At first glance, this seems unlikely, since ADAM-10 and -17 proteases, metalloproteases unrelated to rhomboids, are known to be the main executors of EGFR ligand shedding in mammals. Nevertheless, it has been shown that rhomboids can also contribute to this process, but this can only be detected when ADAM metalloproteases activity is blocked [9–11]. EGFR activation is crucial at different stages of development, and it also has important pathological significance: its aberrant activation is well established to be involved in carcinoma progression [12, 13]. Therefore, any agent involved in EGFR signaling could be a potential therapeutic target. Consistent with this idea, it has been demonstrated that rhomboids participate in EGFR activation, with studies in human and mouse that have established links with cancer for RHBDL2 and RHBDL4 [10, 14].

Much of the work aimed at identifying new rhomboid substrates have based their results on methods similar to the one described here: a rhomboid-based secretion assay for the detection of cell surface shedding of proteins [1, 10, 14]. In this protocol, COS-7 cells (or different cell lines) are transfected with plasmids to express a tagged version of the potential substrate in question, plus or minus a plasmid expressing the relevant rhomboid protease. After transfection, a secretion assay is performed in serum-free medium for 30 h, allowing time for the possible shedding fragments to accumulate. Cells and supernatants are processed, and the presence of cleaved peptides is detected by Western blotting (Fig. 1).

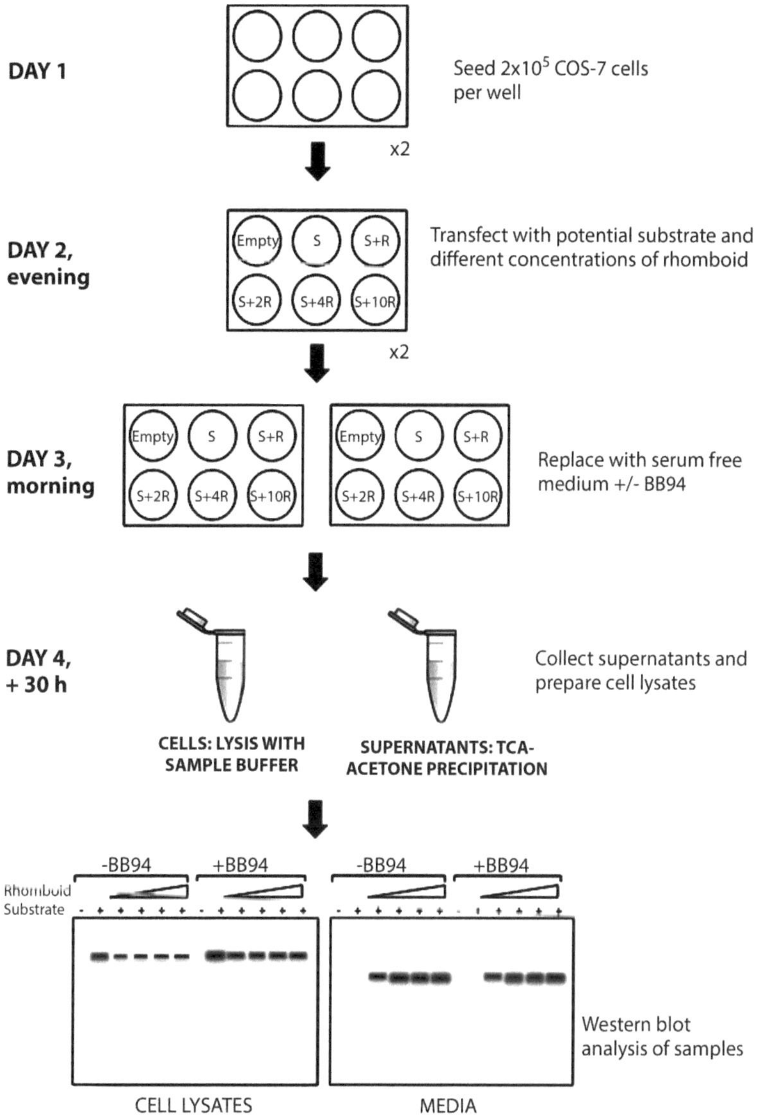

Fig. 1 Schematic diagram of the protocol. The whole protocol should take 5 days, divided into three main sections of work: plating and transfection of cells, incubation in assay medium, and processing and analysis of samples

2 Materials

1. Complete medium: Dulbecco's Modified Eagle Medium (DMEM) supplemented with 10% fetal bovine serum (FBS), 100 U/mL penicillin, 100 µg/mL streptomycin, and 2 mM L-glutamine.
2. Serum-free medium: DMEM plus 100 U/mL penicillin, 100 µg/mL streptomycin, and 2 mM L-glutamine.

3. TrypLE™ or any other dissociation reagent for adherent cells.
4. Phosphate-buffered saline (PBS).
5. Plasmids for expression in mammalian cells (*see* **Note 1**).
6. FuGENE®6 or any other optimized transfection reagent.
7. 10 mM batimastat/BB94 prepared in dimethyl sulfoxide (DMSO), to be used at 10 μM.
8. SDS-PAGE sample buffer.
9. 100% (w/v) trichloroacetic acid (TCA).
10. 100% acetone.

3 Methods

3.1 Cell Culture and Transfection

1. Maintain COS-7 (*see* **Note 2**) cells in complete medium in a humidified incubator at 37 °C and 5% CO_2. Use tissue culture-treated plates, and perform all work with living cells in cell culture hoods to maintain sterility.
2. 24 h before transfection, seed 2 × 10^5 COS-7 cells per well on 6-well plates in 2 mL complete medium. To count cells, remove medium from plates, wash once with PBS, add TrypLE™ or any other dissociating reagent, incubate at 37 °C until cells detach, add complete medium, and use the required volume for counting. As an example, if 10 cm diameter plates are used for maintenance, wash with 10 mL PBS, dissociate with 1 mL TrypLE™, and stop the reaction with 3 mL complete medium (*see* **Note 3**). If starting from a confluent plate, use a 1:10 dilution of cells to determine concentration. Cells can be counted using a Neubauer chamber or any other counting device (*see* **Note 4**).
3. On the day of transfection, ideally in the evening, prepare tubes for the different transfection mixtures in the tissue culture hood. Mix 50 μL serum-free medium (*see* **Note 5**) with 3 μL FuGENE®6 (*see* **Note 6**) per tube/reaction; mix immediately by vortexing for 5–10 s, and incubate at room temperature for 5 min. Add 250 ng vector DNA coding for the tested substrate, plus/minus different amounts of vector coding for the rhomboid to be evaluated (normally between 25 and 250 ng) (*see* **Note 7**). Balance the total amount of DNA to 500 ng with the required amount of empty vector. Mix immediately (vortex 5–10 s) and incubate 15 min at room temperature. Add to the corresponding well with 2 mL complete medium (*see* **Note 8**).

Secretion Assay

4. The morning after transfection, pre-warm serum-free medium at 37 °C.

5. Take plates out of the incubator, remove medium, and wash once with 1 mL PBS per well.
6. Remove PBS and add 750 μL (*see* **Note 9**) pre-warmed serum-free medium, with or without 10 μM of batimastat (BB94), an inhibitor of metalloproteases. Batimastat will stop metalloproteases from cleaving the potential substrates, and thus the shedding detected in the presence of this drug will correspond to rhomboid protease activity. This serum-free medium will be the assay-conditioned medium.
7. Leave the cells in the incubator for 30 h in assay-conditioned medium. The potential shedding products will accumulate in the medium over this time.

3.2 Preparation of Samples and Western Blotting

1. After 30 h of incubation (this would correspond to early afternoon if the assay was started in the morning the day before), place the plates on ice.
2. Collect the supernatant (assay-conditioned medium) in 1.5 mL tubes and put on ice.
3. Centrifuge supernatants at maximum speed (~20,000 × *g*) on a bench centrifuge for 5 min at 4 °C, to remove any cell debris.
4. During the centrifugation step, lyse the monolayer of cells remaining on the plates. Start by washing with 1 mL ice-cold PBS and then add 100 μL SDS-PAGE sample buffer. Use a cell scraper to detach the cells. Pipette up and down a few times and transfer lysates to clean 1.5 mL tubes. Keep on ice throughout.
5. Transfer clean supernatants (assay-conditioned media) to new tubes; avoid taking any debris from the bottom.
6. Add 150 μL 100% TCA to precipitate proteins (~12–15% final concentration). Protein precipitation is needed to concentrate the products to be detected in the medium.
7. Incubate for 10 min on ice.
8. Centrifuge supernatants at maximum speed at 4 °C for 10 min.
9. Carefully aspirate supernatant; this can be done by using a vacuum aspirator or by pipetting carefully.
10. Wash the pellet by adding 180 μL ice-cold pure acetone and rocking the tube gently twice.
11. Centrifuge at maximum speed at 4 °C for 2 min.
12. Carefully remove all acetone by pipetting.
13. (Optional) Repeat **steps 8–10** one further time.
14. Leave the tubes open and allow to air-dry. This should take ~10–15 min at room temperature (*see* **Note 10**).

15. Resuspend the protein pellet by adding 30 μL SDS-PAGE sample buffer and pipette up and down several times.
16. Incubate all samples (cell lysates and supernatants) at 95 °C for 10 min to denature proteins (*see* **Note 11**). Samples can be used directly for loading on an SDS-PAGE gel or stored at −20 °C until use.
17. Electrophorese 15 μL of each sample on SDS-PAGE gels, as standard (*see* **Note 12**).
18. If using tagged versions of substrates, use the indicated anti-tag antibodies for detection of proteins. If using untagged substrates, antibodies able to detect the cleaved fragment can be used (*see* **Note 13**).
19. A positive result (identification of substrate shedding by the rhomboid protease) is considered when smaller (cleaved) versions of the substrate are seen in the supernatant only when co-expressed with the particular rhomboid. If an inactivated rhomboid protease with the catalytic serine or histidine mutated to alanine has been included, the cleavage product should not be present in the medium.

4 Notes

1. In this protocol, rhomboid proteases and potential substrates are exogenously overexpressed after transfection. Mammalian expression plasmids containing the cDNA sequence for the relevant rhomboids and substrates either tagged or untagged might be used. If untagged, specific antibodies recognising the different proteins will be necessary. It is important to note that, if using tagged proteins, the tag must be different for the protease and the substrate. The tag or the epitope recognised by the antibody of the substrate should be at the extracellular portion of the protein, so that both intact and shed protein can be detected. It is critical to demonstrate the detection of the shed substrate is directly due to active proteolysis by rhomboids. For this reason, plasmids that express catalytically dead mutants of the rhomboid protease in question should be used as controls. To render a rhomboid protease inactive, the catalytic serine and/or histidine can be mutated to alanine.
2. Different cell lines can also be used for these secretion assays. If so, cell culture and transfection protocols may require adaptation.
3. TrypLE™ was used in this example; any alternative dissociation reaction can be used.
4. Follow the manufacturer's instructions if using a Neubauer or equivalent manual counting system. Automatised cell counters

might also be used. As an alternative to counting cells, a 1:5 dilution of COS-7 cells starting from a confluent well will suffice.

5. Opti-MEM can be used instead of serum-free medium.
6. FuGENE®6 was used for transfection in this protocol; any other transfection reagents and systems (polyethylenimine, lipofectamine, etc.) might be used after optimisation.
7. If the volume of any of the plasmids is too small to dispense accurately and it is not possible to pool several reactions, predilute the plasmid solutions 1:10 and pipette a tenfold volume.
8. The media mixtures used for transfection do not have to be removed and can remain on the cells until the next morning. Alternative transfection reagents, such as polyethylenimine, will give better results if transfecting in serum-free medium and would need replacement with complete medium after 3–6 h.
9. A smaller volume than that typically used for culture in 6-well plates (2 mL/well) is used to increase the concentration of cleavage products. Care should be taken to ensure the monolayer of cells is completely covered with liquid.
10. Residual acetone will make resuspension more difficult, so it needs to be entirely removed. For faster acetone evaporation, tubes can be left at 65 °C for up to 1 min. A vacuum evaporator might also be used.
11. If cell protein lysates are too viscous, samples can be sonicated to break DNA and facilitate loading.
12. Concentration of SDS-PAGE gels and running time should be chosen based on the expected size of full length potential substrates and cleaved fragments.
13. The antibodies employed for detection should recognise a tag or antigen that remains in the cleaved soluble fragment after shedding. In this way, both the full-length and the cleaved products will be detected in the Western blotting.

References

1. Urban S, Lee JR, Freeman M (2001) Drosophila rhomboid-1 defines a family of putative intramembrane serine proteases. Cell 107(2):173–182
2. Koonin EV, Makarova KS, Rogozin IB et al (2003) The rhomboids: a nearly ubiquitous family of intramembrane serine proteases that probably evolved by multiple ancient horizontal gene transfers. Genome Biol 4(3):R19
3. Wang Y, Zhang Y, Ha Y (2006) Crystal structure of a rhomboid family intramembrane protease. Nature 444(7116):179–180. https://doi.org/10.1038/nature05255
4. Freeman M (2014) The rhomboid-like superfamily: molecular mechanisms and biological roles. Annu Rev Cell Dev Biol 30:235–254. https://doi.org/10.1146/annurev-cellbio-100913-012944

5. Lemberg MK, Menendez J, Misik A et al (2005) Mechanism of intramembrane proteolysis investigated with purified rhomboid proteases. EMBO J 24(3):464–472. https://doi.org/10.1038/sj.emboj.7600537
6. Urban S (2010) Taking the plunge: integrating structural, enzymatic and computational insights into a unified model for membrane-immersed rhomboid proteolysis. Biochem J 425(3):501–512. https://doi.org/10.1042/BJ20090861
7. Lastun VL, Grieve AG, Freeman M (2016) Substrates and physiological functions of secretase rhomboid proteases. Semin Cell Dev Biol 60:10–18. https://doi.org/10.1016/j.semcdb.2016.07.033
8. Urban S, Lee JR, Freeman M (2002) A family of rhomboid intramembrane proteases activates all Drosophila membrane-tethered EGF ligands. EMBO J 21(16):4277–4286
9. Lohi O, Urban S, Freeman M (2004) Diverse substrate recognition mechanisms for rhomboids; thrombomodulin is cleaved by mammalian rhomboids. Curr Biol 14(3):236–241. https://doi.org/10.1016/j.cub.2004.01.025
10. Adrain C, Strisovsky K, Zettl M et al (2011) Mammalian EGF receptor activation by the rhomboid protease RHBDL2. EMBO Rep 12(5):421–427. https://doi.org/10.1038/embor.2011.50
11. Pascall JC, Brown KD (2004) Intramembrane cleavage of ephrinB3 by the human rhomboid family protease, RHBDL2. Biochem Biophys Res Commun 317(1):244–252. https://doi.org/10.1016/j.bbrc.2004.03.039
12. Arteaga CL, Engelman JA (2014) ERBB receptors: from oncogene discovery to basic science to mechanism-based cancer therapeutics. Cancer Cell 25(3):282–303. https://doi.org/10.1016/j.ccr.2014.02.025
13. Normanno N, De Luca A, Bianco C et al (2006) Epidermal growth factor receptor (EGFR) signaling in cancer. Gene 366(1):2–16. https://doi.org/10.1016/j.gene.2005.10.018
14. Song W, Liu W, Zhao H et al (2015) Rhomboid domain containing 1 promotes colorectal cancer growth through activation of the EGFR signalling pathway. Nat Commun 6:8022. https://doi.org/10.1038/ncomms9022

Chapter 7

Functional Production of Catalytic Domains of Human MMPs in Escherichia coli Periplasm

Dong Hyun Nam, Ki Baek Lee, and Xin Ge

Abstract

Due to their central roles in tumor growth and invasion, milligram-level amounts of active MMPs are frequently required for cancer research and development of chemical or biological MMP inhibitors. Here we describe methods for functional production of catalytic domains of MMPs (cdMMPs) in *E. coli* periplasm without refolding or activation process. We demonstrate applications of this straightforward approach for cdMMP-9, cdMMP-14, and cdMMP-14 mutants.

Key words Periplasmic expression, MMP, Catalytic domain

1 Introduction

MMPs (matrix metalloproteases) are multi-domain zinc-dependent endopeptidases that share a basic structural organization comprising propeptidic, catalytic, hinge, and hemopexin-like domains [1] (Fig. 1a, b). Besides functioning in normal physiological processes, many MMPs correlate with cancer progression, including cancer cell invasion, proliferation and apoptosis, and tumor angiogenesis and vasculogenesis [2–4]. Taking these preclinical and clinical evidences together, some MMPs such as MMP-2/MMP-9/MMP-14, etc. have been considered as important regulatory enzymes for cancer research and predominant therapeutic targets for cancer treatments [5–7]. Therefore, the consistent supply of active MMPs at mg scales is essential for cancer biology research and for the developments of novel diagnostic and therapeutic agents. Applications include identification of physiological substrates of MMPs, characterization of extracellular matrix remolding in vitro and in vivo, and screening for highly selective MMP inhibitors.

Recombinant overexpression of many human MMPs and their catalytic domains in *E. coli* exclusively results in the formation of inclusion bodies [8]. After solubilization and purification, the denatured MMPs can be refolded to their active form via multiple

Santiago Cal and Alvaro J. Obaya (eds.), *Proteases and Cancer: Methods and Protocols*, Methods in Molecular Biology, vol. 1731, https://doi.org/10.1007/978-1-4939-7595-2_7, © Springer Science+Business Media, LLC 2018

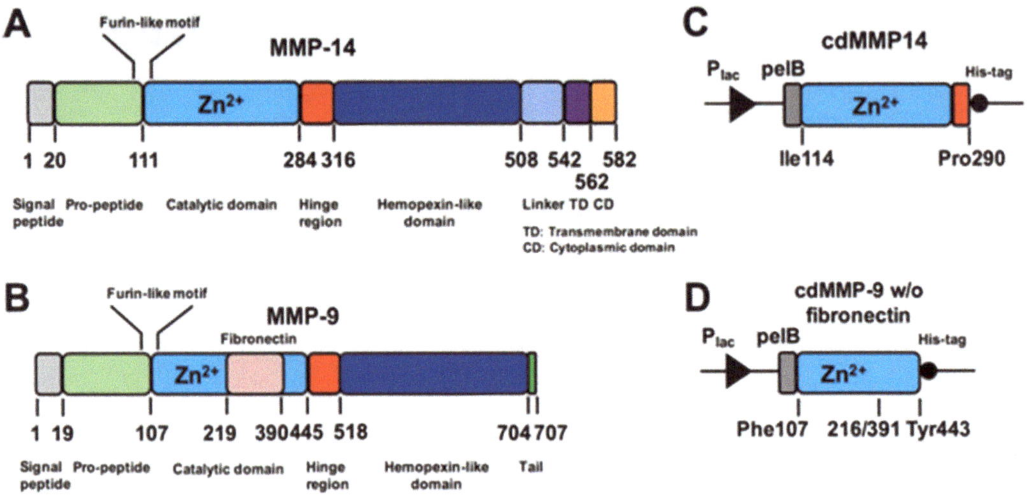

Fig. 1 Gene structures for (**a**) full-length MMP-14 and (**b**) full-length MMP-9, and periplasmic expression cassettes for (**c**) MMP-14 catalytic domain and (**d**) MMP-9 catalytic domain without fibronectin domain. Plac promoter and pelB leader peptide were used for cdMMP expression

steps of gradient dialysis, which are often labor-extensive and time-consuming. Besides low yields (typically <35%) and uncontrollable lot-to-lot variation, during the refolding process, autoproteolysis occurs at both termini with various degrees thus generating heterogeneous mixtures [9]. Alternatively, MMP with its propeptidic domain, e.g., pro-MMP-14, has been periplasmically expressed in *E. coli* by fusing with a signal peptide [10]. However, after purification, pro-MMP-14 was treated with 4-aminophynylmercuric acetate (APMA) or trypsin to yield the functional enzyme [11]. As an organomercury compound, APMA is toxic, and complete activation of pro-MMP-14 using APMA is difficult [12]. In addition to cleavage of the propeptide, trypsin treatment also digests the C-terminus of MMP-14 at the putative furin cleavage site (RRKR/YAIQ) resulting in truncated products [11].

Taking advantages of a slow processing rate controlled by secretion machineries and multiple periplasmic molecular chaperons that enhance proper protein folding, we develop a method to directly express functional MMP catalytic domains in the periplasmic space of *E. coli* [13]. This straightforward method avoids the problematic activation and tedious refolding processes associated with inclusion bodies. Here we demonstrate this method for producing catalytic domains of both a secreted MMP (cdMMP-9) and a membrane-based MMP (cdMMP-14). We further expand this method to produce cdMMP-14 mutants. A facile approach to obtaining milligrams of active cdMMPs is beneficial for MMP related studies, particularly for the development of therapeutic drugs targeting important MMPs for cancer treatments.

2 Materials

2.1 Construction of cdMMP Genes

1. Plasmid pMopac16 [14].
2. DNA fragments encoding cdMMPs.
3. Jude-I [DH10B F′[proAB lacI^Q lacZ ΔM15 Tn10(Tet^R)]] competent cells.

2.2 Periplasmic Expression and Purification of cdMMPs

1. BL21 [*E. coli* B F$^-$ *ompT gal dcm lon hsdS*$_B$($r_B^- m_B^-$) [*malB*$^+$]$_{K\text{-}12}$(λ^S)].
2. 2×YT/Chlor: 2×YT, 34 μg/mL chloramphenicol.
3. LB/Chlor agar: LB, 1.5 g/L agar, 34 μg/mL chloramphenicol.
4. Periplasmic buffer: 200 mM Tris–HCl, pH 7.5, 20% sucrose, 50 μg/mL lysozyme.
5. 0.45 μm filter units, 90 mm, 500 mL.
6. Ni-NTA agarose (Qiagen).
7. Ni-NTA column equilibrium buffer: 50 mM Tris–HCl, pH 8.0, 300 mM NaCl.
8. Ni-NTA column washing buffer: 50 mM Tris–HCl, pH 8.0, 300 mM NaCl, 20 mM imidazole.
9. Ni-NTA column elution buffer: 50 mM Tris–HCl, pH 8.0, 300 mM NaCl, 200 mM imidazole.
10. Ultrafiltration centrifugal units, 3 kDa MWCO.
11. SnakeSkin dialysis tubing, 3.5 kDa MWCO, 16 mm (Thermo Scientific).
12. Dialysis buffer: 50 mM Tris–HCl, pH 7.5, 150 mM NaCl, 5 mM $CaCl_2$, 0.1 mM $ZnCl_2$.

2.3 Characterizations of cdMMPs

2.3.1 Activity Measurement by FRET

1. Peptide M-2350 (Bachem): Mca-Lys-Pro-Leu-Gly-Leu-Dap(Dnp)-Ala-Arg-NH_2.
2. Peptide XV (AnaSpec): QXL®520-γ-Abu-Pro-Glu-Gly-Leu-Dab(5-FAM)-Ala-Lys-NH_2.
3. GM6001 (Millipore).
4. N-Tissue inhibitor of metalloproteinases 2 (nTIMP-2).
5. Black flat-bottom polystyrene NBS 96-well microplate (Corning).
6. 20% dimethyl sulfoxide (DMSO).
7. Assay buffer: 50 mM Tris–HCl, pH 7.5, 150 mM NaCl, 5 mM $CaCl_2$, 0.1 mM $ZnCl_2$.

2.3.2 Analysis by Gel Permeable Chromatography

1. Ovalbumin.
2. Lysozyme.
3. Superdex 75 10/300 GL size-exclusion column.
4. Equilibrium buffer: 50 mM HEPES-NaOH, pH 7.5, 150 mM NaCl.

3 Methods

3.1 Construction of cdMMP Genes

1. Synthesize DNA fragments encoding catalytic domains of human MMP-14 (Ile114-Pro290) and human MMP-9 (fibronectin domain removed, Ile107-Val216 fused with Glu391-Tyr443) (Fig. 1c, d).
2. Following standard molecular biology techniques, clone cdMMP genes to the periplasmic expression plasmid pMopac16 [14], which carries a *Lac* promoter, a pelB leader peptide, and a C-terminal His-tag (Fig. 1c, d).
3. Construct cdMMP-14 mutant genes by overlapping PCRs, in which the site-specific mutagenesis is introduced by oligonucleotides.
4. Confirm all cloning results by DNA sequencing (*see* **Note 1**). Transform constructed cdMMP periplasmic expression plasmids to Jude-I component cells. Incubate on LB/Chlor agar plates.

3.2 Periplasmic Expression and Purification of cdMMPs

1. Inoculate a single colony of Jude-I or BL21 cells carrying pMopac-cdMMP to 5 mL 2×YT/Chlor. Culture at 30 °C overnight (*see* **Note 2**).
2. Add 5 mL overnight pre-culture to 500 mL 2×YT/Chlor. Culture overnight at 30 °C without IPTG (*see* **Note 3**).
3. Measure OD_{600}. Centrifuge cells at 4500 × *g*, 4 °C for 15 min. Decant supernatant.
4. Add periplasmic buffer (*see* **Note 4**) at a volume of 20 μL per OD_{600}. Suspend collected cells by vortex.
5. Incubate for 5 min at room temperature with gentle shaking.
6. Add ice-cold DDW at volume of 20 μL per OD_{600}. Incubate on ice for 10 min with gentle shaking.
7. Centrifuge 4500 × *g*, 4 °C for 15 min. Filtrate supernatant through 0.45 μm membranes. Osmotic shocked supernatants are ready for cdMMP purification.
8. Purify cdMMPs by Ni-NTA resin. Use 20 and 200 mM imidazole in 50 mM Tris–HCl, pH 8.0, 300 mM NaCl as the washing and elution buffers.
9. Concentrate eluted samples using ultrafiltration units (3 kDa MWCO) by centrifugation at 4000 × *g* 4 °C for 15 min.
10. Dialyze concentrated cdMMP samples at 4 °C overnight (*see* **Note 5**).
11. On the next day, measure cdMMP concentrations. Analyze by SDS-PAGE (typical results shown in Fig. 2). Store in 20% glycerol at −80 °C.

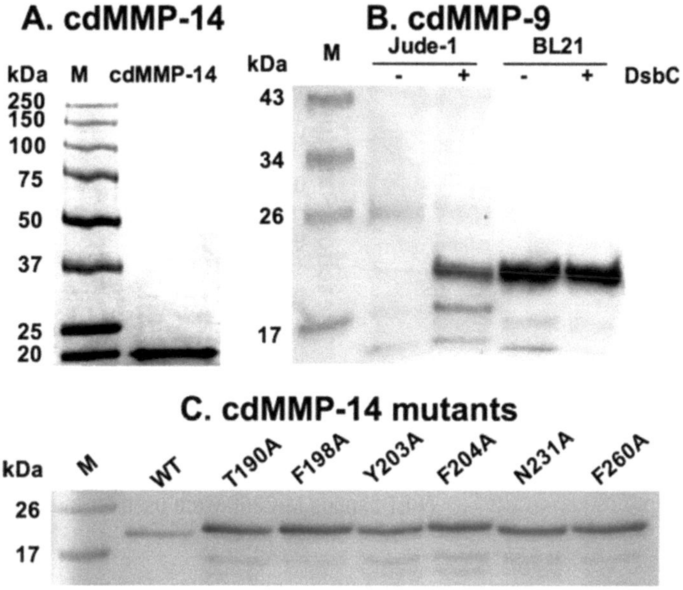

Fig. 2 SDS-PAGE of purified (**a**) cdMMP-14, (**b**) cdMMP-9, and (**c**) cdMMP-14 mutants

3.3 Characterizations of cdMMPs

K_m and k_{cat} values of purified cdMMPs and their mutants can be measured (Subheading 3.3.1). In addition to enzymatic kinetics, the periplasmic preparation without purification can be directly applied for activity tests (Subheading 3.3.2), which are particularly useful in screening of MMP inhibitors [15].

3.3.1 Enzymatic Kinetics Measurement

1. Dissolve fluorogenic substrate peptide M-2350 in 20% DMSO to concentrations of 62.5–2000 μM.
2. Add 50 μL 1–10 nM cdMMP to a 96-well black assay plate.
3. To start the reaction, add 1 μL substrate peptide stock solutions into wells to give final concentrations of 1.25–40 μM.
4. Monitor the hydrolysis of peptide M-2350 with excitation at 328 nm and emission at 393 nm.
5. Triplicate the experiments. Fit Michaelis-Menten equation to find K_m and k_{cat} (Fig. 3).

3.3.2 Periplasmic FRET Assays

1. Suspend 2–3 OD_{600} overnight cultures (Subheading 3.2) in 100 μL periplasmic buffer. Incubate on ice for 5 min.
2. Add same volume ice-cold DDW. Incubate on ice for 10 min to release periplasmic fraction.
3. Centrifuge 13,000 × *g*, RT for 2 min.

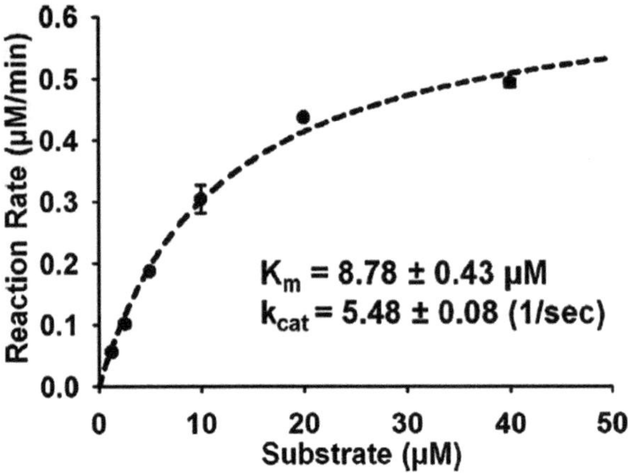

Fig. 3 Enzyme kinetics of cdMMP-14. 1–10 nM cdMMP-14 and 1.25–40 μM FRET peptide M-2350 were used for measurements of K_m and k_{cat}

4. Add 50–100 μL periplasmic fraction to a 96-well black assay plate.
5. To start the reaction, add peptide XV to a final concentration of 1 μM (*see* **Note 6**). Monitor hydrolysis with excitation at 490 nm and emission at 520 nm.
6. For inhibitor screening, add 0–1000 nM compound inhibitors (e.g., GM60001), 0–2000 nM nTIMP-2, or 0–8000 nM Fabs (e.g., 3A2, [16]) into the periplasmic fraction before adding the peptide substrate (*see* **Note 7**).

3.3.3 Analysis by Gel Permeable Chromatography

1. Equilibrate superdex 75 10/300 GL size-exclusion column with 50 mM HEPES pH 7.5, 150 mM NaCl.
2. Inject 200 μL 500 μg/mL cdMMP-9 at a flow rate of 0.5 mL/min.
3. Monitor chromatograms of absorbance at 280 nm (Fig. 4).
4. Estimate the molecular mass of cdMMP-9 based on the retention times of ovalbumin (43 kDa) and lysozyme (14 kDa).

4 Notes

1. In addition to DNA sequencing, correct in-frame cdMMP clones can also be identified by measuring their proteolytic activities ([15]; also *see* Subheading 3.3.2).
2. Expression of cdMMP-9 in Jude-I resulted in truncated products likely due to endogenous proteases. Using protease deficient host BL21 reduced the amount of unwanted truncations.

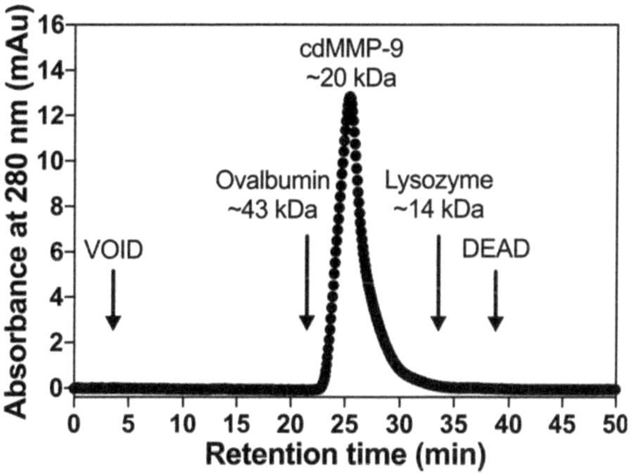

Fig. 4 Gel permeation chromatography result of purified cdMMP-9. Chromatograms were obtained by monitoring absorbance at 280 nm. Ovalbumin (43 kDa) and lysozyme (14 kDa) were used as controls for molecular weight comparison

In addition, although cdMMPs do not have disulfide bonds, we found that co-expression of molecular chaperon DsbC (a disulfide isomerase) significantly improved the yields of cdMMPs (Fig. 2b), a similar observation for TIMPs [17].

3. Although cdMMPs are regulated under a *Lac* promoter, experimental results indicate that the highest activity was achieved without IPTG induction [13].
4. EDTA treatment, a step of standard periplasmic fraction protocol [18], should be avoided due to its ability to chelate Ca^{2+} and Zn^{2+} ions which are essential for MMP structure and activity.
5. Dialysis is required to remove imidazole (a weak inhibitor of MMPs) for downstream applications.
6. Certain FRET substrates, e.g., M-2350 peptide, cannot be used for periplasmic activity assays due to its proteolysis by homologous endopeptidases present in *E. coli* periplasm.
7. Other than adding purified Fabs into periplasmic fraction, the Fab clone of interest can also be co-expressed with cdMMP for inhibitor screening [13].

Acknowledgments

This work was supported by National Science Foundation the Faculty Early Career Development (CAREER) Program 1453645 and National Institutes of Health Grant R01 GM115672 to X.G.

References

1. Sela-Passwell N, Rosenblum G, Shoham T et al (2010) Structural and functional bases for allosteric control of MMP activities: can it pave the path for selective inhibition? Biochim Biophys Acta 1803(1):29–38
2. Jiang A, Lehti K, Wang X et al (2001) Regulation of membrane-type matrix metalloproteinase 1 activity by dynamin-mediated endocytosis. Proc Natl Acad Sci U S A 98(24):13693–13698
3. Tetu B, Brisson J, Wang CS et al (2006) The influence of MMP-14, TIMP-2 and MMP-2 expression on breast cancer prognosis. Breast Cancer Res 8(3):R28
4. Mimori K, Ueo H, Shirasaka C et al (2001) Clinical significance of MT1-MMP mRNA expression in breast cancer. Oncol Rep 8(2):401–403
5. Genís L, Gálvez BG, Gonzalo P et al (2006) MT1-MMP: universal or particular player in angiogenesis? Cancer Metastasis Rev 25(1):77–86
6. Morrison CJ, Butler GS, Rodríguez D et al (2009) Matrix metalloproteinase proteomics: substrates, targets, and therapy. Curr Opin Cell Biol 21(5):645–653
7. Devy L, Dransfield DT (2011) New Strategies for the next generation of matrix-metalloproteinase inhibitors: selectively targeting membrane-anchored MMPs with therapeutic antibodies. Biochem Res Int 2011:191670
8. Koo HM, Kim JH, Hwang IK et al (2002) Refolding of the catalytic and hinge domains of human MT1-mMP expressed in Escherichia coli and its characterization. Mol Cells 13(1):118–124
9. Lichte A, Kolkenbrock H, Tschesche H (1996) The recombinant catalytic domain of membrane-type matrix metalloproteinase-1 (MT1-MMP) induces activation of progelatinase A and progelatinase A complexed with TIMP-2. FEBS Lett 397(2–3):277–282
10. Baneyx F, Mujacic M (2004) Recombinant protein folding and misfolding in Escherichia coli. Nat Biotechnol 22(11):1399–1408
11. Will H, Atkinson SJ, Butler GS et al (1996) The soluble catalytic domain of membrane type 1 matrix metalloproteinase cleaves the propeptide of progelatinase A and initiates autoproteolytic activation. Regulation by TIMP-2 and TIMP-3. J Biol Chem 271(29):17119–17123
12. Knäuper V, Will H, López-Otin C et al (1996) Cellular mechanisms for human procollagenase-3 (MMP-13) activation. Evidence that MT1-MMP (MMP-14) and gelatinase a (MMP-2) are able to generate active enzyme. J Biol Chem 271(29):17124–17131
13. Nam DH, Ge X (2016) Direct production of functional matrix metalloproteinase-14 without refolding or activation and its application for in vitro inhibition assays. Biotechnol Bioeng 113(4):717–723
14. Hayhurst A, Happe S, Mabry R et al (2003) Isolation and expression of recombinant antibody fragments to the biological warfare pathogen Brucella melitensis. J Immunol Methods 276(1–2):185–196
15. Nam DH, Ge X (2013) Development of periplasmic FRET-based screening method for protease inhibitory antibodies. Biotechnol Bioeng 110(11):2856–2864
16. Nam DH, Rodriguez C, Remacle AG et al (2016) Active-site MMP-selective antibody inhibitors discovered from convex paratope synthetic libraries. Proc Natl Acad Sci U S A 113(52):14970–14975
17. Lee KB, Nam DH, Nuhn J et al (2017) Direct expression of active human tissue inhibitors of Metalloproteinase by periplasmic secretion in Escherichia coli. Microb Cell Factories 16:73
18. Goldman ER, Hayhurst A, Lingerfelt BM et al (2003) 2,4,6-Trinitrotoluene detection using recombinant antibodies. J Environ Monit 5(3):380–383

Chapter 8

Autophagy and Proteases: Basic Study of the Autophagic Flux by Western Blot

Álvaro F. Fernández

Abstract

Autophagy is a catabolic process triggered in the cell by a wide range of stress stimuli, both external (including nutrient deprivation) and internal (like the presence of protein aggregates or damaged organelles). First described in yeast, this pathway has recently gained major importance due to its role in several pathologies, from inflammatory processes to cancer or aging. However, its analysis can be easily misinterpreted if it is not done properly, leading to conflicting results. Here, the classical autophagy flux study by Western blot is described, as a first and basic analysis of the status of autophagy in a given system.

Key words Autophagy, Western blot, LC3, p62, Bafilomycin A1

1 Introduction

Originally described in yeast, autophagy (term derived from the Greek for "self-eating") is an evolutionary conserved pathway characterized by the transport of cytoplasmic components to a lysosome [1]. There, they are degraded into their basic building blocks (like amino acids or lipids) that will return to the cytoplasm to be further reused. Cells can use three different ways to complete this transfer to the lysosome: by invaginations of the lysosomal membrane (microautophagy), by the action of chaperones associated with the lysosomal membrane that recognize specific targets (chaperone-mediated autophagy, or CMA), or by sequestering cytoplasmic portions into double-membrane vesicles called autophagosomes that eventually fuse with the lysosome (macroautophagy, or "autophagy" for simplicity). The latter is the most studied pathway to date, and it requires a complex molecular machinery that is not fully understood yet [2]. Nevertheless, autophagy is intimately related with different groups of proteases of potential interest [3] (Fig. 1). For instance, there are several proteinases that can modulate the process by cleaving important regulators like beclin-1 or ATG5 [4], proteases that are targeted

Santiago Cal and Alvaro J. Obaya (eds.), *Proteases and Cancer: Methods and Protocols*, Methods in Molecular Biology, vol. 1731,
https://doi.org/10.1007/978-1-4939-7595-2_8, © Springer Science+Business Media, LLC 2018

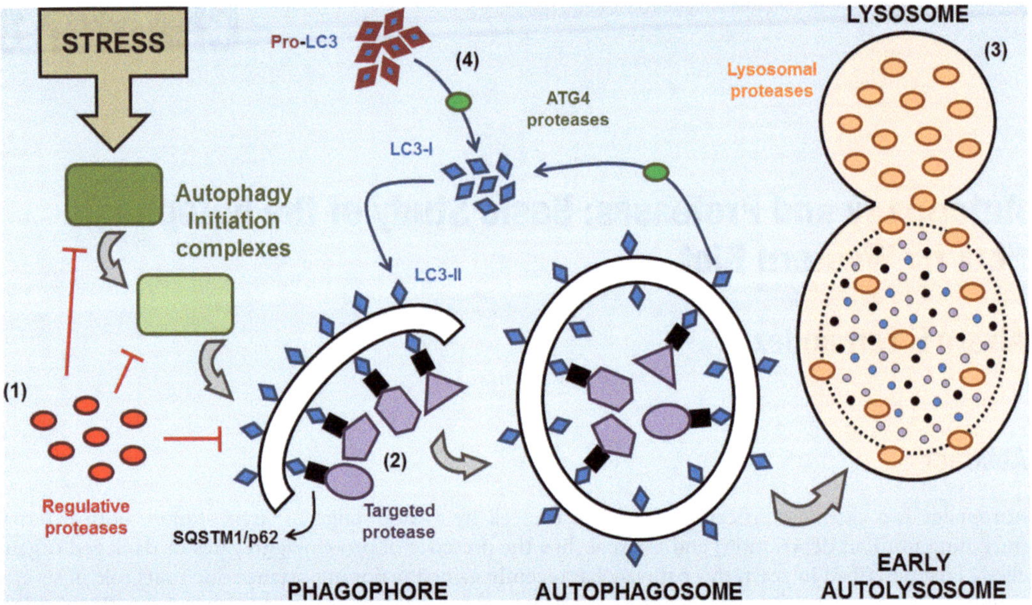

Fig. 1 Proteases in macroautophagy. Different groups of proteases are involved throughout the autophagy process, including proteinases that regulate key effectors of autophagy initiation (1), proteases that are degraded within other cytoplasmic components (2), and lysosomal hydrolases that mediate the final step (3). Moreover, there is a specific group of cysteine proteases, called ATG4s or autophagins, which are responsible for the activation and recycling of LC3. Notice LC3 cycle (going from LC3-I to LC3-II and vice versa) and the degradation of the adaptor p62 during the process

for degradation by autophagy as part of their own regulation [5], and lysosomal hydrolases that mediate the last step of the pathway [6]. Moreover, there is a cysteine proteinase crucial for the formation of the autophagosome in yeast (called Atg4) that has evolved into a family of four different orthologues in mammals, termed autophagins [7].

Even though autophagy was first considered to be a catabolic pathway aimed to recycle unspecific cargos in response to starvation and other bioenergetics demands, it is now clear that this process can be very specific and tightly regulated, being triggered by an extensive range of stress stimuli [8]. Moreover, it has recently gained increased relevance due to its importance in different pathologies, like cancer, inflammation, and aging-associated diseases [9–12]. Thus, it is now essential to correctly assess the status of the "autophagy flux" in those scenarios where the pathway may be playing an important role.

While there are different publications summarizing the wide set of experiments traditionally used in autophagy research [13] or detailing specific assays to analyze Atg4 activity [14, 15], the main goal of this chapter is the analysis of the autophagy flux by Western blot in mammalian cell lines. This procedure is based on the dynamic status of two autophagic proteins during the process: MAP1-LC3B (herein simply referred to LC3) and SQSTM1/p62. The former is one of the six mammalian orthologues of yeast Atg8 described to date. Similarly to its yeast counterpart, these proteins must be activated by Atg4 (or, in this case, autophagins) so they are lipidated and transferred to the growing autophagosome membrane. For this reason, a rise in the amounts of lipidated LC3 (that shows increased electrophoretic mobility in SDS-PAGE gels) is in most cases related to autophagy induction. On the other hand, SQSTM1/p62 (or just p62) is an adaptor that recognizes cytoplasmic components that have been marked by ubiquitination for autophagy degradation. In fact, p62 acts as a link between the target and LC3 molecules in the inner surface of the autophagosome structure, being degraded with them in the last step of the pathway. Thus, protein levels of p62 negatively correlate with an increased autophagy flux. Though basic, this technique is the most important way to primarily assess autophagy in a working system. Unfortunately, it is uncommonly performed in a suitable way, resulting in misleading data and inaccurate conclusions.

2 Materials

2.1 Cell Culture

1. 6-well tissue culture plates (*see* **Note 1**).
2. Dulbecco's phosphate-buffered saline (PBS).
3. Nutrient-rich medium: Use regular growing medium for the cell line to be tested.
4. Starvation medium: Earle's balanced salt solution (EBSS) or Hank's balanced salt solution are the most used for this procedure (*see* **Note 2**).
5. Bafilomycin A1: Prepare a stock solution of 100 μM in DMSO (*see* **Note 3**).

2.2 Sample Preparation

1. Cell scraper.
2. Microcentrifuge tubes (1.5 mL).
3. Lysis buffer: 1 mM EDTA, 1% Triton X-100, 0.1% sodium dodecyl sulfate (SDS), and 140 mM NaCl in 20 mM Tris–HCl buffer (pH 7.4). Store at 4 °C until use, when Complete® protease inhibitor cocktail and Halt phosphatase inhibitor cocktail must be added. Keep in ice during the experiment (*see* **Note 4**).
4. Microcentrifuge in cold room or with temperature control.
5. Reagents for protein quantification, e.g., bicinchoninic acid assay (BCA).

6. Loading buffer (2×): 5% 2-mercaptoethanol in 2× Laemmli sample buffer (4% SDS, 20% glycerol, 0.004% bromophenol blue in 125 mM Tris–HCl, pH 6.8) (*see* **Note 5**).
7. Heat block.

2.3 SDS-PAGE

1. 13% SDS-polyacrylamide gels (*see* **Note 6**).
2. Protein standards.
3. Running buffer (10×): 250 mM Tris–HCl, 1.92 M glycine and 1% SDS in H_2O (pH 8.3).

2.4 Immunoblotting

1. Spatula.
2. Plastic containers.
3. Methanol.
4. Polyvinylidene difluoride (PVDF) membrane (*see* **Note 7**).
5. Blotting filter paper for protein transfer.
6. Transfer buffer: 60 mM Tris–HCl, 40 mM CAPS, 15% methanol in H_2O (pH 9.6) (*see* **Note 8**).
7. Transfer system (for either tank or semidry blotting).
8. Washing buffer: TBS-T (50 mM Tris–HCl pH 7.4, 150 mM NaCl, and 0.1% Tween20) (*see* **Note 9**).
9. Blocking and diluent buffer: 5% nonfat dried milk in TBS-T (*see* **Note 10**).
10. Primary antibodies to recognize LC3, p62, and "housekeeping" proteins, e.g., β-actin (*see* **Note 11**).
11. Specific HRP-conjugated secondary antibodies.
12. Chemiluminescent substrate for detection of horseradish peroxidase (HRP) activity.
13. Plastic wrap.
14. X-ray film or chemiluminescence imager.
15. ImageJ software.

3 Methods

3.1 In Vitro Autophagy Induction

1. Seed the cells in 6-well plates so the confluence by the time of the experiment is 80–90% approximately (*see* **Note 12**).
2. Warm nutrient-rich and starvation media in 37 °C water bath prior to use. Thaw an aliquot of bafilomycin A1, and add it to tubes with nutrient-rich or starvation medium for a final concentration of 100 nM.
3. Discard the growing medium from the wells, and carefully wash the cells with PBS to further remove remaining nutrients.

4. Add the corresponding treatments (nutrient-rich or starvation medium, with or without bafilomycin A1) to the cells, and incubate for 3 h at 37 °C in a cell incubator (*see* **Note 13**).

3.2 Preparation of the Samples

1. Discard the medium, rinse the cells with PBS twice, and add cold lysis buffer to the wells (*see* **Note 14**). Detach the cells with a scrapper, collect them in 1.5 mL tubes, and place them in ice.
2. Lyse the cells for 1 h in ice or, preferably, using a rotator at 4 °C. Next, centrifuge the samples at 1300 × *g* at 4 °C, and collect the supernatants to get rid of debris.
3. Determine protein concentration in the samples by any standard protein quantification (i.e., BCA). Mix the samples with loading buffer so 15–50 μg of protein can easily be loaded to a SDS-polyacrylamide gel.
4. Boil the samples for 10 min, spin them, and let them temper before loading the gel (*see* **Note 15**).

3.3 Western Blot Analysis

1. Load 15–50 μg of protein per lane (along with protein standards as molecular weight markers) in a 13% SDS-polyacrylamide gel. Run the gel in running buffer (1×) until the dye front reaches the bottom.
2. Separate the gel from the plates (using a spatula or similar), and discard the stacking part of it before washing the remaining portion with transfer buffer for no more than 5 min (*see* **Note 16**).
3. Activate a PVDF membrane by immersing it in methanol and washing it vigorously in transfer buffer until it sinks. Also submerge other components required for the transfer in the same buffer.
4. Blot the proteins of the gel into the PVDF membrane by electrophoretic transfer using transfer buffer.
5. Recover the membrane and, without letting it dry (*see* **Note 17**), incubate it with blocking buffer for 1 h at room temperature.
6. While still in blocking buffer, cut the membrane in three pieces using the protein standards as a reference of the size of the proteins included in each part. One gel can be used to analyze p62 (62 kDa), housekeeping proteins like β-actin (44 kDa), and LC3-I/LC3-II (16 and 14 kDa, approximately) at once.
7. Incubate the membranes with the corresponding primary antibodies diluted in blocking buffer overnight at 4 °C.
8. Wash the membranes three times with TBS-T in agitation, 5–10 min each (*see* **Note 18**).

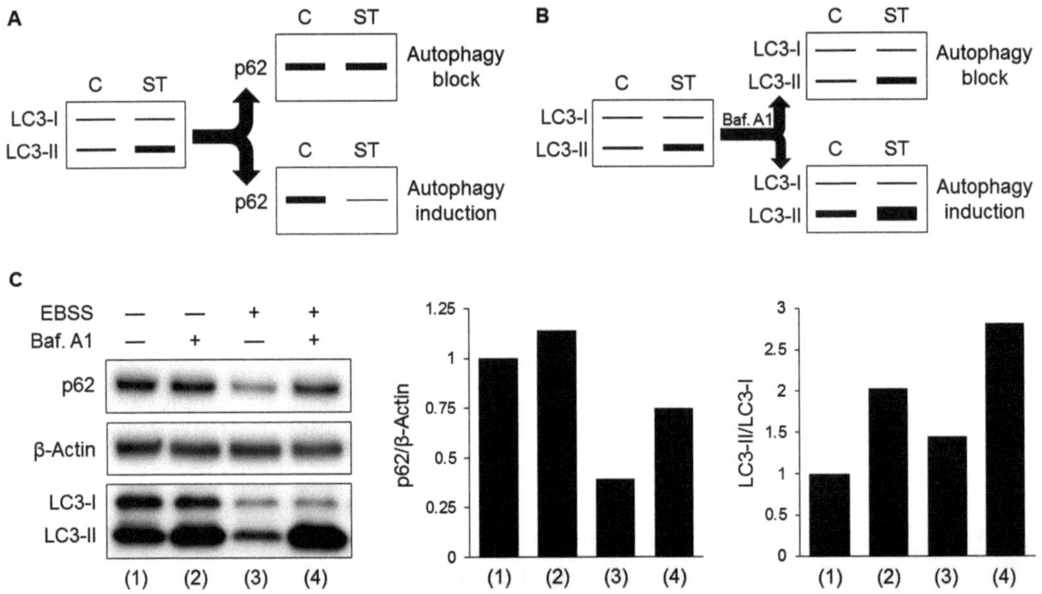

Fig. 2 Interpreting the autophagy flux analysis by Western blot. Most of the times, a simple Western blot of LC3 is shown to confirm autophagy induction upon stimulation of the process. However, this assumption may be incorrect. An accumulation of LC3-II, for example, can also mean a block in the last step of the process that diminishes its degradation. To avoid this mistake, an additional analysis of p62 is always recommended to discern these two possibilities (**a**). Nevertheless, a complete study of the autophagy flux using inhibitors like bafilomycin A1, when possible, is the best way to establish a first assessment of autophagy as it further clarifies the reasons why LC3-II may be accumulated (**b**). A real case is displayed in (**c**), where a complete study in HeLa cells treated with EBSS and bafilomycin A1 shows how these cells are capable of triggering a correct autophagy process. In this example, the ratio LC3-II/LC3-I turns out to be necessary, as LC3-II levels decreased after starvation due to its intense degradation

9. Incubate the membranes with the corresponding secondary antibodies diluted in blocking buffer for 1 h at room temperature.
10. Wash the membranes three times with TBS-T in agitation, 5–10 min each.
11. Cover the membranes with the chemiluminescent substrate, and incubate for 5 min in dark at room temperature. Then, wrap them in transparent plastic for signal detection using an X-ray film or a chemiluminescence imager (*see* **Note 19**).
12. Perform a densitometry analysis of the intensity of the resulting bands using ImageJ. Relativize the values of p62, LC3-I, and LC3-II to those of β-actin, and calculate the ratio between LC3-II and LC3-I (*see* **Note 20**).
13. Interpret the results accordingly (Fig. 2).

4 Notes

1. Some cell lines with high protein expression would allow working with 12-well culture plates. However, using 6-well plates ensures having enough sample to perform different analysis.
2. Though specific nutrient deficiency (like using glucose-free or amino acid-free medium) is also of interest in autophagy research, complete nutrient deprivation has been traditionally used for autophagy flux analysis.
3. Other inhibitors of the last step of autophagy, like chloroquine or leupeptin, are frequently used for in vivo analysis of the autophagy flux. However, bafilomycin A1 is generally the preferred choice in vitro.
4. Different lysis buffers may be also suitable for this procedure. Nevertheless, the presence of SDS will always help the recovery and detection of the lipidated form of LC3.
5. Always handle 2-mercaptoethanol and SDS under a hood to avoid being exposed to it.
6. A high concentration of polyacrylamide is required to better separate the two forms of LC3. Alternatively, gradient gels can help to obtain a good separation.
7. Nitrocellulose membrane can also be used. However, LC3 detection is highly increased in PVDF membranes, though they require special handling (methanol activation and avoidance of dryness).
8. If LC3 blotting is problematic, try to increase methanol concentration up to 20% in the transfer buffer, as it helps the blotting of small proteins.
9. PBST (PBS with 0.05% Tween20) is another valid option in this case, as phospho-specific antibodies are not required in this procedure.
10. Blocking the membrane with bovine serum albumin (BSA) is also acceptable if the antibodies require it.
11. It is important to keep in mind that some LC3B antibodies can also recognize other isoforms, mostly LC3A. Moreover, LC3-II appears to be more sensitive to detection by some commercially available antibodies, giving more importance to the complete study of the autophagy flux.
12. Be sure that the cells grow evenly throughout the surface, ensuring a uniform effect of the treatment. Vibrations in the incubator may sometimes cause cell accumulation in the center of the well and cell isolation in the periphery, protecting the former from the treatment and overexposing the latter to it.

Place water bottles over the trays in the incubator to minimize these vibrations.

13. Do not treat the cells for extended periods of time. Prolonged starvation would increase cell death, and long treatments with inhibitors like bafilomycin A1 have additional effects in cell homeostasis that may increase autophagy rather than block it.
14. Proceed as quickly as possible during this step to avoid cellular stress that may alter the results. Discard by sudden inversion of the plate, and add the PBS or the lysis buffer quickly while keeping the plate over ice.
15. Complete sample preparation is recommended before freezing and storing the samples as LC3-I is more easily degraded by freeze-thaw cycles, affecting to LC3-II/LC3-I ratios.
16. Washing the gel before the transfer removes SDS that interferes with the blotting of small proteins like LC3.
17. A new methanol activation is required if the membrane dries. However, it can deliberately be dried to stop the procedure and storage. Interestingly, drying the membrane before continuing with the immunoblot increases the binding of the proteins and improves the detection of small proteins like LC3.
18. This is a commonly underrated step, though it is important to get clean and clear bands, even more in the case of the double signal of LC3.
19. Do not overexpose the signal, as this reduces differences in the intensity of the bands between lanes. The aim of this experiment is analyzing quantitative, rather than qualitative, variations. Thus, it is important to discern even the smallest changes. Even more in the case of β-Actin, as the intensity of the other bands will be normalized to the amount of this protein.
20. In some cases, relative amounts of LC3-II are enough to assess autophagy status in samples. However, extended induction times may result in lower levels of LC3-II due to high degradation, which could be mistaken with autophagy block. Thus, LC3-II/LC3-I ratios (within p62 degradation) are always useful to assess the autophagy flux.

Acknowledgments

I thank Dr. Salwa Sebti for helpful comments on the manuscript. My work in the laboratory is supported by Leducq Foundation.

References

1. Galluzzi L, Baehrecke EH, Ballabio A et al (2017) Molecular definitions of autophagy and related processes. EMBO J 36(19):2809–2924. https://doi.org/10.15252/embj.201796697
2. Feng Y, He D, Yao Z et al (2014) The machinery of macroautophagy. Cell Res 24(1):24–41. https://doi.org/10.1038/cr.2013.168
3. Kaminskyy V, Zhivotovsky B (2012) Proteases in autophagy. Biochim Biophys Acta 1824(1):44–50. https://doi.org/10.1016/j.bbapap.2011.05.013
4. Norman JM, Cohen GM, Bampton ET (2010) The in vitro cleavage of the hAtg proteins by cell death proteases. Autophagy 6(8):1042–1056
5. Tsapras P, Nezis IP (2017) Caspase involvement in autophagy. Cell Death Differ 24(8):1369–1379. https://doi.org/10.1038/cdd.2017.43
6. Repnik U, Stoka V, Turk V et al (2012) Lysosomes and lysosomal cathepsins in cell death. Biochim Biophys Acta 1824(1):22–33. https://doi.org/10.1016/j.bbapap.2011.08.016
7. Fernandez AF, Lopez-Otin C (2015) The functional and pathologic relevance of autophagy proteases. J Clin Invest 125(1):33–41. https://doi.org/10.1172/JCI73940
8. Kroemer G, Marino G, Levine B (2010) Autophagy and the integrated stress response. Mol Cell 40(2):280–293. https://doi.org/10.1016/j.molcel.2010.09.023
9. Choi AM, Ryter SW, Levine B (2013) Autophagy in human health and disease. N Engl J Med 368(7):651–662. https://doi.org/10.1056/NEJMra1205406
10. Galluzzi L, Pietrocola F, Bravo-San Pedro JM et al (2015) Autophagy in malignant transformation and cancer progression. EMBO J 34(7):856–880. https://doi.org/10.15252/embj.201490784
11. Cadwell K (2016) Crosstalk between autophagy and inflammatory signalling pathways: balancing defence and homeostasis. Nat Rev Immunol 16(11):661–675. https://doi.org/10.1038/nri.2016.100
12. Lopez-Otin C, Blasco MA, Partridge L et al (2013) The hallmarks of aging. Cell 153(6):1194–1217. https://doi.org/10.1016/j.cell.2013.05.039
13. Klionsky DJ, Abdelmohsen K, Abe A et al (2016) Guidelines for the use and interpretation of assays for monitoring autophagy (3rd edition). Autophagy 12(1):1–222. https://doi.org/10.1080/15548627.2015.1100356
14. Lopez-Otin C, Marino G (2017) Tagged ATG8-coding constructs for the In vitro and in vivo assessment of ATG4 activity. Methods Enzymol 587:189–205. https://doi.org/10.1016/bs.mie.2016.11.001
15. Li M, Fu Y, Yang Z et al (2017) Measurement of the activity of the Atg4 cysteine proteases. Methods Enzymol 587:207–225. https://doi.org/10.1016/bs.mie.2016.10.024

Chapter 9

Gel-Based Gelatin Zymography to Examine Matrix Metalloproteinase Activity in Cell Culture

Aastha Chhabra and Vibha Rani

Abstract

Gelatin zymography, first described by Heussen and Dowdle in the 1980s, is a widely used valuable tool in research and diagnostics. The technique identifies gelatinases by the degradation of their preferential substrate as well as by their molecular weight (kDa). We here describe detailed methodology for the detection of pro- and active- forms of both MMP-2 (gelatinase A) and MMP-9 (gelatinase B) in cells using norepinephrine-stimulated H9c2 cardiomyoblasts as model. An easy to follow step-by-step protocol has been carefully written for reliable results. We also suggest an acceptable method for quantification of gelatin zymograms.

Key words Cell culture, Extracellular matrix, MMPs, Gelatinases, Gelatin zymography, Proteolytic activity

1 Introduction

Matrix metalloproteinases (MMPs) are a family of at least 26 endopeptidases (23 identified in humans) that act as key players in extracellular matrix (ECM) remodeling in various physiological and pathological conditions [1]. This class of Zn^{2+}- and Ca^{2+}-dependent proteases is intricately involved in physiological processes such as embryogenesis and angiogenesis as well as pathological conditions including tumor metastasis, inflammation, arthritis, chronic obstructive pulmonary disease (COPD), and cardiovascular complications like hypertrophy, stroke, and heart failure [2]. These regulatory proteases have been subdivided into collagenases (MMP-1, MMP-8, MMP-13, and MMP-18), gelatinases (MMP-2 and MMP-9), stromelysins (MMP-3, MMP-10, MMP-11, and MMP-12), matrilysins (MMP-7 and MMP-26), membrane-type MMPs (MMP-14, MMP-15, MMP-16, and MMP-25), and others, based on their substrate specificity [3]. Structurally, MMPs are multi-domain proteins consisting of four distinct domains: an

Santiago Cal and Alvaro J. Obaya (eds.), *Proteases and Cancer: Methods and Protocols*, Methods in Molecular Biology, vol. 1731, https://doi.org/10.1007/978-1-4939-7595-2_9, © Springer Science+Business Media, LLC 2018

amino terminal hydrophobic pro-domain, a Zn^{2+}-containing catalytic domain, a flexible hinge region, and a carboxy terminal hemopexin-like domain which determines its substrate-specific nature [4]. They are produced in latent inactive form and are hence called "zymogens." Activation of MMPs requires cleavage of its inhibitory N-terminal domain (~10 kDa) [5]. MMP activity is closely regulated by tissue inhibitors of matrix metalloproteinases (TIMPs), a group of four endogenous MMP inhibitors which bind to the catalytic site of MMPs in a 1:1 ratio. An imbalance in MMP-TIMP levels consequently disrupts ECM integrity and thus affects associated biological functions [6, 7].

Gelatinases, MMP-2 and MMP-9, are two members of the MMP family that have been extensively studied owing to their consistent association with a number of physiological and pathological processes. These were originally described as type IV collagenases because of their ability to promote hydrolysis of collagen IV, a major component of ECM [8, 9]. However, they were also found to hydrolyze denatured collagen I (gelatin) efficiently and thus began to be referred as "gelatinases" [10]. This ability of MMP-2 and MMP-9 was suitably harnessed to develop "gelatin zymography," a relatively easy yet powerful technique for detection of MMP activity in biological samples [11]. This technique was utilized by our group, and the important role of curcumin in suppressing gelatinase B mediated norepinephrine induced cardiac stress in H9c2 cells was established [12].

Gelatin zymography is an electrophoretic technique which utilizes sodium dodecyl sulfate-polyacrylamide gel electrophoresis (SDS-PAGE) wherein gelatin is impregnated in the polyacrylamide gel matrix. The samples are prepared under nonreducing conditions, i.e., without boiling, and any reducing agent like β-mercaptoethanol or dithiothreitol. After the electrophoretic run, the gel is washed off SDS by incubation in nonionic detergent, Triton X-100. The gel is digested in calcium-containing buffer for an optimized length of time such that the partially renatured enzymes degrade gelatin leaving a clear zone on the gel. Subsequently, the gel is stained with Coomassie Brilliant Blue to distinguish areas of digestion against a darkly stained background [13]. A number of zymography techniques have been developed over years and are tabulated in Table 1.

This protocol holds the advantage of detecting both latent and active forms of gelatinases (72 and 64 kDa for MMP-2, 92–95 and 82 kDa for MMP-9). The denaturation in the presence of SDS followed by partial renaturation in the presence of Triton X-100 allows the pro-form to activate and exhibit gelatinolytic activity. Difference in molecular weight between the two forms (pro-form migrates lesser than active form) permits activity by both to be seen on gel. SDS also helps to disrupt any non-covalent interactions

Table 1
Types of zymography and its associated MMPs/TIMPs

S. No.	Zymography	MMP/TIMP	Remarks
Substrate zymography			
1.	Gelatin zymography	MMP-2, MMP-9; MMP-1, MMP-8, and MMP-13 to a lesser extent	Simplest and most widely used type of zymography
2.	Casein zymography	MMP-11, also for MMP-1, MMP-3, MMP-7, MMP-12, and MMP-13	Pre-running of gel to avoid casein gradient in the zymogram is important
3.	Collagen zymography	MMP-1, MMP-13; MMP-2 and MMP-9 may also be detected	Incorporation of native collagen fibers in gel is challenging
4.	Carboxymethylated (CM) transferrin zymography	MMP-3, MMP-7	Usually accompanied with addition of heparin to samples
5.	Fibronectin zymography	MMP-3	Vitronectin and laminin zymography may be done along with it
Modified substrate zymography			
1.	Heparin-enhanced substrate zymography	MMP-7, MMP-1, MMP-13	Addition of heparin to samples during or prior to electrophoresis improves the detection limit for MMP
2.	Reverse zymography	TIMP family (TIMP-1, TIMP-2, TIMP-3, and TIMP-4)	Both substrate (gelatin) and MMP (MMP-2) are incorporated in gel
3.	In situ zymography	Usually performed for MMPs whose fluorophore-conjugated substrates are easily available like FITC-gelatin	Assessment of functional activity on site within the histochemical or cytochemical sections
4.	Real-time zymography	Holds advantage over conventional protocol	Utilizes fluorophore-conjugated substrate to monitor proteolytic activity in real time
5.	Real-time reverse zymography	Holds advantage over conventional protocol	Similar to real-time zymography, gel contains specific MMP along with fluorescent-labeled substrate

between gelatinases and TIMPs [14]. Gelatin zymography is very useful as a qualitative tool for the detection and analysis of the level and type of gelatinases expressed in different cell types/tissues at any time point or after a treatment; however, it lacks the ability to be classified as quantitative. Despite this, owing to its ease-of-conduct and the useful information it generates, it remains a method of choice among researchers involved in the field of matrix biology [15]. Moreover, a few methods have been devised to quantify zymograms utilizing image processing softwares like Image J, and thus, the technique may be considered as semiquantitative [16].

Here, we provide a detailed protocol to set up gel-based gelatin zymography and guide on sample preparation from cells. We also discuss the detailed procedure for quantification of gelatin zymogram as accepted and used widely.

2 Materials

Make all solutions in ultrapure water by purifying deionized water to attain a sensitivity of 18 MΩ cm at 25 °C (dH_2O). Prepare and store all reagents at room temperature (unless indicated otherwise). Ensure adherence to good laboratory practices (GLPs) while conducting the experiment.

2.1 Cell Culture Components

1. Cell line: Rat heart-derived H9c2 cardiomyoblasts obtained from National Centre for Cell Science (NCCS), Pune (*see* **Note 1**).
2. Growth media (Dulbecco's modified eagle medium (DMEM, pH 7.4)): 25 mM glucose, 4 mM L-glutamine, 1 mM sodium pyruvate, 44 mM sodium bicarbonate, and 11 mM HEPES, supplemented with antibiotic (100 units/mL penicillin and 100 μg/mL streptomycin) and 10% fetal bovine serum (FBS). Prepare, filter, and sterilize the media with a 0.22 μm filter. Store at 4 °C (*see* **Note 2**).
3. Trypsin-EDTA solution: 0.25%, sterile-filtered, suitable for cell culture, 2.5 g porcine trypsin, and 0.2 g EDTA-4NA per liter of Hanks' balanced salt solution (HBSS), with phenol red, pH 7.0–7.6.
4. 1× Phosphate-buffered saline (PBS): 137 mM NaCl, 2.7 mM KCl, 4.3 mM Na_2HPO_4, and 1.47 mM KH_2PO_4. Adjust to a final pH of 7.4, autoclave, and store at 4 °C for long-term use. Warm to 37 °C before usage.
5. Cell culture flask: Surface area 75 cm^2, canted neck, vented cap, sterile, rectangular bottom, surface treated, polystyrene.
6. Culture dish: Surface area 55 cm^2, inside D (diameter) × H (height) 100 mm × 20 mm, sterile, round bottom, surface treated, polystyrene.
7. Humidified CO_2 incubator: 5% CO_2, 37 °C.
8. Inverted microscope.

2.2 Total Protein Extraction and Estimation Components

1. Protein extraction buffer: 20 mM HEPES-NaOH (pH 7.9), 20% glycerol, 500 mM NaCl, 1.5 mM $MgCl_2$, 0.1% Triton X-100, and protease inhibitor cocktail (without metalloprotease inhibitors).
2. Protease inhibitor cocktail: For use with mammalian cell and tissue extracts, does not contain EDTA, inhibits serine, cysteine, and acid proteases, and aminopeptidases but not metalloproteinases. Contains individual components, including 104 mM AEBSF (serine protease inhibitor), 80 μM aprotinin (serine protease inhibitor), 4 mM bestatin (aminopeptidase inhibitor), 1.4 mM E-64 (cysteine protease inhibitor), 2 mM leupeptin (serine and cysteine protease inhibitor), and 1.5 mM pepstatin A (acid protease inhibitor). Store at −20 °C.
3. Bradford reagent: Ready to use or prepared as described. For Bradford reagent (1×, 1000 mL), dissolve 100 mg Coomassie Brilliant Blue G250 in 50 mL of 95% ethanol (C_2H_5OH). Add 100 mL of 85% (w/v) *o*-phosphoric acid (H_3PO_4). Now, add 500 mL H_2O to this solution and mix well. Filter the solution using Whatman filter paper and make up the volume to 1000 mL. Store the reagent in amber-colored bottle at 4 °C (*see* **Note 3**).
4. BSA (bovine serum albumin): To be used as standard. Dissolve BSA in ultrapure water to prepare a stock solution of 2000 μg/mL. Serially dilute the stock in water to make BSA dilutions (used as standards)—1500, 1000, 750, 500, 250, 125, and 0 μg/mL (blank). The dilutions can be stored at 4 °C for long (*see* **Note 4**).
5. Refrigerated benchtop microcentrifuge.
6. Ice.
7. 96-well microplate: With/without lid, sterile/non-sterile, flat bottom, polystyrene, capacity ≥300 μL/well.

2.3 Gelatin Zymography Components

1. SDS-PAGE gel: 30% acrylamide, dH_2O, 1.5 M Tris–HCl (pH 8.8)/1 M Tris–HCl (pH 6.8), 10% ammonium persulfate (APS), TEMED, 10% sodium dodecyl sulfate (SDS). For 500 mL acrylamide solution, add 145 g acrylamide (29 parts) and 5 g bis-acrylamide (1 part) to 350 mL dH_2O in the dark and stir the solution until the components dissolve completely. Filter and store at 4 °C in amber-colored bottle. For 100 mL of 1.5 M Tris–HCl (pH 8.8), weigh 18.17 g Trizma base and dissolve in 50 mL water. Set pH to 8.8 with HCl and make up the volume to 100 mL. Similarly, for 100 mL of 1 M Tris–HCl (pH 6.8), weigh 12.114 g Trizma base and adjust pH to 6.8 with HCl. For 10% APS, dissolve 0.5 g APS in 5 mL of dH_2O and store at 4 °C in amber-colored tube. For 10% SDS, add 10 g SDS to 50 mL dH_2O and make up the volume to 100 mL

once the detergent dissolves completely. Composition for 10% resolving gel (20 mL)—6.6 mL of 30% acrylamide, 8 mL dH_2O, 5 mL of 1.5 M Tris–HCl pH 8.8, 200 μL of 10% SDS, 160 μL of 10% APS, and 16 μL TEMED. Composition for 4% stacking gel (5 mL)—650 μL of 30% acrylamide, 3.7 mL dH_2O, 625 μL of 1 M Tris–HCl pH 6.8, 50 μL of 10% SDS, 50 μL of 10% APS, and 5 μL TEMED.

2. Gelatin: From porcine skin, for electrophoresis, Type A (*see* **Note 5**).
3. Lab hot plate: With uniform heating and maintenance of temperature.
4. 1-D protein electrophoresis unit (casting stand, electrophoresis tank along with suitable power pack).
5. 1× SDS-PAGE running buffer (pH 8.3): 192 mM glycine, 25 mM Tris base, 0.1% SDS. Store the buffer at room temperature.
6. Pre-stained protein ladder: 10–250 kDa, for use in SDS-PAGE (*see* **Note 6**).
7. Zymogram sample buffer (2×): 62.5 mM Tris–HCl, pH 6.8, 25% glycerol, 4% SDS, and 0.005% bromophenol blue. Contains no reducing agent. Use one part sample with one part of this dye.
8. Triton X-100: Add 2.5 mL of detergent to 97.5 mL dH_2O to make a final volume of 100 mL (2.5% v/v). Vortex thoroughly to dissolve the detergent (*see* **Note 7**).
9. Zymography digestion buffer: 50 mM Tris–HCl (pH 7.4), 150 mM NaCl, 5 mM $CaCl_2$, and 0.1% Brij-35. Weigh the components and dissolve in dH_2O. Make up the volume of buffer once all salts dissolve completely. Add 0.1% Brij-35 (nonionic detergent) with a cut tip in the final solution. Use freshly prepared buffer (*see* **Note 8**).
10. Gel rocker/incubator shaker.
11. Coomassie Brilliant Blue staining solution (500 mL): Dissolve 1.25 g Coomassie Brilliant Blue R250 in 225 mL methanol. Add 50 mL of glacial acetic acid and 225 mL of water to the solution. Stir the solution for 2–3 h and filter through a Whatman filter paper. Store the solution at room temperature.
12. Destaining solution (500 mL): Mix methanol (150 mL), glacial acetic acid (50 mL), and water (300 mL) in a ratio of 3/1/6 (v/v/v). Store the solution at room temperature.
13. White light transilluminator.

3 Methods

Carry out all procedures at room temperature unless otherwise specified.

3.1 Cell Culture

Follow GLP guidelines for cell culture techniques (*see* **Note 9**).

1. Seed the suspension of H9c2 cells covering the entire surface of 100 mm culture dish containing 12 mL of growth media (*see* **Note 10**).
2. Gently swirl the plate to allow the cell suspension to settle uniformly in the dish with growth media.
3. Allow the cells to adhere to the surface of culture dish and grow to a confluency of about 60–70% in a humidified CO_2 incubator maintained at 37 °C and 5% CO_2.
4. Give suitable treatment to the cells as per the plan of experiment to be conducted.
5. Harvest the cells for total protein extraction after the treatment. Aspirate the media and add 5 mL of pre-warmed 1× PBS per dish to wash the cells.
6. Remove PBS and add 600 μL pre-warmed trypsin-EDTA solution to each dish. Incubate the dish in the CO_2 incubator at 37 °C for 3–4 min until the attached cells begin to round off and fall from the surface of the dish.
7. Add 5 mL of complete growth media (DMEM with 10% FBS) to stop trypsin activity and flush all the cells to clear the surface.
8. Transfer the cell suspension in a 15 mL centrifuge tube and spin at 200 × *g* for 10 min (*see* **Note 11**).
9. Decant the supernatant and break the pellet before resuspending it in 1 mL of ice-cold PBS. Transfer the contents in a 1.5 mL microfuge tube and spin in a refrigerated centrifuge at 400 × *g* for 10 min to remove traces of any media.

3.2 Total Protein Extraction and Estimation

1. Carefully decant supernatant from the tube and break the pellet before adding prechilled protein extraction buffer (with protease inhibitor cocktail) (*see* **Note 12**).
2. Incubate in ice for 30 min and tap the tube intermittently after every 10 min.
3. Centrifuge at 9600 × *g* for 15 min at 4 °C and collect the supernatant in fresh tube.
4. Aliquot the extracted protein in ice and store at −80 °C for long-term use (*see* **Note 13**).

5. Estimate the protein concentration using the standard protocol followed for Bradford assay using BSA as standard (*see* **Notes 14–16**).

3.3 Gelatin Zymography

1. Prepare zymography sample to be loaded in gel (20–40 μL). Calculate the volume of protein sample in μL required to load at least 30 μg protein in gel based on the estimated concentration. Mix it with suitable amount of zymogram sample buffer so as to bring the dye at 1× working concentration (with respect to the total volume of zymography sample being loaded on gel). Make up the remaining volume with protein extraction buffer. Do not boil the samples. Keep them in ice until loaded (*see* **Note 17**).
2. For gel preparation, weigh 20 mg gelatin and allow it to swell for 15 min in 8 mL of dH_2O being used to prepare 20 mL of 10% resolving gel. Warm it on hot plate at 40–50 °C for 2–3 min or until it dissolves completely. Allow it to cool down before adding rest of the components to prepare the resolving gel (10%). Pour the gel between the plates for casting and allow it to polymerize. Overlay the gel with water-saturated butanol (*see* **Note 18**).
3. Decant the top layer and immediately pour the stacking gel (4%) in the space between the casting plates. Insert a comb so as to make deep wells and allow the gel to polymerize. Ensure there are no air bubbles and at least 1 cm of space for sample to stack properly in the stacking gel.
4. Put the casting unit in the electrophoresis tank filled with SDS-PAGE running buffer and remove the comb carefully. Flush the wells with a syringe before loading the protein sample.
5. Load the samples and pre-stained protein ladder. Run the gel at desirable voltage and current specifications recommended for the electrophoresis unit.
6. Transfer the gel to a box (12 × 10 cm) without cutting the stacking and wash it in 2.5% Triton X-100 (around 50–75 mL for one gel of 8 × 8 cm) for 1 h at room temperature by gently rocking the gel on a rocker (*see* **Note 19**).
7. Transfer the gel to a fresh box (12 × 10 cm) containing zymography digestion buffer (50–75 mL) with/without inhibitor and incubate it at 37 °C for 24 h with constant gentle rocking. Cover the gel box with aluminum foil during incubation (*see* **Notes 20** and **21**).
8. Stain the gel with Coomassie Brilliant Blue staining solution followed by destaining until distinct white bands of MMP activity on gelatin are observed against a blue background of the gel when placed over a white light transilluminator.

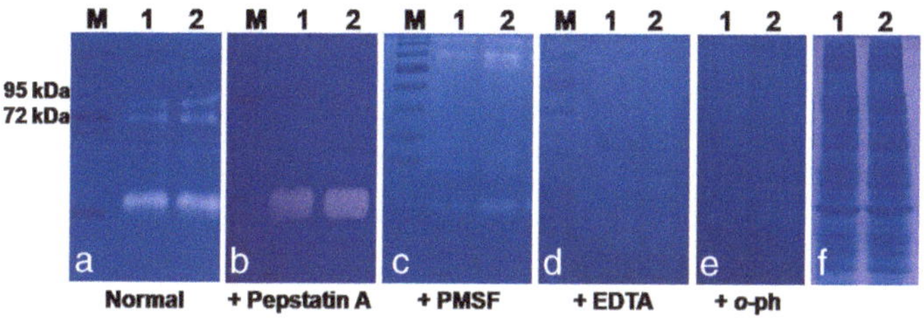

Fig. 1 Gelatin substrate zymography: Total protein samples were subjected to electrophoresis on 10% SDS-PAGE gel containing gelatin (1 mg/mL). Gelatinolytic activity was observed as distinct white bands against a blue background on the gel (M, pre-stained protein ladder; 1, control; 2, norepinephrine treated). (**a**) Gelatin zymogram showing MMP-2 and MMP-9 activity at 72 kDa and 92 kDa, respectively. (**b**) Gelatin zymogram with pepstatin A (aspartyl protease inhibitor) in sample and gel. (**c**) Gelatin zymogram containing PMSF (serine protease inhibitor) in sample and gel. (**d**) Gelatin zymogram with EDTA (divalent cation chelator) in sample and gel. (**e**) Gelatin zymogram with *o*-phenanthroline (zinc chelator) in sample and gel. (**f**) 25 μg of total protein was run on 10% SDS PAGE gel and used as a reference for equal loading

9. Identify the MMP (pro- and active form) based on the molecular weight close to which the activity is observed on the gelatin zymogram (use pre-stained protein ladder as the reference). Also, analyze the zymogram for any difference in MMP activity between the experimental groups taking equal loading SDS-PAGE gel for the same set of samples as a reference/loading control (Fig. 1).

3.4 Gel Scan and Quantification

1. Carefully remove the zymogram from water and place it in a plastic sheet protector.
2. Scan the gel at a resolution of 300 dpi or higher and save the image in ".jpg" format.
3. Open Image J (software can be freely downloaded from http://rsbweb.nih.gov/ij/) and go to "File," then "Open" and select the image to be analyzed. Zoom in or out to an appropriate size.
4. Visualize the image in black and white by setting it to 8-bit format. Go to "Image," then "Type" and select "8-bit."
5. Select the "Rectangular tool" from the tool bar and draw a rectangle along Lane 1 starting from the top of the gel to the bottom.
6. Go to "Analyze," then "Gels" and "Select first lane."
7. Click in the middle of the box drawn over the first lane and move it over to the next lane. Go to "Analyze," then "Gels" and "Select next lane." Repeat this process and make a box along all lanes. All boxes will be at same level vertically.

However, do ensure that there is no spilling over of the box into the next lane horizontally and each box must cover the lane completely.

8. Now, go to "Analyze," then "Gels" and "Plot lanes." A new window showing a plot with intensity profile of the entire lane for each box selected appears on the screen. The area of drop in intensity (light pixels correspond to digested area on gel) is represented as a peak. Identify the peak corresponding to the band of interest and draw a straight line across its base to enclose the area completely. Repeat this process for all lanes.
9. Select "Wand tool" on the tool bar and determine area of each closed peak by clicking on the same. If a lane shows no band at the desired position (absence of MMP activity in the sample), consider the area of peak to be zero.
10. Copy the data in excel, write the lane number and group label across the value and plot it as a bar graph. The data can be normalized to an MMP standard to avoid any gel-gel variation especially when values are being pooled from replicate gels to determine statistical significance of the result.

4 Notes

1. This protocol has been described utilizing embryonic rat heart-derived H9c2 cardiomyoblasts. However, any other adherent/suspension cell type may be used for extraction of total cell protein and conduct of gelatin zymography.
2. The standard guidelines for maintenance of each cell line are detailed by the concerned cell culture repository like American Type Culture Collection (ATCC). DMEM growth medium with the formulation as described in Subheading 2 has been prescribed for H9c2 cells.
3. Bradford solution must be prepared and stored in the dark. The reagent has a reddish brown color at acidic pH (when prepared) which changes to blue on binding to protein. The presence of detergent or alkali in glassware can lead to the reagent turning blue at the time of preparation itself. Such a solution must not be used.
4. BSA standards: Apart from being abundant, affordable, and relatively stable, this protein offers desirable biochemical reactivity with protein estimation methods including BCA, Bradford, and Lowry. It is an intermediately sized protein (66 kDa) containing 607 amino acids which represent all amino acids in a balanced form.
5. Gelatin is a heterogeneous mixture of water-soluble proteins of high average molecular masses, present in collagen. These

proteins are extracted by boiling the relevant skin, tendons, ligaments, bones, or tissue in water. Dry gelatin must be stored in air-tight container at room temperature to maintain its shelf life for years. It is soluble in warm-to-hot water than cold.

6. Pre-stained protein ladder is a mixture of color-stained proteins which are used as size standards in protein electrophoresis (SDS-PAGE). The ready-to-use ladder is supplied in a loading buffer and is directly loaded on gel without boiling. A pre-stained protein marker helps to monitor the progress of gel during electrophoresis and is also visible after Coomassie staining of zymogram which stains the entire gel blue due to the presence of gelatin in the gel. Ensure that the ladder has at least 2–3 red/orange/green bands rather than blue for clarity in gel visualization. The ladder will help estimating the approximate size of separated proteins (MMPs) which have digested gelatin present in the gel and made it visible in the form of white band against blue background.
7. Triton X-100: It is a nonionic mild surfactant that breaks protein-lipid, lipid-lipid associations but not protein-protein interactions. It does not denature protein and thus help obtain it in its native and active form. The detergent is viscous, and hence, a cut tip must be used to add the detergent.
8. Brij-35 is a nonionic light detergent that ensures enzyme stabilization and minimizes the risk of nonspecific interactions.
9. The key for good laboratory practice in cell culture is to ensure that all procedures are carried out to a standard that precludes microbial contamination as well as cross-contamination with other cell lines. Some of the basic precautions are listed as follows: (a) Surface sterilize the work space, materials, and equipments with 70% ethanol and UV before beginning work. (b) Ensure that the growth media and other reagents are sterile and used inside the biosafety cabinet only. Screw the cap of reagent bottle tightly and seal the neck after use. (c) Disinfect all materials before removing them from the hood. Also, surface sterilize the work area with 70% ethanol and UV, after use. (d) Routinely examine the cultures and growth media for evidence of any gross microbial contamination. (e) Clean the cell culture facility regularly. (f) Follow appropriate guidelines for disposal of biological waste (infectious and noninfectious) that include sharps contaminated with biological waste, liquid as well as solid waste.
10. Use ≥3 culture dishes (100 mm) per group in an experiment to get sufficient amount of protein after extraction.
11. The speed of centrifuge must not exceed 400 × *g* for mammalian cells.

12. Add ~150 μL of protein extraction buffer to cell pellet obtained by pooling cells from 3 × 100 mm dishes (60–70% confluent) of each group. Use 1 μL of protease inhibitor cocktail for every 100 μL of protein extraction buffer used or as recommended in the reagent usage instructions.
13. The samples may be stored for long, if aliquoted and stored properly at −80 °C. Avoid freeze thaw cycles. However, it is better to use the protein as fresh as possible. Long-term storage of samples may affect MMP activity.
14. Bradford assay: The basic principle of this colorimetric test lies in complexing of proteins present in the sample with Coomassie Brilliant Blue G under acidic conditions resulting in a color change of the reagent from reddish brown to blue, marked as a shift in the absorption spectrum maximum from 470 nm (cationic/unbound form) to 595 nm (anionic/bound form). The increase in absorption at 595 nm is proportional to the amount of bound dye and thus, to the amount of protein in the sample. Reducing agents such as DTT and β-mercaptoethanol do not cause interference with this reagent. However, the presence of SDS in extraction buffer may affect the assay.
15. Bradford assay protocol: Add 5 μL of BSA standard/sample to each well of 96-well microplate followed by quick addition of 200 μL of 1× Bradford reagent per well in dark. Wrap the plate with aluminum foil and incubate it at 37 °C for 15 min. Read the plate on a spectrophotometer and record A_{595} (absorbance at 595 nm) values. Plot the scatter diagram of the absorbance values obtained for BSA dilutions and use linear regression to determine the standard curve for Bradford assay. This curve will show the relation between protein concentration and A_{595} values in $y = mx + c$ form ($y = A_{595}$; m = slope of the line; x = protein concentration in μg/mL; c = intercept on y-axis). Use this equation to calculate the protein concentration for all unknown samples. Multiply the calculated concentration with appropriate dilution factor, if used.
16. Adjust the initial seeding concentration of cells/number of dishes to be plated per group and protein extraction buffer volume in such a way that the total protein obtained is at a concentration of 6–7 μg/μL. This will ensure that ≥30 μg protein can be conveniently loaded on gel.
17. Also, prepare protein samples using Laemmli sample buffer to run an SDS-PAGE gel in parallel to the zymogram. This buffer contains β-mercaptoethanol and theses samples are boiled before loading. The gel serves as a reference for loading equal amount of protein in all the lanes.

18. Water-saturated butanol (or any organic solvent) helps cut contact of resolving gel with air and thus prevents oxidation. It avoids mixing of trace water with gel, its evaporation leading to shrinkage of gel. This produces a smooth and completely level surface on the top of resolving gel so that bands are straight and uniform.
19. It is advised not to cut the stacking gel after the electrophoresis and retain it till the end of experiment. This portion of gel will help indicate if the gel has been completely destained since it does not contain gelatin and will get clear upon destaining. On the other hand, the resolving gel (containing gelatin) shall be entirely blue even after destaining.
20. *o*-Phenanthroline (1,10-phenanthroline monohydrate) is a metalloproteinase inhibitor that chelates divalent metals like zinc and iron. It is soluble in methanol and can be prepared at a stock concentration of 200 mM. The stock remains stable at −20 °C for months. Effective concentration: 10 mM in sample and 50 mM in digestion buffer. EDTA is also a metalloproteinase inhibitor that chelates divalent ions like Ca^{2+}. It is used at a concentration of 10 mM in sample and 50 mM in digestion buffer. Zinc- and calcium-dependent MMPs show no activity in the presence of these inhibitors.
21. Enzyme (MMP) activity is best observed at 37 °C. Keep the gels in an incubator shaker with controlled temperature and speed if the room temperature is not suitable. Increasing the length of incubation in digestion buffer may also be of help.

Acknowledgment

This work is supported by the research grant awarded to Dr. Vibha Rani by the Science and Engineering Research Board (SERB), Department of Science and Technology (DST), Government of India (EMR/2016/005914).

References

1. Jaiswal A, Chhabra A, Malhotra U et al (2011) Comparative analysis of human matrix metalloproteinases: emerging therapeutic targets in diseases. Bioinformation 6(1):23–30
2. Kupai K, Szucs G, Cseh S et al (2010) Matrix metalloproteinase activity assays: importance of zymography. J Pharmacol Toxicol Methods 61(2):205–209
3. Cathcart J, Pulkoski-Gross A, Cao J (2015) Targeting matrix metalloproteinases in cancer: bringing new life to old ideas. Genes Dis 2(1):26–34
4. Sternlicht MD, Werb Z (2001) How matrix metalloproteinases regulate cell behavior. Annu Rev Cell Dev Biol 17:463–516
5. Nagase H (1997) Activation mechanisms of matrix metalloproteinases. Biol Chem 378(3–4):151–160
6. Brewa K, Nagase H (2010) The tissue inhibitors of metalloproteinases (TIMPs): an ancient

family with structural and functional diversity. Biochim Biophys Acta 1803(1):55–71
7. Visse R, Nagase H (2003) Matrix metalloproteinases and tissue inhibitors of metalloproteinases: structure, function, and biochemistry. Circ Res 92(8):827–839
8. Collier IE, Wilhelm SM, Eisen AZ et al (1988) H-ras oncogene transformed human bronchial epithelial cells (TBE-1) secrete a single metalloprotease capable of degrading basement membrane collagen. J Biol Chem 263(14):6579–6587
9. Wilhelm SM, Collier IE, Marmer BL et al (1989) SV40-transformed human lung fibroblasts secrete a 92-kDa type IV collagenase which is identical to that secreted by normal human macrophages. J Biol Chem 264(29):17213–17221
10. Murphy G, Crabbe T (1995) Gelatinases A and B. Methods Enzymol 248:470–484
11. Toth M, Sohail A, Fridman R (2012) Assessment of gelatinases (MMP-2 and MMP-9) by gelatin zymography. Methods Mol Biol 878:121–135
12. Kohli S, Chhabra A, Jaiswal A et al (2013) Curcumin suppresses gelatinase B mediated norepinephrine induced stress in H9c2 cardiomyocytes. PLoS One 8(10):e76519
13. Troeberg L, Nagase H (2003) Zymography of metalloproteinases. Curr Protoc Protein Sci 33:21.15.1–21.15.12
14. Toth M, Fridman R (2001) Assessment of Gelatinases (MMP-2 and MMP-9) by Gelatin Zymography. Methods Mol Med 57:163–174
15. Manchenko GP (2003) Handbook of detection of enzymes on electrophoretic gels, 2nd edn. CRC, Boca Raton, pp 1–39
16. Hu X, Beeton C (2010) Detection of functional matrix metalloproteinases by zymography. J Vis Exp 8(45):pii: 2445

Chapter 10

Analysis of Enzymatic Activity of Matrix Metalloproteinase (MMP) by Collagen Zymography in Melanoma

Vijay Walia and Yardena Samuels

Abstract

Protein zymography is the most commonly used technique to study the enzymatic activity of matrix metalloproteinases (MMPs) and their inhibitors. MMPs are proteolytic enzymes that promote extracellular matrix degradation. MMPs are frequently mutated in malignant melanomas as well as other cancers and are linked to increasing incidence of tumor metastasis. Substrate zymography characterizes MMP activity by their ability to degrade preferred substrates. Here we describe the collagen zymography technique to measure the active or latent form of MMPs using MMP-8 as an example, which is a frequently mutated MMP family member in malignant melanomas. The same technique can be used with the modification of substrate to detect metalloproteinase activity of other MMPs. Both wild-type and mutated forms of MMPs can be analyzed using a single gel using this method.

Key words Collagen zymography, Matrix metalloproteinases, MMP-8, Malignant melanoma

1 Introduction

Zymography involves a protein separation in a polyacrylamide gel containing a specific substrate under nonreducing, denaturing conditions [1]. This technique is vital in the field of proteomics as it is a simple, sensitive, and quantifiable assay to analyze proteolytic enzymes. MMP activity can be analyzed using multiple zymographic techniques based on the substrate specificity. MMPs are calcium-dependent, zinc-containing endopeptidases that are involved in cell migration, wound healing, tissue remodeling during embryogenesis, and tooth development [2]. Since MMPs degrade extracellular matrix and basement membranes, they are closely associated with the promotion of cancer metastasis [3]. Although clinical trials of small-molecule inhibitors of MMPs were relatively unsuccessful, the new literature suggests that MMP's activity can be harnessed for diagnosis, prognosis, and therapeutic benefits [4, 7].

MMPs are classified according to the substrate specificity, sequence similarity, and organization of the peptide domains [2].

Santiago Cal and Alvaro J. Obaya (eds.), *Proteases and Cancer: Methods and Protocols*, Methods in Molecular Biology, vol. 1731, https://doi.org/10.1007/978-1-4939-7595-2_10, © Springer Science+Business Media, LLC 2018

Bonding between a cysteine residue (Cys^{73}) of the propeptide domain and an active Zn^{2+} site in the catalytic domain stabilizes MMP in the inactive conformation. Binding of a water molecule to the Zn^{2+} releases cysteine residue and causes intermediate activation of the enzyme. This phenomenon is referred to as "cysteine switch" [8]. The removal of prodomain of the MMP by other proteases or by autolytic cleavage results in full activation of the enzyme [8]. Physical and chemical changes such as low pH, heat, or treatment with amino-phenylmercuric acetate can also fully activate MMPs. Here we describe a substrate zymography technique to study the activity of wild-type and mutant MMP. We used MMP-8 as an example to describe this technique. MMP-8 is a MMP family member that is commonly mutated in malignant melanomas. We previously discovered five mutations in MMP-8 that reduces its enzymatic activity [9]. Most of the substrate zymography techniques are very similar except that the substrates (e.g., gelatin, casein, albumin, or hemoglobin) used are unique for different type of MMPs. For MMP-8, we used collagen as the substrate. Thus, this approach can be used to measure the activity of a variety of MMPs with substrate modification.

In zymography, MMPs are separated by molecular mass using the sodium dodecyl sulfate-polyacrylamide gel electrophoresis (SDS-PAGE) under nonreducing conditions (no boiling and no reducing agent) (Fig. 1). SDS-PAGE gels are copolymerized using collagen. SDS inactivates and denatures MMPs during electrophoresis. Washing gel with Triton X-100 buffer renatures and autoactivates MMPs without any cleavage. Concentrated MMPs in the gel digest substrate, which can be detected as clear band against the blue background due to Coomassie blue staining of the intact substrate. We used recombinant purified MMP-8 as a positive control to measure the sensitivity of the procedure and quantify activity in test samples.

We can use this technique for analyzing the activity of wild-type and mutant MMP in a single gel. A positive control such as purified recombinant MMP and a negative control such as lysates from the untransfected cells or culture medium, along with the test samples, could potentially help in the detection of false-positive and false-negative bands (Fig. 2). Several other laboratories have obtained similar results using our protocol or by minor modification of our protocol.

2 Materials

Prepare all solutions using analytical grade reagents and ultrapure water purified by deionization to attain a sensitivity of 18 mΩ-cm at 25 °C. Prepare and store all the reagents and solutions in Subheading 2 at room temperature unless stated in the protocol.

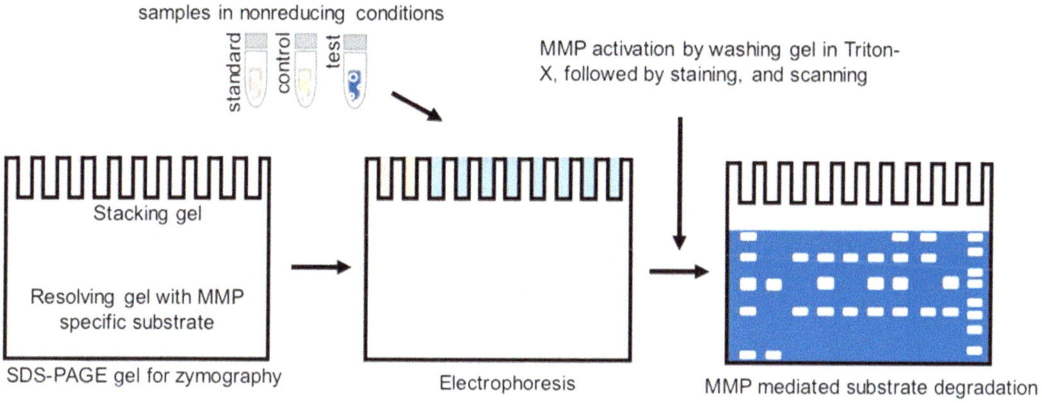

Fig. 1 Flowchart showing steps involved in *in-gel* zymography. Substrate such as collagen is incorporated in the resolving part of the SDS-PAGE gel. The samples along with appropriate controls and standards are separated according to the relative molecular weight during electrophoresis. The gel is then washed in Triton X-100 containing buffer at appropriate pH and temperature. Activated MMP cleaves its substrate in the gel, which appears as a white band on the dark blue background after Coomassie blue staining. The gel is then scanned, and band densities are quantified using the NIH Image J software

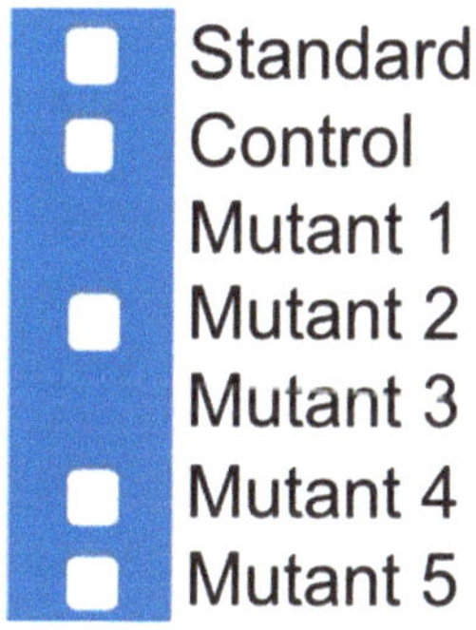

Fig. 2 A typical region of interest in the gel showing substrate cleavage by MMP. A known standard, along with wild-type control and mutant proteins 1–5 are shown. Mutant proteins 1–5 represent various mutations in the protein to be tested. If the mutation inhibits MMP activity, as shown in the mutants 1 and 3, we expect no substrate degradation. We previously showed collagen zymography to assess the activity of wild-type and altered MMP-8 proteins in malignant melanomas [9]. In the experiment shown in our past manuscript, conditioned media from HEK 293T cells expressing wild-type MMP-8 or mutant MMP-8 were immunoprecipitated and were subjected to type I collagen substrate gel zymography [9]

Follow all safety and disposal protocols for the chemicals and solutions used in the protocol.

2.1 Cell Culture

1. HEK 293T cells: Purchase HEK 293T cells from ATCC, Manassas, VA.
2. Cell culture medium: Culture cells in DMEM supplemented with 10% fetal bovine serum, 0.075% sodium bicarbonate, 1× nonessential amino acids, and 2 mM L-glutamine in a T-75 flask.

3. Lipofectamine™ 2000 Transfection Reagent.
4. Amicon Ultra-15 centrifugal filter unit with Ultracel-30 membrane.

2.2 Buffers for Cell Lysis

1. EBC medium: 50 mM Tris–HCl, pH 7.5, 100 mM NaCl, 0.5% NP40, and protease and phosphatase inhibitors (add just before lysing the cells). Add about 100 mL water to a 1 L graduated cylinder or a glass beaker. Weigh 6.06 g Tris base and 5.84 g NaCl and transfer to the cylinder. Add water to a volume of 900 mL. Add 5 mL of NP40 solution (supplied as 10% solution in water). Mix and adjust pH with concentrated HCl. Make up to 1 L of the buffer with water. Store at 4 °C. Keeping water in 37 °C water bath before dissolving Tris base allows quick dissolution. Bring the solution to room temperature before adjusting the pH with HCl. Use HCl with a series of ionic strength such as 1 N, 5 N, and 12 N (concentrated HCl) to adjust the pH and to prevent a sudden drop in pH of the Tris buffer.
2. Protease and phosphatase inhibitor cocktail: 50 mM NaF (working concentration), 0.2 mM Na_3VO_4 (working concentration), and 5% protease inhibitor. Na_3VO_4 needs to be activated before use for maximum inhibition of phosphotyrosyl phosphatases. Prepare a 200 mM stock solution of Na_3VO_4 and adjust pH to 10.0. Boil the solution for 10 min until it turns colorless and bring it to room temperature. Adjust the pH to 10.0 if the solution turns yellow, and redo the boiling until the solution becomes colorless. Store the aliquots at −20 °C.
3. A stock solution of 0.1 N HCl and 10 mM 1,10-phenanthroline monohydrate (10×): Add about 100 mL water to a 1 L graduated cylinder or a glass beaker. Weigh 0.002 g of phenanthroline and transfer to the cylinder. Add water to a volume of 900 mL. Add 8.33 mL of 12 M HCl. Make up to 1 L of the buffer with water. Store at 4 °C.
4. Blocked EBC: 5% milk in EBC medium. Store at 4 °C. To prepare 5% milk in EBC medium, dissolve 5 g of reduced fat milk powder in 100 mL of EBC medium in a beaker. Use a magnetic stirrer for efficient dissolving and store in 4 °C. We recommend the use of freshly prepared milk solution immediately before use.

2.3 Immunoprecipitation

1. ANTI-FLAG® M2 Affinity Gel: Store at 4 °C. Anti-flag affinity gel is used for immunoprecipitating flag-tagged substrate in the cell lysate and culture medium.
2. TBS solution (1×): 25 mM Tris–HCl pH 8 and 150 mM NaCl in water. Store at 4 °C.
3. Nonreduced SDS sample buffer.

2.4 SDS-Polyacrylamide Gel for Zymography

1. Stock collagen: Rat tail collagen I, 100 mg. Neutralized collagen is used for the preparation of resolving gel.
2. Phosphate-buffered saline (PBS) 7.4 (10×).
3. Sodium hydroxide (NaOH): 1 M NaOH in water. Dissolve 40 g of NaOH in 500 mL water in a 1 L graduated cylinder or a glass beaker. Make up the volume to 1 L with water.
4. Resolving gel buffer: 1.5 M Tris–HCl, pH 8.8. Dissolve 181.7 g of Tris base in 100 mL water in a 1 L graduated cylinder or a glass beaker. Add water to a volume of 900 mL. Mix the solution and adjust pH with HCl. Make up the volume to 1 L with water. Store at 4 °C.
5. Stacking gel buffer: 0.5 M Tris–HCl, pH 6.8. Weigh 60.6 g Tris base and prepare a 1 L solution as described in the previous step. Store at 4 °C.
6. Thirty percent acrylamide/Bis solution (29:1).
7. Ammonium persulfate: 10% solution in water. Dissolve 10 g of ammonium persulfate in 100 mL of deionized water in a beaker. Use a magnetic stirrer for efficient dissolving and store small aliquots at −20 °C.
8. *N*,*N*,*N*,*N′*-Tetramethylethylenediamine (TEMED). Store at 4 °C.
9. SDS-PAGE running buffer: 25 mM Tris base, 192 mM glycine, and 0.1% SDS, pH 8.3.
10. Nonreducing SDS sample buffer: Laemmli solution (nonreducing).
11. SDS solution: 10% UltraPure™ SDS Solution, 100 mL.
12. Human recombinant MMP-8: Purchase recombinant purified MMP-8 from Millipore (CC067), 10 μg.

2.5 Zymogram Solutions

1. Zymogram Renaturing Buffer (1×) (Invitrogen, Carlsbad, CA), 100 mL.
2. Zymogram Developing Buffer (1×) (Invitrogen, Carlsbad, CA), 100 mL.
3. Coomassie Blue R-250 (0.05%). Alternatively, dissolve 0.50 g of Coomassie Brilliant Blue R-250 to a final volume of 1 L of methanol/acetic acid/dH_2O solution (40:10:50).
4. Methanol/acetic acid/dH_2O solution (40:10:50): Add 100 mL of glacial acetic acid to 400 mL of methanol. Dilute the solution to a final volume of 1 L with water.

3 Method

Carry out all procedures at room temperature unless otherwise specified. All solutions in Subheading 3 must be prepared in advance.

3.1 Preparation of Cell Lysates Containing MMPs

1. Transfect confluent HEK 293T cells using Lipofectamine™ 2000 Transfection Reagent with 2.5 μg of empty vector (control) or with a vector containing wild-type *MMP-8* or mutant *MMP-8* DNA (*see* **Note 1**).
2. Harvest cells and medium after 24 h of transfection.
3. Harvesting growth medium: Collect growth media from a T-75 flask and placed into Amicon Ultra-15 centrifugal filter unit with Ultracel-30 membrane and spun as per manufacturers instructions at 4 °C.
4. Harvesting transfected cells: Wash the transfected cells with phosphate-buffered saline, lyse for 20 min on ice by using 810 μL EBC medium and 90 μL of 1,10 phenanthroline in 0.1 N HCl per T-75 flask. Remove cell lysates from the flask and centrifuge at 1600 × *g* at 4 °C for 10 min. As the cells are lysing, prepare anti-flag beads for immunoprecipitation.
5. Mix the supernatant from the growth medium and lysed cells with 100 μL blocked EBC (EBC medium + 5% milk).

3.2 Anti-flag M2 Agarose Beads for Immunoprecipitation

1. Use the 30 μL flag suspension beads per sample with a cut tip and place in a 1.5 mL Eppendorf tube.
2. Spin resin at 2000 × *g* for 5 s and let resin settle at the bottom of the tube for 1–2 min.
3. Remove supernatant by aspiration with a narrow syringe.
4. Wash beads with 500 μL TBS and go to **step 2**. Wash beads three times before using.
5. Suspend beads in the blocked EBC and aliquot 100 μL per sample with the cut tip into labeled 1.5 Eppendorf tubes containing a mixture of concentrated growth medium and lysed cells.
6. Rotate the mixtures overnight at 4 °C.

3.3 Sample Preparation for the Zymography

Spin samples at 2000 × *g* for 5 s and then aspirate supernatant off the beads with a narrow syringe. Beads contain immunoprecipitated MMPs.

1. Wash beads three times with 500 μL EBC medium, spin at 2000 × *g* for 5 s, and aspirating off the medium with each wash.
2. Add nonreduced SDS sample buffer to each sample (amount depends on number of times sample loading is required).
3. Incubate at room temperature for 10 min. Do not heat the samples and do not use any reducing agents such as beta-mercaptoethylene.
4. Load 15 μL of sample (avoid loading of the beads) into the zymogram.

5. *Controls samples*: Purified MMP-8 is diluted to achieve a final concentration of 0.002, 0.004, 0.006, 0.008, and 0.01 μg per lane.

3.4 Neutralizing Collagen for the Collagen Gel

1. Place the following on ice: collagen, 10× PBS, dH_2O, and 1 M NaOH.
2. Determine the final concentration and volume of collagen solution for making one gel as per the table. The final concentration of collagen in 2 mL solution is 3 mg/mL for one gel. The concentration of the stock solution of commercially purchased collagen used for calculation is 3.41 mg/mL (*see* **Note 2**).

	Volume for 1 gel	Volume for *x* gels
10× PBS	0.2 mL	0.2*x* mL
Collagen (3.41 mg/mL stock)	1.76 mL	1.76*x* mL
NaOH (1 M)	0.04 mL	0.04*x* mL
dH_2O	0	0
Total volume	2 mL	2*x* mL

3. Add ice cold 1 M NaOH to 10× PBS.
4. Add dH_2O and then add collagen. Since collagen is very viscous, be careful when aliquoting and allow sufficient time for collagen to run out of pipet.
5. Vortex to mix and then divide into Eppendorf tubes (1 mL/tube). Heat collagen to 60 °C for 5 min.
6. Substitute heated collagen for dH_2O in the resolving gel mixture described below.

3.5 Sodium Dodecyl Sulfate-Polyacrylamide Gel Electrophoresis

1. *Resolving gel:* In a 50 mL conical, add all the components listed in the following order for pouring the resolving gel. The collagen mixture is substituting the dH_2O. Remember, to add the 10% ammonium persulfate and TEMED just before pouring the gels in the cassette. The gel will begin to polymerize as soon as these two components are added (*see* **Notes 3** and **4**).

10% resolving collagen zymogram	1 gel	*x* gels
1.5 M Tris–HCl (pH 8.8)	1.3 mL	1.3*x* mL
Collagen mixture	1.9 mL	1.9*x* mL
30% acrylamide mix	1.7 mL	1.7*x* mL
10% SDS	50 μL	50*x* μL
10% ammonium persulfate	50 μL	50*x* μL
TEMED	2 μL	2*x* μL

2. Mix gently by swirling and load into Pasteur pipet with the bulb. Fill rig up to the bottom of the marking and then layer water to the top of the glass. Save the remaining gel in the conical so that you know when it has polymerized (20–40 min). When ready, pour off the water by inverting the rig, and pour the stacking gel on it.
3. Pour stacking gel without collagen substrate after resolving gel has polymerized. Mix the following ingredients in the following order.

4% stacking gel	1 gel	*n* gels
dH_2O	3.05 mL	3.05*n* mL
0.5 M Tris-HCl (pH 6.8)	1.25 mL	1.25*n* mL
10% SDS	50 μL	50*n* μL
30% acrylamide mix	650 μL	650*n* μL
10% ammonium persulfate	25 μL	25*n* μL
TEMED	5 μL	5*n* μL

4. Mix the stacking gel mixture gently and load on Pasteur pipet with the bulb. Fill up to the top of the glass and then insert the comb. Clean any gel mix that spills over. Save the remaining gel in the conical so that you know when it has polymerized. The gel will be ready for use in 20–40 min (*see* **Note 5**).
5. After the gel has polymerized, load the samples, protein ladder, and control samples. Run gel at typical volts used for running a Western blot (~125 V). Run time will be 60–120 min depending on the gel percentage (*see* **Note 6**).

3.6 Developing, Staining, and Analyzing the Zymogram

1. Dilute Novex Zymogram Renaturing Buffer (10×) and Novex Zymogram Developing Buffer (10×) in the ratio of 1:9 with dH_2O. Prepare up to 100 mL of Novex Zymogram Renaturing Buffer and 200 mL of Novex Zymogram Developing Buffer for 1 gel.
2. After electrophoresis, remove gel and incubate the gel in 100 mL of 1× Zymogram Renaturing Buffer for 30 min at room temperature with gentle agitation.
3. Decant the Zymogram Renaturing Buffer and add 100 mL of 1× Zymogram Developing Buffer to the gel.
4. Equilibrate gel for 30 min at room temperature with gentle agitation.
5. Decant buffer and add fresh 100 mL 1× Zymogram Developing Buffer to gel.
6. Incubate gel at 37 °C for at least 4 h or overnight for maximum sensitivity.

7. Next day, stain the gel with 100 mL of 0.5% Coomassie Blue R-250 solution for 30 min with gentle agitation.
8. Destain the gel with 100 mL destaining solution with gentle agitation (*see* **Note 7**).
9. Areas of protease activity will appear as clear bands against a dark blue background.
10. Once the clear bands are visible, tightly wrap the gel with saran wrap.
11. Scan the gel using an image scanner and analyze the band density as the measure of enzyme activity using Image J software.
12. The gel can also be dried and stored by placing the gel in between two blotting papers and drying in the gel dryer for 30 min.

4 Notes

1. We recommend both negative and positive controls in the experimental setup. Negative controls can be untransfected cells, untransfected cells with vector alone, or the culture medium. As a positive control, we prefer using a purified recombinant MMP. FBS in the culture medium may contain MMPs that may interfere with the reading in this assay. Alternatively, you may grow cells in low serum-containing medium.
2. Calculation for preparing 2 mL of the neutralized collagen for the zymogram. This calculation is based on the stock concentration of collagen (3.41 mg/mL):
   (a) Volume of 10× PBS = final volume (mL)/10 = 2/10 = 0.2 mL.
   (b) Volume of Collagen = [final volume × final concentration of collagen (mg/mL)]/stock concentration of collagen = (2 × 3)/3.41 = 1.76.
   (c) Volume of 1 M NaOH = Volume of Collagen × 0.023 = 1 .76 × 0.023 = 0.04 mL.
   (d) Volume of water = final volume − (Volume of 10× PBS + Volume of Collagen + Volume of 1 M NaOH) = 2 − (0.2 + 1.76 + 0.04) = 0.
3. Use fume hood and avoid skin contact with unpolymerized acrylamide as it is a potent neurotoxin. We use commercial solution of acrylamide from BioRad. Alternatively, powdered acrylamide can be used to prepare solution for large batches. Freeze acrylamide solution in aliquots, and use as needed to avoid day-to-day variability.

4. While pouring gels, seal the bottom of the cassettes using a saran wrap or 1% agarose and layer with 1 mL deionized water to avoid contact with air. Atmospheric oxygen prevents acrylamide polymerization. Let the gel polymerize for 1 h before decanting dH_2O and before pouring stacking gel.
5. We prefer using freshly prepared zymography gels as the substrate concentration can be adjusted in the pilot experiments as per the requirements. A careful gel preparation is required; otherwise, there will be significant experimental variables due to gel-to-gel variability.
6. While applying samples to the zymogram gel, we recommend varying concentrations of the samples and the controls. A ladder can be used to predict the molecular weight to the bands.
7. We recommend changing solutions several times and using folded Kimwipes to absorb excessive solution while destaining. The timing for destaining may vary from 60–120 min and can be optimized as per requirements.

Acknowledgments

Y.S. is supported by the ERC (StG-335377), by the MRA Young Investigator Award #402024 by the Henry Chanoch Krenter Institute for Biomedical Imaging and Genomics, the estate of Alice Schwarz-Gardos, the estate of John Hunter, the Knell Family, the Peter and Patricia Gruber Award, and the Hamburger Family.

References

1. Leber TM, Balkwill FR (1997) Zymography: a single-step staining method for quantitation of proteolytic activity on substrate gels. Anal Biochem 249(1):24–28. https://doi.org/10.1006/abio.1997.2170
2. Nagase H, Woessner JF Jr (1999) Matrix metalloproteinases. J Biol Chem 274(31):21491–21494
3. Egeblad M, Werb Z (2002) New functions for the matrix metalloproteinases in cancer progression. Nat Rev Cancer 2(3):161–174
4. Freije JM, Balbin M, Pendas AM, Sanchez LM, Puente XS, Lopez-Otin C (2003) Matrix metalloproteinases and tumor progression. Adv Exp Med Biol 532:91–107
5. Shay G, Lynch CC, Fingleton B (2015) Moving targets: emerging roles for MMPs in cancer progression and metastasis. Matrix Biol 44-46:200–206. https://doi.org/10.1016/j.matbio.2015.01.019
6. Coussens LM, Fingleton B, Matrisian LM (2002) Matrix metalloproteinase inhibitors and cancer: trials and tribulations. Science 295(5564):2387–2392
7. Lopez-Otin C, Matrisian LM (2007) Emerging roles of proteases in tumour suppression. Nat Rev Cancer 7(10):800–808
8. Springman EB, Angleton EL, Birkedal-Hansen H et al (1990) Multiple modes of activation of latent human fibroblast collagenase: evidence for the role of a Cys73 active-site zinc complex in latency and a "cysteine switch" mechanism for activation. Proc Natl Acad Sci U S A 87(1):364–368
9. Palavalli LH, Prickett TD, Wunderlich JR et al (2009) Analysis of the matrix metalloproteinase family reveals that MMP8 is often mutated in melanoma. Nat Genet 41(5):518–520

Chapter 11

Measurement of Protease Activities Using Fluorogenic Substrates

Salvatore Santamaria and Hideaki Nagase

Abstract

Matrix metalloproteinases and the related metalloproteases are implicated in cancer progression. They are endopeptidases that require several defined amino acid residues in both N-terminal and C-terminal sides of the scissile bond. Fluorogenic Förster resonance energy transfer (FRET) substrates that harbor a fluorophore and a quencher on opposite sides of the scissile bond are conveniently used to measure their activities. In this chapter, we describe the principle of FRET substrates and how to use them to measure activities and kinetic parameters of endopeptidases.

Key words ADAM, ADAMTS, Enzyme kinetics, FRET peptide substrates, Inner filter effect, MMP

1 Introduction

Proteases hydrolyze peptide bonds of proteins and peptides. They are involved in numerous biological processes such as embryonic development, morphogenesis, fertilization, processing of peptide hormones, antigen processing, angiogenesis, bone remodeling, release of cytokines and growth factors, blood clotting, apoptosis, intestinal digestion of protein diet, etc. [1]. Their aberrant activities have been implicated to diseases such as arthritis, cancer, cardiovascular diseases, disorders in the central nervous system, etc. In cancer, the involvement of matrix metalloproteinases (MMPs) [2], cysteine cathepsins [3], caspases [4], and proteasome [5] has been well established. Because of the importance of proteases in physiology and pathology, measuring their protease activities is one of the basic practices in research. For these measurements, the use of native protein or peptide substrates is ideal, but often they are not readily available. This has led to develop synthetic peptide substrates, which are labeled with a fluorogenic/chromogenic group for easier and rapid detection of the products. The synthetic substrates may not be specific, as they may be cleaved by a number of structurally homologous enzymes which share similar substrate

Santiago Cal and Alvaro J. Obaya (eds.), *Proteases and Cancer: Methods and Protocols*, Methods in Molecular Biology, vol. 1731, https://doi.org/10.1007/978-1-4939-7595-2_11, © Springer Science+Business Media, LLC 2018

binding sites or even by different class of proteases. Within this limitation, the determination of kinetic parameters (k_{cat}, K_m, k_{cat}/K_m values) gives useful values that are specific to each enzyme.

In this chapter, we describe, as an example, the procedures to measure metalloproteinase activities (MMPs, ADAMs, and ADAMTSs) in vitro using synthetic fluorogenic substrates. These metalloproteinases are endopeptidases, and they require several defined amino acid residues both at the N-terminal and C-terminal sides of the scissile bond. Thus, the Förster resonance energy transfer (FRET) substrates that harbor a fluorophore and a quencher on opposite sides of the scissile bond are conveniently used. Fluorescence-based assays for other proteases may be found in other volumes of the Methods in Molecular Biology series [6, 7].

1.1 Principle of FRET Substrates

FRET occurs between a fluorescent donor group and a quenching acceptor, which are coupled by a dipole-dipole interaction. FRET substrates are synthesized by incorporating the donor and acceptor fluorophores on opposite sides of the scissile bond, at a distance which allows for efficient energy transfer (between 15 and 60 Å) [8]. The hydrolysis of the substrate and the separation of both fluorophores abolish the energy transfer and lead to an increase of fluorescence (Fig. 1). FRET substrates have been widely used for both in vitro enzymatic assays and as probes to measure protease activities in vivo [10–12]. An optimal FRET substrate requires a fluorescent donor (fluorophore) that has a high quantum yield and an acceptor (quencher) that absorbs the emitted fluorescence of the donor within the donor fluorescence emission wavelength. Examples of donor/quencher pairs are shown in Table 1.

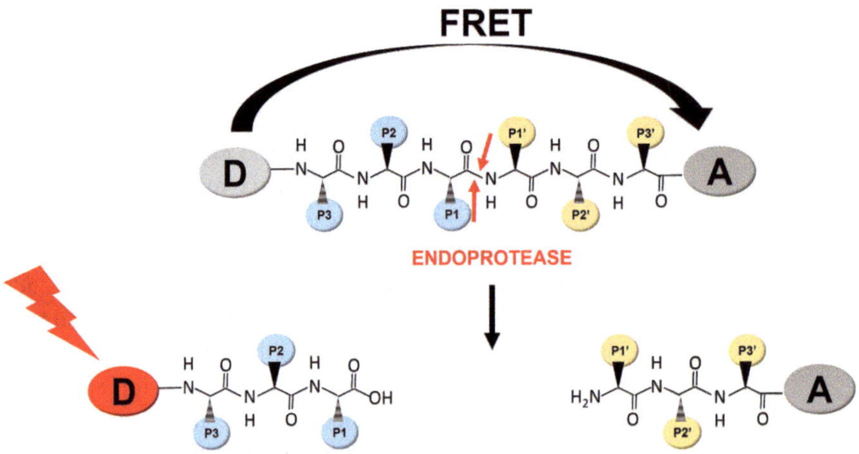

Fig. 1 Schematic diagram of cleavage of a FRET peptide by an endoprotease. D, FRET donor group; A, acceptor group (quencher). P1, P2, P3 indicate the amino acid residues on the N-terminal side of the scissile bond, whereas P1',P2', P3' indicate the residues on the C-terminal side [9]. Note that the both the donor and the acceptor group can be conjugated to the side chain of an internal amino acid

Table 1
Examples of common fluorophore/quencher pairs used in FRET substrates. λ_{ex}, excitation wavelength, λ_{em}, emission wavelength

Fluorophore	Quencher	λ_{ex} (nm)	λ_{em} (nm)
Trp	*N*-2,4-Dinitrophenyl (Dnp)	280	346
(7-Methoxycoumarin-4-yl)acetyl (Mca)	*N*-3-(2,4-Dinitrophenyl)-L-2,3-diaminopropionyl diaminopropionic amide (Dpa)	328	420
2-Aminobenzoic acid (Abz)	*N*-3-(2,4-Dinitrophenyl)-L-2,3-diaminopropionyl diaminopropionic amide (Dpa)	300	430
2-Aminobenzoic acid (Abz)	3-Nitrotyrosine	320	405
5-[(2-Aminoethyl)amino] naphthalene-1-sulfonic acid (Edans)	4-[4-(Dimethylaminophenylazo)benzoic acid (Dabcyl)	360	460
Lucifer yellow	Carboxytetramethylrhodamine (Tamra)	420	530
Coumarin 343	Carboxytetramethylrhodamine (Tamra)	450	490
5-Carboxyfluorescein (5-Fam)	(Tamra)	485	538
4-(4-Methylaminophenylazo)benzoyl (Dabcyl)	Fluorescein	485	538

An important physical parameter of a substrate is its quenching efficiency, i.e., the change in fluorescence between the cleaved product and the intact substrate. The higher the quenching efficiency, the higher the increase in signal upon cleavage, thus giving lower background fluorescence of the uncleaved substrate. For instance, upon cleavage, the fluorescence of the MMP substrate FS6 (7-methoxycoumarin-4-yl)acetyl-KPLGL(*N*-3-(2,4-dinitrophenyl)-L-2,3-diaminopropionyl diaminopropionic amide) AR-NH_2) increases 62.5-fold, corresponding to a quenching efficiency of 98.4% [13]. Such a high quenching efficiency is typical of the 7-methoxycoumarin-4-yl (Mca)/2,4 dinitrophenyl (Dnp) pair [13, 14]. Another factor to consider when choosing a fluorogenic substrate is its solubility. Since most fluorophores and quenchers are hydrophobic, FRET substrates typically display poor solubility in aqueous environments. If the protease under study shows a broad substrate specificity, hydrophilic residues can be introduced to enhance solubility [13].

1.2 Measuring of Initial Velocity

An enzymatic reaction can be followed by using discontinuous or continuous assays. A discontinuous assay involves running many reactions individually and stopping them at a specific time point by adding a reagent that stops the enzyme reaction without destroying

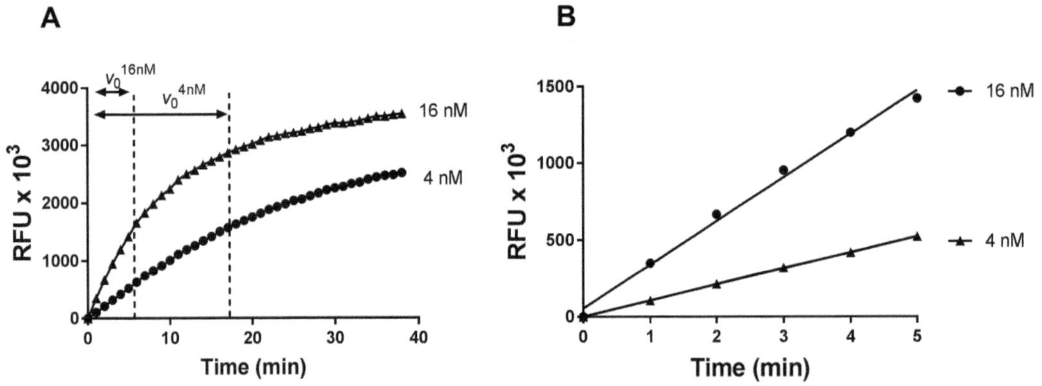

Fig. 2 Example of an enzyme reaction curve. (**a**) Cleavage of FRET substrate Fam-AE~LQGRPISIAK-Tamra (0.5 μM) at two different concentrations (16 and 4 nM) of ADAMTS4-2 (16 nM). Fluorescence was detected (λ_{ex} = 485 nm, λ_{em} = 520 nm) every minute for 40 min at 37 °C fluorometer and reported as relative fluorescence units (RFU). The linear portion of the curve corresponding to the initial velocities for the two enzyme concentrations (v_0^{16nM} and v_0^{4nM}) is indicated by vertical dotted lines. (**b**) Linear portion of the curves fitted with linear regression (r^2 = 0.993 for 16 nM and r^2 = 0.9998 for 4 nM)

the product that has been formed. For example, addition of glacial acetic acid stops the reaction of enzymes which require a pH above 5.0. A continuous assay involves directly monitoring the reaction for a period of time. This requires a fluorometer capable of rapidly collecting data at multiple time points (kinetic mode). Generally, discontinuous assays involve performing multiple reactions in parallel, and this tend to lead to more variable data than continuous assays.

Figure 2a shows an example of curves generated by continuous assay, where the FRET substrate, 5-carboxyfluorescein-AE~LQGRPISIAK-carboxytetramethylrhodamine (the tilde indicate the site cleaved) was incubated with ADAMTS-4 (a disintegrin and metalloproteinase with thrombospondin motif 4) and measured with λ_{ex} = 485 nm and λ_{em} = 538 nm. The increase in fluorescence was linear up to 5 min (Fig. 2b) and then reaches a plateau. Since the reaction was monitored within the dynamic range of the instrument (*see* **Note 1**), this plateau may be originated by various factors, such as (1) substrate depletion; (2) product inhibition, i.e., enzyme inhibition by the vast amount of product formed; and/or (3) enzyme inactivation (*see* **Note 2**).

At a fixed substrate concentration, the initial velocity is linearly proportional to the enzyme concentration (*see* **Note 3**). However, higher enzyme concentrations reach a plateau early, due to substrate depletion, while lower enzyme concentrations extend the time for linear kinetics (Fig. 2a). A compromise should be reached between signal detection (the lower the enzyme concentration, the lower the signal) and time (the lower the enzyme concentration, the longer the linear phase of the reaction). Provided that the enzyme is stable under the assay conditions, all enzyme concentrations should eventually reach the same maximum signal.

We define the initial velocity (v_0) as the change in the fluorescence F (generally displayed as relative fluorescence units or RFU) divided by the change in time observed in the linear portion of the reaction curve:

$$\Delta \text{RFU} / \Delta t = v_0 \quad (1)$$

where $\Delta\text{RFU} = \text{RFU}_1 - \text{RFU}_0$ and $\Delta t = t_1 - t_0$.

Graphically, the initial velocity is equivalent to the slope of the linear portion of the reaction curve and can be calculated using linear regression. Under these conditions, we can assume that the substrate concentration does not significantly change (i.e., substrate cleavage <10%); therefore, the factors mentioned above (substrate depletion, product inhibition, and enzyme inactivation) would not affect the reaction. If initial velocities are not measured, the formation of product will not be linear with respect to the amount of enzyme. Thus, the steady-state or rapid equilibrium kinetic studies will not be valid (the concentration of substrate is unknown since a non-negligible amount of it is consumed).

1.3 Determination of k_{cat}, K_m, and k_{cat}/K_m

When the initial rate of the enzyme reaction is measured with various concentrations of a substrate at a fixed enzyme concentration, it initially increases as the substrate concentration increases (Fig. 3). At low substrate concentrations, only a small percentage of the enzyme is bound to the substrate. At higher substrate concentrations, a larger portion of the enzyme is bound to the substrate, and eventually all of the enzyme is saturated with the substrate, giving the maximum velocity V_{max} of the enzyme. The substrate concentration that gives 50% of the V_{max} is defined as K_m. This represents a useful working definition of the K_m.

However, the K_m is actually a kinetic constant (expressed in molarity, M), involving the three rate constants in the following scheme:

$$\text{E} + \text{S} \underset{k_{off}}{\overset{k_{on}}{\rightleftarrows}} \text{ES} \xrightarrow{k_{cat}} \text{E} + \text{P} \qquad \text{Scheme1}$$

$$K_m = (k_{off} + k_{cat}) / k_{on} \quad (2)$$

where k_{on} is the bimolecular association rate constant for the formation of the enzyme-substrate (ES) complex, k_{off} is the unimolecular dissociation rate constant of the ES complex to give free enzyme (E) and substrate (S), and k_{cat} is the unimolecular rate constant of the *ES* complex to give free enzyme and the product (P).

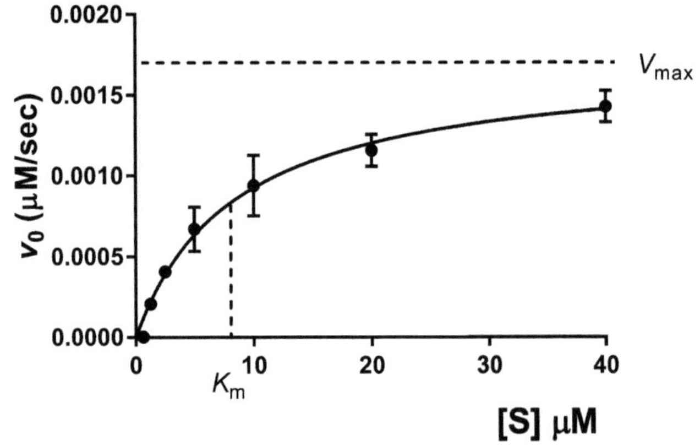

Fig. 3 Plot of initial velocity as a function of substrate concentration for an enzyme-catalyzed reaction. Cleavage of the FRET substrate 5-carboxyfluorescein-AE~LQGRPISIAK-Tamra by ADAMTS-4 (5 nM) is shown. Data were fitted to the Michaelis-Menten equation by GraphPad Prism. Values for K_m, V_{max}, and k_{cat} were 8.5 μM, 1.7×10^{-3} μM/s, and 0.34 s^{-1}, respectively. Results are mean ± s.e

The higher the K_m, the lower the affinity of the enzyme for the substrate. The k_{cat} (commonly referred as the turnover number) represents the turnover rate of the enzyme to hydrolyze the substrate (the number of substrate molecules converted to the product by one molecule of the enzyme in time, which is often expressed as *per second*, s^{-1}) and can be calculated by dividing V_{max} by the enzyme concentration $[E]$:

$$k_{cat} = V_{max} / [E] \tag{3}$$

Therefore, the higher the k_{cat}, the quicker the enzyme will release the product from the ES complex. The k_{cat}/K_m ratio (referred to as specificity constant) indicates the specificity of the substrate for a particular enzyme, expressed as $s^{-1}\ M^{-1}$. These parameters are useful as they are unique to each enzyme with the specific substrate. Some examples of k_{cat}, K_m, and k_{cat}/K_m values reported for representative FRET substrates of MMPs and ADAMs (a disintegrin and metalloproteinase) are shown in Tables 2 and 3.

From an experimental point of view, enzymatic reactions are studied under steady-state conditions, i.e., under conditions where the concentration of enzyme-substrate complex is kept constant by having a large excess of substrate versus enzyme. Under steady-state conditions, the enzyme velocity, v, as a function of substrate concentration is described by the Michaelis-Menten equation:

$$v = [E][S]k_{cat} / (K_m + [S]) \tag{4}$$

Since $k_{cat} = V_{max}/[E]$, this equation can be rearranged to give:

$$v = V_{max}[S] / (K_m + [S]) \tag{5}$$

Table 2
Specificity constants (k_{cat}/K_m) for cleavage of FRET substrate FS6 ((Mca)-KPLG~L(Dpa)AR-NH_2) by members of the MMP and ADAM families

Enzyme	k_{cat} (s^{-1})	K_M (M)	k_{cat}/K_M (s^{-1} M^{-1})	Reference
MMP-1	2.5	28×10^{-6}	9.2×10^4	[13]
MMP-2	ND	$>3 \times 10^{-5}$	6.9×10^5	[13]
MMP-3	ND	ND	2.0×10^4	[13]
MMP-7	ND	ND	3.0×10^5	[13]
MMP-8	ND	ND	4.2×10^5	[13]
MMP-9	ND	$>3 \times 10^{-5}$	6.2×10^5	[13]
MMP-12	17.0	1.3×10^{-4}	1.3×10^5	[15]
MMP-13	5.9	5.2×10^{-6}	1.1×10^6	[13]
MMP-14	9.9	7.9×10^{-6}	1.3×10^6	[13]
ADAM-10	ND	ND	1.1×10^3	[13]
ADAM-17	ND	ND	7.8×10^5	[13]

Table 3
Specificity constants (k_{cat}/K_m) for cleavage of FRET substrate 5-((2-aminoethyl)amino)naphthalene-l-sulfonic (Edans)EPLAQGA~VRSSSK(Dabcyl)-NH_2 by members of the ADAM family [16]

Enzyme	k_{cat} (s^{-1})	K_M (M)	k_{cat}/K_M (s^{-1} M^{-1})
ADAM-8	0.01	46×10^{-6}	2.2×10^2
ADAM-9	0.06	49×10^{-6}	1.2×10^3
ADAM-10	0.28	12×10^{-6}	2.5×10^4
ADAM-12	0.01	12×10^{-6}	8.5×10^2
ADAM-17	0.14	12×10^{-6}	1.2×10^4

This equation describes a rectangular hyperbola. Linear transformations, such as a double reciprocal Lineweaver-Burk plot (i.e., $1/[S]$ versus $1/v_0$), which were used before computation was routine, should not be used for calculating the K_m and V_{max} from substrate saturations experiments, since they tend to distort the errors involved with the measurement [17]. Instead, it is recommended to fit the data to a rectangular hyperbola using nonlinear regression analysis. Software packages are commonly used for the determination of kinetic parameters and the most popular of them are listed in Subheading 2.4.

From simple mathematical manipulations of Eq. 4 follows that when $[S] \ll K_m$ (pseudo-first-order conditions)

$$k_{cat} / K_m = v / [E][S] \quad (6)$$

Under these conditions, once the initial velocity is measured, it is possible to derive the combined value of the specificity constant k_{cat}/K_m. Subheading 3.3 shows how to calculate independently the value of k_{cat} and K_m by measuring the initial velocity of the enzymatic reaction at different substrate concentrations.

1.4 Considerations when Choosing the Substrate Concentration for Routine Enzyme Assays

To choose a substrate concentration for an enzyme assay, several considerations should be taken into account:

1. If the substrate concentration is much lower than the K_m ($[S] \ll K_m$), the initial velocity is very sensitive to changes in substrate concentrations. On the other hand, if $[S] \gg K_m$, then the velocity is insensitive to changes in substrate concentrations.
2. Substrate inhibition may occur at high substrate concentrations.
3. Solubility of the substrate may decrease at high substrate concentrations. This will lead to a decrease in enzyme activity due to aggregation/precipitation of the substrate.
4. At high substrate concentrations, inner filter effects are more pronounced (*see* Subheading 1.5).

Generally, the inner filter effect and the solubility of the substrate are the main factors affecting the choice of the substrate concentrations. For this reason, most of the assays involving FRET peptides are performed at substrate concentrations well below the K_m value.

1.5 Inner Filter Effect

Under conditions of high optical densities when the absorption spectra of the fluorophore and quencher dyes overlap [8], some of the emitted light may be absorbed by quencher groups on neighboring substrates or cleaved products. This effectively reduces the amount of emitted light being detected by the fluorometer. As a result, the experimentally measured fluorescence intensities are not proportional to the concentration of free donor group. This phenomenon is commonly called "inner filter effect." The magnitude of the inner filter effect depends on the Stoke shift, path length, and substrate concentration, with higher substrate concentrations producing greater inner filter effect. This typically becomes significant with 10–20 μM of FRET substrate [15, 18]. As a result, high rates will be estimated if a correction factor is not introduced (Fig. 4). Subheading 3.4 describes a method widely used to correct inner filter effects [18].

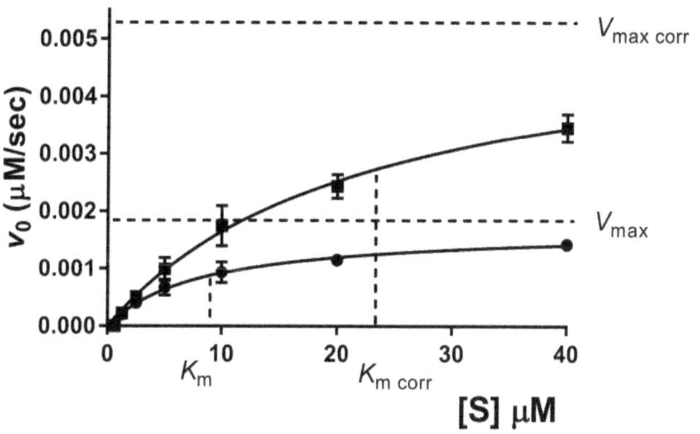

Fig. 4 Effect of inner filter on the estimate of kinetic parameters. Cleavage of FRET substrate Fam-AE~LQGRPISIAK-Tamra by ADAMTS4-2 (5 nM) is shown. Data were fitted to the Michaelis-Menten equation by GraphPad Prism. Curve (filled circle) shows uncorrected value as shown in Fig. 3. Curve (filled square) shows values corrected with inner filter effect using 5(6)-carboxyfluorescein (Fam) as free fluorophore as described in Subheading 3.4. Note that at low substrate concentrations the corrected rate values do not differ much from the uncorrected rates. Corrected values for K_m, V_{max}, and k_{cat} were 23 µM, 5.4×10^{-3} µM/s, and 1.1 s^{-1}, respectively. Results are mean ± s.e.

2 Materials

The following protocols describe a continuous ADAMTS-4 assay using FRET substrate in a total volume of 200 µL for detection in a 96-well plate reader. For analysis requiring smaller/larger volumes, decrease/increase proportionally. It is necessary to adapt the concentrations of enzyme and substrate to each particular protease under study. For example, to test MMP activities, use substrate Mca-Pro-Leu-Gly~Leu-Dpa-Ala-Arg-NH_2 [14] (excitation wavelength, 325 nm; emission wavelength, 393 nm) or its derivative FS-6 [13] at a final concentration of 1.5 µM and 1–10 nM of the particular MMP under study. All assays must be carried out at least in duplicate.

2.1 Apparatus

1. Micro-well plate fluorometer equipped with temperature controller and interfaced with a compatible personal computer.

2.2 Materials

1. 96-well black polypropylene or non-binding polystyrene microplates with U-bottom (final volume 200 µL).
2. Eppendorf tubes.

2.3 Reagents

1. Assay buffer (TNC): 50 mM Tris–HCl pH 7.5, 150 mM NaCl, 10 mM $CaCl_2$, 0.02% NaN_3, and 0.05% (v/v) Brij® 35. In a glass bottle, dissolve Trizma Base (6.055 g), NaCl (8.766 g), $CaCl_2 \cdot 2H_2O$, and NaN_3 (0.2 g) in ~900 mL of deionized water and adjust to pH 7.5 with HCl. Add 1.667 mL 30% Brij® 35 solution and make up to 1000 mL. The assay buffer can be stored at room temperature and used for a month.
2. ADAMTS-4: cloning, expression, and purification procedures are available in the literature [19, 20]. Active concentrations of enzyme were determined by titration against known concentrations of tissue inhibitor of metalloproteinase (TIMP)-3. The data shown here are for the ADAMTS-4 deletion mutant lacking the spacer domain (ADAMTS4-2) [20].
3. Enzyme stock solution in TNC. The solution should be freshly prepared, mixed carefully, and stored on ice till used.
4. 5 μM FRET substrate Fam-AE~LQGRPISIAK-Tamra in TNC. Prepare it by diluting 1:1000 from a 5 mM solution in DMSO, previously prepared by weighing the lyophilized substrate powder (*see* **Note 4**). Substrate solutions have a red color.
5. Free fluorophore 5-FAM or, whenever possible, peptide corresponding to the cleavage product covalently linked to the fluorophore (Fam-AE). Free fluorophore solutions have a yellow color.
6. Dimethyl sulfoxide (DMSO).

2.4 Software Packages Used for Fitting Enzyme Kinetics Data

1. GraFit (http://www.erithacus.com/grafit/).
2. GraphPad Prism (http://www.graphpad.com/scientific-software/prism/).
3. OriginLab (http://www.originlab.com/).
4. SigmaPlot (http://www.sigmaplot.co.uk/products/sigmaplot/sigmaplot-details.php).

3 Methods

3.1 Determination of Initial Velocity

1. Dispense 160 μL of TNC buffer into a 96-well plate. In control wells (not containing the enzyme), dispense 180 μL of buffer.
2. Prepare a 50 nM ADAMTS-4 solution (10× the final concentration, 5 nM) from the stock solution. Dispense 20 μL (*see* **Note 5**).
3. Equilibrate the solution at 37 °C for 5–10 min in the plate reader.

4. Start the reaction by adding 20 μL of the 5 μM substrate solution (final concentration of 0.5 μM). Since ideally this step should be simultaneous for every well, try to be as quick as possible and use a multichannel pipette. If using a continuous assay, set up a 5-s stir prior to measurement to allow proper mixing of the solution.
5. Start recording the fluorescence every min for 1 h. The excitation wavelength for the FRET pair used here is 485 nm and the emission wavelength is 520 nm.
6. Calculate the initial velocity by using Eq. 1. Most of the microwell plate fluorometers reading in continuous mode allow the researcher to choose the time interval of the reaction and then automatically calculate the initial velocity. If an increase in fluorescence is observed in the well containing only buffer and substrate, a rate should be calculated and subtracted from the rates measured in the presence of the enzyme.

3.2 Conversion of the Recorded Fluorescence to the Actual Amount of Product Formed by the Enzyme

For determination of kinetic parameters, it is necessary to convert the initial velocities from RFU/min to μM/s. For this purpose, it is necessary to record the fluorescence from a reaction where the substrate has been completely digested with enzyme.

1. Incubate 0.5 μM of substrate with 5 nM ADAMTS-4 for 16 h (*see* **Note 6**). After this incubation time, all the substrate is converted into product. Record the fluorescence.
2. To convert the initial velocities from RFU/s to μM/s, divide the initial velocity by the fluorescence corresponding to complete hydrolysis of 0.5 μM substrate (RFU_{tot}) and then multiply it by the concentration of digested substrate:

   Rate (μM/s) = $(RFU/RFU_{tot}) \times s^{-1} \times$ [substrate]. For example, complete digestion of 0.5 μM of substrate gives a fluorescence of 10,000 RFU. If we measured an initial velocity of 2000 RFU/s, this corresponds to 2000 RFU/10,000 RFU × s^{-1} × 0.5 μM = 0.1 μMx s^{-1}.

3.3 Determination of Kinetic Parameters (k_{cat}, K_m)

1. Dispense 160 μL of TNC buffer into a 96-well plate. In control wells (not containing the enzyme), dispense 180 μL of buffer.
2. Dispense 20 μL of the 50 nM enzyme solution (final concentration of 5 nM).
3. Equilibrate the solution at 37 °C for 5–10 min.
4. Prepare a 400 μM solution of the FRET substrate. Use this solution to prepare various dilutions (10× the final concentration) in TNC. Use at least three substrate concentrations above and three below the theoretical K_m value (in the case of ADAMTS-4 the value reported in literature is 16 μM [21]).

If the approximate K_m value is not known, use a broad range of substrate concentrations with the maximum final concentration being high enough to provide saturation of the enzyme (e.g., 50 μM). It should be also tested if the substrate is unstable and is cleaved in the absence of enzyme. In this case, a separate blank rate should be determined and subtracted for each substrate concentration.

5. Start the reaction with the addition of 20 μL of each substrate solution.
6. Record the fluorescence and, for each reaction, measure the initial velocity.
7. Fit the data to the Michaelis-Menten equation using any of the software packages listed in Subheading 2.4 (*see* **Note 7**). They calculate directly values of K_m and V_{max}. To calculate k_{cat} use the formula $k_{cat} = V_{max}/[E]$ (Eq. 3).

3.4 Correction of Inner Filter Effects

The initial velocities measured in Subheading 3.3 should be corrected for the presence of inner filter effect (*see* Subheading 1.5). The following protocol is based on the measurement of the fluorescence from a fixed concentration of free fluorophore (*see* **Note 8**) in the absence and presence of various concentrations of FRET substrate [18]. The fluorescence from the fluorophore is decreased in the presence of the substrate due to the ability of its quencher groups to absorb a part of the emitted light. The higher the concentration of substrate, the lower the fluorescence from the free fluorophore due to inner filter effect. The difference between the values measured in the absence and presence of the substrate will give an estimate of how much the fluorescence from the released fluorogenic cleavage product is decreased by the substrate.

1. Dispense 190 μL TNC buffer in the wells which will contain either substrate or FAM and 180 μL buffer in the well which will contain both substrate and FAM. Prepare a blank containing buffer only.
2. Prepare an 80 μM solution of free fluorophore (20× the final concentration 4 μM) and add 10 μL to the wells.
3. Prepare an 800 μM solution of FRET substrate. Use this solution to prepare various dilutions (20× the final concentration) in TNC buffer corresponding to the substrate concentrations used in Subheading 3.3. Add 10 μL of substrate dilutions to the wells.
4. Record fluorescence at a single point using the excitation of 485 nm and emission wavelength of 520 nm.
5. Subtract the fluorescence from the blank.
6. Subtract the fluorescence recorded in the presence of a certain substrate concentration from the fluorescence recorded in the

presence of substrate plus free fluorophore. This value will give the fluorescence of the free fluorophore in the presence of a certain concentration of substrate. The reduction in the observed fluorescence of the free fluorophore in the presence of various substrate concentrations reflects the inner filter effect at those substrate concentrations.

7. Calculate the correction factor by dividing the fluorescence measured in the presence of the free fluorophore alone by the fluorescence measured in the presence of both free fluorophore and substrate.
8. Divide the enzymatic velocity measured at each substrate concentration as described in Subheading 3.3 by the corresponding correction factor. Table 4 shows an example of experimental layout and the correction factors for the FRET substrate Fam-AE~LQGRPISIAK-Tamra.

4 Notes

1. When measuring the rate of an enzymatic reaction, it is important that the measured fluorescence is within the dynamic range of the fluorometer, as determined by the minimum and maximum detection limits (photon/seconds). The dynamic range is typical for each instrument and operating conditions and is generally provided by the manufacturer.
2. It is generally assumed that no changes in pH and temperature occur during the course of the reaction. Changes in pH can be avoided by adequate buffering of the reaction mixture. Most of instruments are equipped with a built-in thermostat that can control the temperature during the course of the reaction.
3. This linear relationship is valid within a limited range of enzyme concentrations and incubation time. At extremely low and high enzyme concentrations, the researcher's ability to measure the initial velocity is compromised by detection limits and sensitivity. Moreover, the enzyme may be unstable at extremely low concentrations or aggregate at extremely high concentrations.
4. For this reason, the substrate stock solution (1–10 mM) is generally prepared in an organic solvent such as DMSO. However, enzymes may be sensitive at relatively high concentrations of nonaqueous solvents; therefore, their effect should be tested by incubating increasing concentrations of the organic solvent (0–10% v/v) with the enzyme and then choosing a solvent concentration high enough to guarantee solubility of the substrate and low enough not to affect sensibly the initial rate of the reaction. Once an acceptable concentration

Table 4
Correction factors for the inner filter effect of the FRET substrate Fam-AE~LQGRPISIAK-Tamra

	RFU substrate	RFU substrate + FAM	RFU FAM	Correction factor
[*S*] (μM)	A	B	B − A	
0	175	1490	1315	1.0
0.625	163	1476	1413	1.0
1.25	165	1393	1228	0.93
2.5	169	1188	1019	0.77
5	170	1072	902	0.69
10	170	892	722	0.56
20	173	891	718	0.55
40	165	708	543	0.41

Note how these values are significantly below unity for substrate concentrations higher than 2 μM

of nonaqueous solvent has been fixed, it should be kept constant throughout the experiment, in order to enable comparison of the initial velocities between different conditions.

5. It is recommended to take note of the initial velocity measured each day under identical experimental conditions. This will help identifying a decrease in activity due to decay in the enzyme batch or unusual differences in activity between different batches.

6. A problem with such a long digestion time is the evaporation from the reaction well. Even though it is possible to seal the micro-well plate with appropriate tape films, condensation may occur on these surfaces. In this case, it is necessary to spin down the plate using centrifuges whose rotor is adapted to such plates. Alternatively, perform the reaction in an Eppendorf tube to avoid evaporation, spin it down in a table top centrifuge (10 s at 10,000 × *g*), and then transfer the liquid to the micro-well plate. To confirm that substrate hydrolysis is complete, measure the fluorescence from the reaction at different time points. Upon complete digestion, no further increase in fluorescence should be measured.

7. The nonlinear fitting has greater statistical power if every replicate is used separately for curve fitting instead of being averaged [22].

8. If possible, to better mimic the free donor fluorophore groups, a so-called split peptide (i.e., the fluorophore-labeled peptide corresponding to the C-terminal cleavage product) should be used.

However, it is not recommended to use the FRET substrate which has been completely digested with enzyme, since this will still contain quencher groups. Before measuring inner filter effects, we recommend to measure the fluorescence of different fluorophore concentrations. These values should be linear for a wide range of concentrations. The reader should then choose a fluorophore concentration which allows reproducible and sensitive reading.

Acknowledgments

This work was supported by the National Institutes of Health (grant number AR40994) and the British Heart Foundation (PG/14/63/31036).

References

1. Hooper NM (2002) Proteases in biology and medicine. Portland Press, London
2. Overall CM, Dean RA (2006) Degradomics: systems biology of the protease web. Pleiotropic roles of MMPs in cancer. Cancer Metastasis Rev 25:69–75
3. Mohamed MM, Sloane BF (2006) Cysteine cathepsins: multifunctional enzymes in cancer. Nat Rev Cancer 6:764–775
4. Fulda S, Debatin KM (2004) Signaling through death receptors in cancer therapy. Curr Opin Pharmacol 4:327–332
5. Sterz J, von Metzler I, Hahne JC et al (2008) The potential of proteasome inhibitors in cancer therapy. Expert Opin Investig Drugs 17:879–895
6. Fields GB (2010) Methods Mol Biol 622:393–433
7. Nitsche C, Klein CD (2013) Fluorimetric and HPLC-based dengue virus protease assays using a FRET substrate. Methods Mol Biol 1030:221–236
8. Lakowicz JR (1983) Principles of Fluorescence Spectroscopy. Plenum Press, New York
9. Schechter I, Berger A (1967) On the size of the active site in proteases. Biochem Biophys Res Commun 27:157–162
10. Weissleder R, Tung CH, Mahmood U et al (1999) In vivo imaging of tumors with protease-activated near-infrared fluorescent probes. Nat Biotechnol 17:375–378
11. Chen J, Tung CH, Allport JR et al (2005) Near-infrared fluorescent imaging of matrix metalloproteinase activity after myocardial infarction. Circulation 111:1800–1805
12. Lim NH, Meinjohanns E, Bou-Gharios G et al (2014) In vivo imaging of matrix metalloproteinase 12 and matrix metalloproteinase 13 activities in the mouse model of collagen-induced arthritis. Arthritis Rheumatol 66:589–598
13. Neumann U, Kubota H, Frei K et al (2004) Characterization of Mca-Lys-Pro-Leu-Gly-Leu-Dpa-Ala-Arg-NH_2, a fluorogenic substrate with increased specificity constants for collagenases and tumor necrosis factor converting enzyme. Anal Biochem 328:166–173
14. Knight CG, Willenbrock F, Murphy G (1992) A novel coumarin labelled peptide for sensitive continuous assays of the matrix metalloproteinases. FEBS Lett 296:263–266
15. Palmier MO, Van Doren SR (2007) Rapid determination of enzyme kinetics from fluorescence: overcoming the inner filter effect. Anal Biochem 371:43–51
16. Minond D, Cudic M, Bionda N et al (2012) Discovery of novel inhibitors of a disintegrin and metalloprotease 17 (ADAM17) using glycosylated and non-glycosylated substrates. J Biol Chem 287:36473–36487
17. Cornish-Bowden A (1995) Fundamentals of Enzyme Kinetics. Portland Press, London
18. Liu Y, Kati W, Chen CM et al (1999) Use of a fluorescence plate reader for measuring kinetic parameters with inner filter effect correction. Anal Biochem 267:331–335
19. Gendron C, Kashiwagi M, Lim NH et al (2007) Proteolytic activities of human ADAMTS-5. Comparative studies with ADAMTS-4. J Biol Chem 282:18294–18306

20. Fushimi K, Troeberg L, Nakamura H et al (2008) Functional differences of the catalytic and non-catalytic domains in human ADAMTS-4 and ADAMTS-5 in aggrecanolytic activity. J Biol Chem 283:6706–6716
21. Wayne GJ, Deng SJ, Amour A et al (2007) TIMP-3 inhibition of ADAMTS-4 (Aggrecanase-1) is modulated by interactions between aggrecan and the C-terminal domain of ADAMTS-4. J Biol Chem 282:20991–20998
22. Copeland RA (2003) Mechanistic considerations in high-throughput screening. Anal Biochem 320:1–12

Chapter 12

Targeting the Expression of Cathepsin B Using CRISPR/Cas9 System in Mammalian Cancer Cells

Manu Gnanamony and Christopher S. Gondi

Abstract

Cathepsin B belongs to a family of cathepsins and plays an important role in normal physiological functions in the cell. However, overexpression of cathepsin B has been associated with different malignancies, and this has made it an attractive pharmacological target. The advent of CRISPR-Cas9 technology has allowed researchers to efficiently knock down genes with very less nonspecific activity compared to earlier methods. The protocol described below will enable investigators to develop cathepsin B knockdown stable cells and explains ways to study the knockdown.

Key words Cathepsin B, Cancer therapy, Cancer target, Cathepsin B signaling, RNAi, Antibody, Inhibitor

1 Introduction

Cathepsin B is a lysosomal cysteine protease that was first isolated in 1957 and plays a role in intracellular proteolysis [1]. The cathepsin B gene is located on chromosome 8p22 and belongs to a family of papain proteases. Numerous cathepsins have been identified, and cathepsin B is considered the most significant as it is involved in various pathologic and oncogenic processes [2]. Overexpression of cathepsin B has been reported in several cancers such as brain [3] and colorectal carcinoma [4]. Cathepsin B has also shown potential as a marker of prognosis in hepatocellular carcinoma [5] and human lung squamous cell carcinoma [6].

Multiple methods are possible for targeting cathepsin B: using (1) chemical inhibitors [7, 8], (2) liposomal inhibitors [9], and (3) RNA interference.

We have described here a detailed protocol to efficiently knock down the expression of cathepsin B in mammalian cancer cells using the CRISPR-Cas9 technology. We also present protocols for validation of cathepsin B knockdown at the mRNA level using RT-PCR and protein level using Western blotting.

Santiago Cal and Alvaro J. Obaya (eds.), *Proteases and Cancer: Methods and Protocols*, Methods in Molecular Biology, vol. 1731, https://doi.org/10.1007/978-1-4939-7595-2_12,

2 Materials

2.1 Cell Lines and Culture Conditions

1. MIA PaCa-2 cell line (ATCC). This cell line that we have used for this experiment is a pancreatic carcinoma cell line first isolated in 1977 [10]. It has a doubling time of 40 h and is an easy transfection host. We chose this cell line to demonstrate cathepsin B knockdown because of its inherently high expression of cathepsin B.
2. RPMI 1640 medium with glutamine. Store at +4 °C.
3. Fetal bovine serum. Store at −20 °C.
4. Penicillin streptomycin solution. Store at −20 °C.
5. Complete medium: RPMI 1640 medium, 10% fetal bovine serum, and 1% penicillin streptomycin solution.
6. Puromycin.
7. Selection medium: Complete medium with 1 μg/mL of puromycin.

2.2 Plasmid Isolation and Transfection

1. Cathepsin B guide sequence CTCCACGCTGACGTGCGCAT cloned in vector pSpCas9 BB-2A-Puro (PX459) v2.0 (Genscript).
2. Cathepsin B scrambled guide sequence GCGATTAGCCGCC TCGTACC cloned in vector pSpCas9 BB-2A-Puro (PX459) v2.0 (Genscript) (*see* **Note 1**).
3. Transfection reagent (*see* **Note 2**).

2.3 Protein Extraction and Estimation

1. M-PER Mammalian Protein Extraction Reagent.
2. Protease phosphatase inhibitor cocktail (100×).
3. Pierce™ Bovine Serum Albumin Standard Pre-Diluted Set (BSA): 125, 250, 500, 750, 1000, 1500, 2000 μg/mL.
4. Pierce 660 nm Protein Assay Reagent.

2.4 Western Blotting

1. Resolving gel buffer: 1 M Tris–HCl, pH 8.8. Add 157.6 grams of Tris base to 800 mL of water in a glass beaker. Stir using a magnetic stirrer until Tris base is completely dissolved. Adjust pH to 8.8 with 1 N sodium hydroxide or 1 N hydrochloric acid. Make up the volume to 1 L. Store the solution at +4 °C.
2. Stacking gel buffer: 1 M Tris base, pH 6.8. Add 157.6 g of Tris–HCl to 800 mL of water in a glass beaker. Stir using a magnetic stirrer until Tris base is completely dissolved. Adjust pH to 6.8 with 1 N sodium hydroxide or 1 N hydrochloric acid. Make up the volume to 1 liter. Store the solution at +4 °C.
3. Thirty percent acrylamide/Bis Solution. Store at +4 °C.
4. Sodium dodecyl sulfate solution (SDS): Add 2 g of sodium dodecyl sulfate to 10 mL of water in a ventilated fume hood. Store SDS solution at room temperature.

5. Ammonium persulfate solution (APS): Dissolve 1 g of ammonium per sulfate (APS) in 10 mL of water. Store APS solution in dark at +4 °C.
6. *N*,*N*,*N*,*N*′-Tetramethylethylenediamine (TEMED). Store at +4 °C.
7. Gel cassettes.
8. Gel combs.
9. Running buffer: 10× Tris/Glycine/SDS buffer. Prepare a 1× solution by adding 100 mL of the 10× buffer to 900 mL of water.
10. Sample loading dye (4×): 0.25 M Tris–HCl, pH 6.8, 10% SDS, 10% glycerol, 0.02% bromophenol blue, and 25% β-mercaptoethanol (*see* **Note 3**).
11. Electrophoresis apparatus.
12. Transfer apparatus: iBlot apparatus.
13. Transfer membrane: iBlot® Transfer Stack, PVDF (*see* **Note 4**).
14. Blocking buffer: 5% skimmed milk in 1× PBS with 0.1% Tween 20.
15. Wash buffer: 1× PBS with 0.1% Tween 20.
16. Pierce ECL Western Blotting Substrate Kit.

2.5 Antibodies

1. Cathepsin B: D1C7Y XP Rabbit mAb (Cell signaling).
2. β-Actin: C4 (Santa Cruz).
3. Goat anti-rabbit IgG-HRP.
4. Anti-mouse IgG, HRP linked antibody.

2.6 RNA Isolation

1. TRIzol reagent.
2. Chloroform.
3. Isopropanol, molecular grade.
4. Absolute alcohol, molecular grade.

2.7 cDNA synthesis and RT-PCR

1. Thermal cycler.
2. Real-time PCR.
3. cDNA Synthesis Kit.
4. iTaq Universal SYBR Green Master Mix.
5. Primers: Primers were synthesized commercially by Integrated DNA Technologies at 25 nmol concentration. The sequences of the oligos synthesized are as follows:

   Cathepsin B Forward: 5′-AGAGTTATGTTTACCGAGGACCT-3′.

   Cathepsin B Reverse: 5′-GATGCAGATCCGGTCAGAGA-3′.

   HPRT Forward: 5′-TGACACTGGCAAAACAATGCA-3′.

   HPRT Reverse: 5′-GGTCCTTTTCACCAGCAAGCT-3′.

3 Methods

3.1 Cell Culture

1. Culture the cell line of interest at 37 °C in a humidified CO_2 incubator. Make sure that the cell lines are of low passage number for successful transfection. In this protocol, we seeded about 200,000 MIA PaCa-2 cells in a 10 cm cell culture plate in complete media.

3.2 Plasmid Transfection

1. Day 1: Seed cells in a way that they are 50–60% confluent on the next day. Cell seeding density is different for each cell line, so plate according to the doubling time of the cell line of your interest.
2. Day 2: The following protocol is for cells plated in 10 cm tissue culture plates. Prepare the plasmid mix by adding 15 μg of plasmid with 500 μL of serum-free RPMI medium. Prepare the transfection reagent mix by adding 45 μL of JET PEI transfection reagent to 500 μL of serum-free RPMI medium. Add the transfection reagent mix to the plasmid mix and incubate at room temperature for 30 min. After 30 min, add the mixture dropwise onto cells cultured with 9 mL of complete medium.
3. Incubate the plates in a 37 °C humidified CO_2 incubator for 72 h.
4. Day 5: Replace complete medium in the plate with selection medium and subsequently once every 3 days until resistant cells emerge and start forming colonies (*see* **Note 5**).
5. Expression of cathepsin B can be verified using RT-PCR and by Western blotting to confirm efficient knockdown.

3.3 Protein Isolation and Estimation

1. Prepare cell lysis solution by adding 1 μL of protease phosphatase inhibitor cocktail to every 100 μL of M-PER Mammalian Protein Extraction Reagent to make it a 1× solution (*see* **Note 6**).
2. Remove cell culture plates from CO_2 incubator and place on ice. Remove the medium and wash cells once with ice-cold phosphate-buffered saline (PBS) (*see* **Note 7**).
3. Add 250 μL of cell lysis solution to each 10 cm plate, and scrape the cells with a cell scraper.
4. Transfer the solution to a 1.5 mL microcentrifuge (MCT) tube and incubate on ice for 10 min.
5. Spin the solution at 18,000 × *g* in a + 4 °C refrigerated centrifuge for 30 min.
6. Transfer the supernatants to a fresh 1.5 mL MCT tube and place on ice. If the lysate is not going to be used immediately, store it at −80 °C.
7. For protein estimation, add 10 μL of the cell lysate in a 96-well clear plate. Add 10 μL of each BSA standards to the same plate.

8. Add 150 μL of the protein assay reagent to all the wells, and incubate the plate for 5 min at room temperature.
9. Measure the optical density at 660 nm using a spectrophotometer. The unknown concentration of the sample can be deduced from the generated standard curve. Samples and standards should be tested in duplicate.

3.4 Western Blotting

1. Bring all the solutions needed to prepare the SDS gel to room temperature. The procedure mentioned below is for a 10% SDS gel that is suitable to detect cathepsin B.
2. Resolving gel: Mix 1.9 mL of water; 2.5 mL of acrylamide/bis-acrylamide solution; 3.0 mL of 1 M Tris–HCl, pH 6.8; 38 μL of SDS; 36 μL of APS; and 5 μL of TEMED in a 15 mL conical tube. Mix well and add the mixture into 1.5 mm gel cassettes allowing space for stacking gel. Overlay the gel with water to prevent bubble formation, and let the gel set for 30 min to 1 h. After the gel has set, remove the water layer before preparing the stacking gel.
3. Stacking gel: Mix 1.8 mL water; 330 μL of acrylamide/bis-acrylamide solution; 315 μL of 1 M Tris–HCl, pH 8.8; 12.5 μL of SDS; 12.5 μL of APS; and 2.5 μL of TEMED in a 15 mL conical tube. Mix well and pour on top of the resolving gel. Place the gel comb and let it set for around 30 min. Place the cassette in the electrophoresis apparatus filled with 1× running buffer.
4. Protein sample preparation: Mix 30 μg of protein extract with 6 μL of sample loading dye, and make up the volume to 24 μL with water. Denature the protein at 95 °C for 5 min followed by cooling on ice for 2 min. Spin down the samples briefly and load them in SDS-PAGE gel. Load 3 μL of the pre-stained protein ladder in one of the lanes. Run the gel at 100 V until the bands in the ladder separate completely.
5. Protein transfer: Carefully place the gel onto the PVDF membrane in the gel transfer pack. Close the lid and run for 7 min (*see* **Note 8**).
6. Incubate the membrane with the blocking buffer at room temperature for 1 h in a vertical shaker.
7. Remove blocking buffer and add appropriate primary antibody diluted in blocking buffer. Incubate at room temperature for 4 h or at +4 °C overnight in a shaker (*see* **Note 9**).
8. Wash the membrane five times with wash buffer, 5 min each time.
9. Add appropriate secondary antibody diluted in blocking buffer, and incubate at room temperature for 1 h in a shaker (*see* **Note 9**).
10. Wash membrane five times with wash buffer, 5 min each time.

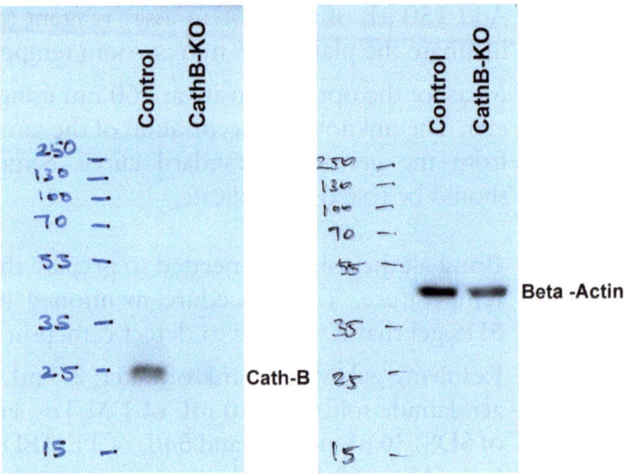

Fig. 1 Cathepsin B and β-actin protein expression is shown using western blotting. Immunoblot shows downregulation of cathepsin B protein expression in MIA PaCa-2 cells with stable expression of cathepsin B CRISPR-Cas9 plasmid compared to cells expressing scrambled sequence

11. Prepare ECL substrate solution by mixing equal volumes of solution A and solution B from the ECL substrate detection kit. Add the substrate solution to the membrane, and incubate at room temperature for 5 min.
12. Blot dry the membrane and place in cassette. In a dark room, expose the membrane to an autoradiography film, and develop the film in an autoradiography equipment (Fig. 1).

3.5 Total RNA Isolation

1. Remove cell culture plate from CO_2 incubator and place on ice. Remove media and wash once with ice-cold 1× PBS. Add 1 mL of TRIzol and gently dislodge the cells by pipetting. Transfer the cells to a 1.5 mL MCT tube.
2. Add 0.2 mL of chloroform, mix well, and incubate at room temperature for 2–3 min. Centrifuge the tube at 18,000 × *g* in a +4 °C refrigerated centrifuge for 15 min.
3. Carefully transfer the top layer containing RNA into a new tube without touching the interphase or the bottom layer. Add 0.5 mL of isopropanol, mix well, and incubate at room temperature for 10 min. Spin the tube at 18,000 × *g* in a + 4 °C refrigerated centrifuge for 10 min. Discard the supernatant, being careful not to disturb the pellet.
4. Wash the pellet with 0.75 mL 75% ethanol. Remove all the residual ethanol by drying the tube at room temperature.
5. Reconstitute the pellet in RNase-free water. Measure concentration and purity of the extracted RNA in a NanoDrop 1000 spectrophotometer. Total RNA can be used immediately or stored at −80 °C until further analysis (*see* **Note 10**).

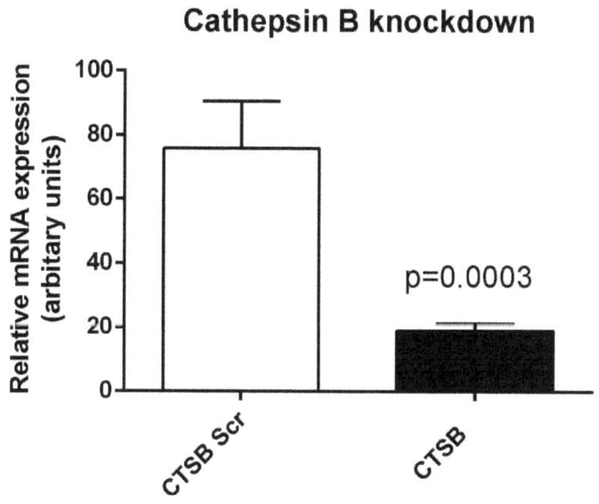

Fig. 2 Real-time PCR results showing significant reduction in cathepsin B mRNA levels in MIA PaCa-2 cells with cathepsin B CRISPR-Cas9 plasmid when compared with cells expressing scrambled sequence

3.6 cDNA Synthesis and RT-PCR

1. Prepare a mix containing 1 μg of RNA, 1× iScript reaction mix, and 1 μL reverse transcriptase enzyme from the iScript cDNA Synthesis Kit, and make up the total volume of 20 μL using RNase-free water.
2. Incubate the mix for 5 min at +25 °C, 30 min at +42 °C, and 5 min at +85 °C in a thermal cycler.
3. The resulting cDNA can be used immediately or stored at −20 °C until further analysis.
4. Prepare PCR mix containing 1× iQ SYBR Green Master Mix, 300 nM forward and reverse primers, and 2 μL cDNA in a total volume of 10 μL.
5. Perform PCR amplification under the following conditions in a real-time PCR: 95 °C for 3 min, 40 cycles of +95 °C for 15 s, and +60 °C for 60 seconds. Melt curve analysis can also be performed at +55 to +95 °C with 0.5 °C increment to validate the primers.
6. All samples have to be tested with cathepsin B using HPRT for normalization. The Ct value is then exported to Excel, and the difference in expression is calculated using the delta delta ct method described by Livak [11] (Fig. 2).

4 Notes

1. Scrambled sequence was generated using the online tool at GenScript (http://www.genscript.com/tools/create-scrambled-sequence). Plasmids were obtained as bacterial stab cultures. We find it more convenient than ordering pure plasmids.

2. From our experience, any liposome-based transfection reagent should work well as long as the manufacturer's instructions are followed.
3. Mix Tris–HCl, SDS, and glycerol in water, and warm it at +37 °C to completely dissolve it. Adding bromophenol blue powder directly will make it difficult to verify if SDS has dissolved. We find it easy to prepare a 1% stock solution of bromophenol blue and adding it after SDS and glycerol have mixed well. Store the buffer without β-mercaptoethanol in aliquots at −20 °C. Add fresh β-mercaptoethanol in a fume hood to one of the aliquots and use it for Western blotting. SDS tends to precipitate at −20 °C, so warm it well at room temperature before using.
4. These are disposable PVDF membrane sets that are compatible with the iBlot transfer apparatus. Using this setup, protein transfer can be accomplished in 7 min. Alternatively, wet transfer can also be done. Nitrocellulose membrane can also be used instead of PVDF membrane.
5. The time it takes for resistant colonies to form can vary for different cell lines. We usually start seeing individual colonies from 3 weeks after selection.
6. Harvest cells for protein and RNA extraction when the cells reach 60–70% growth. Confluent plates give inconsistent results.
7. Sonication can be used to maximize cell lysis, but is not compulsory when used with this lysis solution.
8. Alternatively, wet transfer can also be performed for 1 h at room temperature using appropriate transfer equipment and reagents.
9. A 1/1000 dilution works best for us for most primary antibodies and 1/5000 dilution works well for secondary antibodies. Increase or decrease antibody dilution based on your needs.
10. A 260/280 value close to 2.0 represents pure RNA.

References

1. Greembaum LM, Fruton JS (1957) Purification and properties of beef spleen cathepsin B. J Biol Chem 226(173):173–180
2. Gondi CS, Rao JS (2013) Cathepsin B as a cancer target. Expert Opin Ther Targets 17(3): 281–291
3. Rempel SA, Rosenblum ML, Mikkelsen T et al (1994) Cathepsin B expression and localization in glioma progression and invasion. Cancer Res 54(23):6027–6031
4. Bian B, Mongrain S, Cagnol S et al (2016) Cathepsin B promotes colorectal tumorigenesis, cell invasion, and metastasis. Mol Carcinog 55(5):671–687
5. Ruan J, Zheng H, Rong X et al (2016) Overexpression of cathepsin B in hepatocellular carcinomas predicts poor prognosis of HCC patients. Mol Cancer 15:17
6. Gong F, Peng X, Luo C et al (2013) Cathepsin B as a potential prognostic and therapeutic marker for human lung squamous cell carcinoma. Mol Cancer 12:125
7. Towatari T, Nikawa T, Murata M et al (1991) Novel epoxysuccinyl peptides. A selective

inhibitor of cathepsin B, in vivo. FEBS Lett 280(23):311–315

8. Stern I, Schaschke N, Moroder L et al (2004) Crystal structure of NS-134 in complex with bovine cathepsin B: a two-headed epoxysuccinyl inhibitor extends along the entire active-site cleft. Biochem J 381(Pt 2):511–517
9. Mikhaylov G, Klimpel D, Schaschke N et al (2014) Selective targeting of tumor and stromal cells by a nanocarrier system displaying lipidated cathepsin B inhibitor. Angew Chem Int Ed Engl 53(38):10077–10081
10. Yunis AA, Arimura GK, Russin DJ (1977) Human pancreatic carcinoma (MIA PaCa-2) in continuous culture: sensitivity to asparaginase. Int J Cancer 19(1):128–135
11. Livak KJ, Schmittgen TD (2001) Analysis of relative gene expression data using real-time quantitative PCR and the 2(−Delta Delta C(T)). Methods 25(4):402–408

Chapter 13

Assessing the Influence of a Protease in Cell Migration Using the Barrier-Migration Assay

Tania Fontanil, Yamina Mohamedi, Santiago Cal, and Álvaro J. Obaya

Abstract

Proteases play crucial roles in all steps of tumor progression including cancer cell migration. In fact, uncontrolled proteolytic activity could lead to the degradation of different components of the extracellular matrix which facilitates dissemination of tumor cells. However, numerous studies have revealed that proteases may also exert tumor-protective actions which could impede progression of malignant cells. Consequently, it is crucial to distinguish those situations in which proteases promote tumor growth from those in which exhibit tumor-suppressive effects. In this regard, analysis of the influence of a particular protease on the capacity of a cell line to migrate can be employed as an approach to better understand its involvement in tumorigenesis. Different experimental designs have been developed to investigate cell migration. Herein, we describe a barrier assay to monitor cell migration, which overcomes some disadvantages of traditional methods such as the Boyden chamber or the wound healing assays. The version of the barrier assay explained in this chapter allows to examine cell migration through the analysis of the closure of a premade 500 μm wound. This method also facilitates comparison between two different situations in a given cell line (i.e., gene up- or downregulation) in the same assay and under the same conditions. Additionally, migration can be monitored and measured using a time lapse microscope which facilitates further analysis through different softwares.

Key words Cell migration, Barrier assay, Time lapse, Extracellular matrix

1 Introduction

Motility is an intrinsic property of living cells related to fundamental processes necessary for life including the creation of tissues during embryogenesis, immune surveillance, wound repair, or inflammation [1, 2]. However, this property is very often altered in different pathologies such as cancer. In fact, an increased cell motility is associated with a higher invasion and dissemination of tumor cells thereby facilitating metastasis and confinement of malignant cells in distant tissues. These effects ultimately would contribute to potentiate the lethality of the tumor [1, 3].

Different mechanisms are involved in cell migration. To effectively migrate, one single cell needs to rearrange the cytoskeleton

Santiago Cal and Alvaro J. Obaya (eds.), *Proteases and Cancer: Methods and Protocols*, Methods in Molecular Biology, vol. 1731, https://doi.org/10.1007/978-1-4939-7595-2_13, © Springer Science+Business Media, LLC 2018

in response to external stimuli [4], but ECM surrounding the migratory cell must also be modified to facilitate cell movement and attachment [5]. In this regard, proteolytic enzymes have been largely associated to the remodeling of the ECM components, and their participation in the different stages of tumor progression is broadly documented [6]. First association between proteolytic enzymes and migration of cancer cells was established by Albert Fischer in 1946 [7]. Thus, during the development of the tumor, a proteolytic activity is responsible for the degradation of the cell matrix, which facilitates metastatic process by removing physical barriers and promoting migration and invasion [7, 8]. Since then, a broad number of studies have confirmed the involvement of proteases in tumor development facilitating crucial processes, including cell migration. In this regard, matrix metalloproteinases or MMPs display essential roles in regulating the migratory activity of malignant cells. Thus, pericellular proteolysis mediated by MMP2 [9] increases the migratory capacity of tumor cells, or the increased expression of MMP19 in melanoma potentiates cell dissemination through the cleavage of type IV collagen to generate two main high molecular mass fragments [10]. These and other examples [11] illustrate the influence of MMPs in the migratory capacity of tumor cells.

The ADAMTS (A Disintegrin And Metalloproteinase with ThromboSpondin motifs) family consists of 19 secreted metalloproteases also involved in tumor-related functions including migration process. For instance, ADAMTS-1, the best characterized member of the family, is overexpressed in pancreatic cancer, and it has been proposed to participate in tumor progression by facilitating local invasion and lymph node metastasis [12, 13]. A possible mechanism by which ADAMTS-1 potentiates metastasis is the promotion of cell migration by the cleavage of syndecan 4 and semaphorin 3C [14–16]. Another example of the same family is ADAMTS-12. Exogenous expression of this metalloprotease correlates with an increased migratory capacity of the breast cancer cell line MCF-7 on type IV collagen [17]. However, a growing number of studies highlight the tumor-suppressing effects mediated by ADAMTSs, which are mainly due to the thrombospondin domains identified within their molecular architecture. In conclusion, both MMPs [8] and ADAMTSs [13] show tumor-promoting or tumor-suppressor properties depending on multiple factors which are not fully understood.

To examine the effects that a protease may cause on cell motility, classical cell migration assays, as the Boyden chambers or the wound healing assays, have been successfully employed. Technically, these assays are highly reproducible and easy to handle and analyze. Moreover, these assays have a lower economic cost than those performed in vivo [18]. However, these techniques also show some disadvantages. Boyden chambers consist of a transwell system with a rigid and porous membrane between two cell culture chambers [3]. Cells move from one chamber to another in response to a chemotactic agent. Nonetheless, Boyden chambers are endpoint assays, and it is difficult to examine the movement of the cells during migration. Moreover, this type of assay provides a too simplistic vision of the migration as it analyzes the ability of single cells to directionally respond to the chemotactic agent. However, tumor cells could also be able to move collectively, generate sprouts or branches, or to maintain cell-cell contacts. These and other important morphological properties cannot be properly examined using Boyden chambers [19].

Collective cell migration has been traditionally examined by the wound healing assay, also known as scratch assay [20]. This technique consists of the creation of a scratch in a cell monolayer using a tip or scraper. Then, cells at the leading edges of the scratch will eventually close the gap depending on their migration capacity and proliferation rates [3, 21]. This assay allows to capture images at different times or to record the migration of the cells which, in turn, can permit to calculate migration rates. However, scratches made in this way are very variable in width and can damage not only the cells at the edges but also the extracellular matrix components where cells are attached.

To overcome the drawbacks of the handmade scratches, this technique can be improved by the use of silicone barriers or "inserts," and different versions of this method are currently available. Herein, we describe a version in which the cells are seeded in two compartments separated by a silicone barrier within a culture dish. When cells are attached, this support or insert is removed, and two different cell monolayers separated by a 500 μm wound are created. Moreover, cells cultured in each particular compartment may represent two different situations or conditions [18, 22–24]. For instance, a tumor cell line that overexpresses a particular protease can be grown in one compartment and the same cell line transfected with an empty vector in the other one. Consequently, this technique allows to confront these two different situations within the same assay. In addition, cells can be recorded using a time-lapse microscopy to further compare their ability to migrate on different substrates using diverse softwares [20, 24, 25]. In this chapter, we include some images generated to investigate how the exogenous expression of the ADAMTS-12 metalloprotease affects the migration of the murine melanoma tumor cell line B16F10 when compared with control cells. However, this technique can be easily adapted to other assays in which the researcher needs to evaluate cell migration between two different situations.

2 Materials

Prepare all solutions using analytical grade reagents and ultrapure water deionized (sensitivity of 18.2 MΩ-cm at 25 °C) in sterile conditions and at room temperature (unless otherwise noted).

2.1 Reagent and Chemicals

1. Dish types:

   Coated dish: culture insert (μ-Dish 35 mm, Ibidi).

   Uncoated dish: culture insert (μ-Dish 35 mm, Ibidi).

   Culture inserts for self-insertion (Ibidi).
2. Cell line: B16F10 (ATCC® CRL-6475™).
3. Medium DMEM, supplemented with 10% FBS, 1% penicillin-streptomycin-glutamine (solution contains 10,000 units of penicillin, 10,000 μg of streptomycin, and 29.2 mg/mL of L-glutamine in a 10 mM citrate buffer), and 1% antibiotic-antimycotic (with 10,000 units penicillin, 10 mg streptomycin, and 25 μg amphotericin B per mL, sterile-filtered).
4. Trypan blue.
5. Phosphate-buffered saline (PBS): phosphate-buffered saline 10× (1.36 M NaCl, 26.8 mM KCl, 101.4 mM Na_2HPO_4, 17.6 mM KH_2PO_4, pH 7.4) is diluted in Milli-Q water ten times to obtain a 1× solution.
6. Hank's balanced salt solution (HBSS) 1×: 138 mM NaCl, 5 mM KCl, 0.45 mM KH_2PO_4, 5.6 mM glucose, 0.35 mM Na_2HPO_4 anhyd., 0.8 mM $MgSO_4$, 1.25 mM $CaCl_2$, 4 mM $NaHCO_3$.
7. Trypsin.

2.2 Equipment

1. Laboratory microcentrifuge.
2. Neubauer chamber.
3. Forceps.
4. Zeiss Axiovert 200 M inverted microscope (*see* **Note 1**).
5. Zeiss Incubator XL S1 provides controlled stage and ambient temperature conditions, as well as humidified CO_2 supply.
6. ImageJ-Fiji software [26].

2.3 Dish Coating Procedure

2.3.1 Substrate Preparation

(a) Laminin: commercial solution is gently thawed and diluted in HBSS to a working concentration of 15 μg/mL. For 5 μ-Dish 35 mm Ibidi plates, prepare 2 mL.

(b) Fibronectin: dissolve 1 mg in 1 mL of water for at least 30 min at 37 °C. Once dissolved, dilute this stock in HBSS to a working concentration of 15 μg/mL. For 5 μ-Dish 35 mm Ibidi plates, prepare 2 mL.

(c) Type IV collagen: commercial solution is gently thawed and diluted in HBSS to a working concentration of 15 μg/mL. For 5 μ-Dish 35 mm Ibidi plates, prepare 2 mL.

(d) Vitronectin: prepare a stock solution of 50 μg/mL in sterile water and pass it through a 0.2 μm filter. Dilute to a working concentration of 5 μg/mL in HBSS. For 5 μ-Dish 35 mm Ibidi plates, prepare 2 mL.

2.3.2 Coating Process

1. Add 400 μL of each working solution to each plate. Then:
   (a) For laminin, type IV collagen, and vitronectin, incubate the plates at 37 °C for 2 h.
   (b) For fibronectin, allow the plates to air dry for at least 1 h at room temperature.

2.3.3 Washing

(a) For laminin, type IV collagen, and vitronectin, wash three times each plate with PBS.

(b) For fibronectin remove remaining drops by aspiration.

2.3.4 Storing

Coated plates can be individually stored for approximately 1 month wrapped in sterile conditions at 4 °C.

3 Methods

All procedures should be carried out at room temperature and in sterile conditions unless otherwise specified.

3.1 Cell Seeding

Two methods can be used depending on whether we use plates with the insert already in its position or we use our previously coated dishes in which we put the insert by our own. The first one is very useful if you want to test standard or initial conditions, and the other option is used when you want to check for cell behavior on different substrates (*see* Subheading 2.3 *and* **Note 2**). In any case, once we have the plate ready with the insert in its position, the procedure is as follows:

1. Wash the cells to be used with abundant PBS 1×, and then trypsinize the cells (add approximately 1 mL of trypsin per 100 mm diameter plate; *see* **Note 3**). Once the cells have been removed from the dish surface, neutralize them with complete medium (*see* **Note 4**), and centrifuge at 350 × *g* for 3 min.
2. Remove the supernatant with care in order not to damage the pelleted cells, and add 2 mL of complete medium (volume will depend on the volume of the pellet; *see* **Note 5**).

3. Use a Neubauer camera to count viable cells using trypan blue (in a 1:1 dilution; *see* **Note 6**) according to Strober [27].
4. Once the cells are counted, suspensions of 3–7 × 10^5 cells/mL for each condition to be studied are prepared in complete medium (*see* **Notes** 7 and **8**).
5. To compare two different cellular conditions, 70 μL of each cell suspension is added to each of the compartments of the insert. Leave the dish in the incubator at 37 °C and 5% CO_2 during the required time to allow complete cell adhesion (*see* **Note 9**).
6. Carefully remove the insert with sterile forceps, leaving both cell lines separated by the 500 μm gap (Fig. 1).
7. Wash the dish twice with PBS in order to remove dead cells and cellular debris, and add fresh complete medium (about 2 mL). At this point, the cells and the setup are ready for starting the acquisition of images.

3.2 Time Lapse

1. It is recommended to prepare the microscope (in our example Zeiss Axiovert 200 M type) in the appropriate conditions at least 1 h before performing the assay so that when the cells are inserted in the incubator camera, the acquisition can be started immediately (*see* **Note 10**). For that reason, the first thing to do is to initialize and set up the CO_2 and the temperature control modules.
2. Once the microscope is turned on and ready to be used, load the corresponding software that must be employed to capture images. In our case, we use AxioVision Release 4.7.2 software. With this software we also control the parameters of the culture chamber attached to the microscope (thus, we already checked them to 5% CO_2 and 37 °C).
3. When the CO_2 and 37 °C levels have been reached and the conditions are optimal, place the dish on the appropriate support (there are different dish supports depending on the microscope), and adjust the focus in brightfield so that the two fronts are seen at the same distance from the central point of the image (Figs. 1 and 2 *see* **Note 11**).
4. Use the appropriate software (AxioVision in our case) to fix the conditions of your experiment. Conditions for image acquisition (i.e., exposition time, light intensity), time intervals between each image, and the total duration of the experiment should be fixed at this time (*see* **Note 12**). We routinely take images each 10 min for a period of 24 h.
5. Once the experiment has finished, it will be saved as various formats for posterior analysis (.avi, .zvi, .jpg, depending on the employed software). In the case of the AxioVision software, it

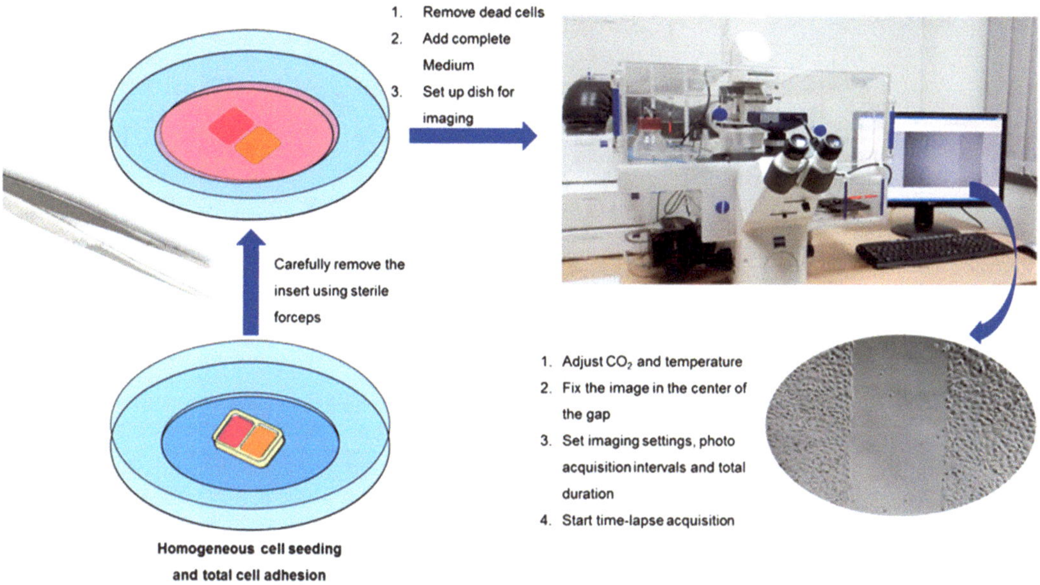

Fig. 1 Workflow of the process. Different steps to monitor cell migration using the barrier-migration assay are indicated

allows you to save each time point photo independently (jpg) as well as to save the whole experiment as a time-lapse movie (zvi).

6. For further analysis we normally use ImageJ software although any other similar program can be used (Fig. 2). We routinely analyzed the area covered by each cell condition at different time points. Advanced distance from the starting edges can also be used taking three or four discretional points.

4 Notes

1. The inverted design has ample room for the samples and their manipulation, facilitating the development of different techniques. It also allows easy fixing of cameras, lasers, specific stages, etc. The whole set allows the realization of experiments that would not be possible with vertical microscopes.
2. Sometimes, differences between various cell conditions are not appreciated on a standard culture dish. However, depending on the cell line and by using different substrates, this difference in cell migration, or cell morphology, can be observed. One important thing to keep in mind is to place and remove carefully the insert so as not to remove the substrate layer from the area of study.
3. Trypsin is usually used to remove adherent cells from a culture surface, especially those cells which are tightly attached. Some

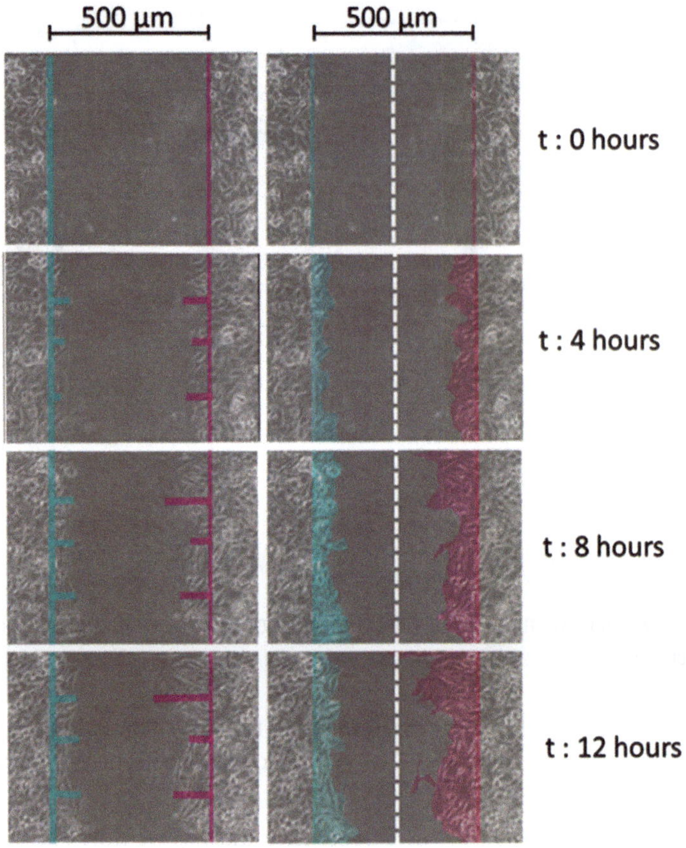

Fig. 2 Cell migratory properties examined at the indicated times. As an illustrative example, migratory capacity of B16F10 mouse melanoma cells overexpressing the ADAMTS-12 metalloprotease (blue) or control cells, transfected with an empty vector (purple). Left, advanced distance from the starting edges is measured using discretionary points; right, covered area by each cell condition at different time points is indicated

cell lines do not require the use of trypsin because they are softly attached and can be easily removed by pipetting PBS.

4. Longtime exposure to trypsin might cause cell damage, so it is important to inhibit trypsin action by adding complete culture medium (trypsin is inhibited by the presence of inhibitors in fetal bovine serum). It is advisable to use twice the volume of trypsin previously used.
5. The volume to resuspend the cells will depend on the size of the pellet, that is to say, the more concentrated cells the harder it will be to count them, so it is advisable to make subsequent dilutions until you have a concentration which you are comfortable with to facilitate cell counting in the Neubauer camera.

6. Trypan blue is a compound that colors blue viable cells and thus prevents the dead cells to be counted as alive. In the calculation, it is important to take into account the dilution made by adding this colorant (1:1) which dilutes the initial number of cells in half.
7. In this type of tests, medium will not interfere with image capture, so it should be the optimal for cell growth in order to avoid any cellular stress.
8. Once the cell suspensions are prepared, it should be noted that the aim is to seed cells so that they occupy the entire surface of the insert compartment. In this setting, when the insert is removed, we will have two different cellular conditions to be compared separated by a strip of about 500 μm with two straight fronts. To be successful, it is necessary to test for each cell line the number of cells to be seeded in order to get the same cell confluency and, thus, straight fronts. This will allow us to observed cellular movement due to the cell migration capacity and not to the number of starting cells.
9. Due to the symmetry of the dish and the absence of any mark for guidance, it is very important to label on which side you are seeding each cellular condition. Furthermore, in order to facilitate the homogenous distribution of the cells, it is very important to be extremely careful pipetting the cell suspension into the compartment to avoid bubble formation or any other disturbance. If the cells are not well distributed, there could be fronts with different migrations under the same conditions.
10. Culture cells require optimum CO_2 level and temperature, which are generally 5% CO_2 and 37 °C (these parameters may vary with cell type or, e.g., under hypoxic conditions). These are the general conditions used in cell culture incubators, so they should be the conditions during the experiment. The microscopes used to perform these assays have a coupled incubation chamber needed for the survival of cells while monitoring their migration. Therefore, it is advisable to adjust the parameters half an hour before starting the experiment so that optimal conditions will be fixed at zero time of the experiment and the cells do not suffer any lack.
11. The Zeiss Axiovert 200 M-type microscope is an inverted microscope, so the image observed on the computer screen is the inverse of the one that is placed in the support. At the time of analyzing your results, make sure you know which condition corresponds to each side of the image.
12. Before setting the final parameters, we recommend to do a first test during a few minutes to check the equipment works correctly and there are no problems when the images are acquired (out of focus, high exposure, etc.).

References

1. Keely P, Nain A (2015) Capturing relevant extracellular matrices for investigating cell migration. F1000Res 4:pii: F1000 Faculty Rev-1408. 10.12688/f1000research.6623.1
2. Durbec P, Franceschini I, Lazarini F et al (2008) In vitro migration assays of neural stem cells. Methods Mol Biol 438:213–225. https://doi.org/10.1007/978-1-59745-133-8_18
3. Polacheck WJ, Zervantonakis IK, Kamm RD (2013) Tumor cell migration in complex microenvironments. Cell Mol Life Sci 70(8):1335–1356. https://doi.org/10.1007/s00018-012-1115-1
4. Yamaguchi H, Condeelis J (2007) Regulation of the actin cytoskeleton in cancer cell migration and invasion. Biochim Biophys Acta 1773(5):642–652. https://doi.org/10.1016/j.bbamcr.2006.07.001
5. Bonnans C, Chou J, Werb Z (2014) Remodelling the extracellular matrix in development and disease. Nat Rev Mol Cell Biol 15(12):786–801. https://doi.org/10.1038/nrm3904
6. Mason SD, Joyce JA (2011) Proteolytic networks in cancer. Trends Cell Biol 21(4):228–237. https://doi.org/10.1016/j.tcb.2010.12.002
7. Fischer A (1946) Mechanism of the proteolytic activity of malignant tissue cells. Nature 157:442
8. Lopez-Otin C, Matrisian LM (2007) Emerging roles of proteases in tumour suppression. Nat Rev Cancer 7(10):800–808. https://doi.org/10.1038/nrc2228
9. Sato H, Takino T (2010) Coordinate action of membrane-type matrix metalloproteinase-1 (MT1-MMP) and MMP-2 enhances pericellular proteolysis and invasion. Cancer Sci 101(4):843–847. https://doi.org/10.1111/j.1349-7006.2010.01498.x
10. Stracke JO, Hutton M, Stewart M et al (2000) Biochemical characterization of the catalytic domain of human matrix metalloproteinase 19. Evidence for a role as a potent basement membrane degrading enzyme. J Biol Chem 275(20):14809–14816
11. Kessenbrock K, Plaks V, Werb Z (2010) Matrix metalloproteinases: regulators of the tumor microenvironment. Cell 141(1):52–67. https://doi.org/10.1016/j.cell.2010.03.015
12. Masui T, Hosotani R, Tsuji S et al (2001) Expression of METH-1 and METH-2 in pancreatic cancer. Clin Cancer Res 7(11): 3437–3443
13. Cal S, Lopez-Otin C (2015) ADAMTS proteases and cancer. Matrix Biol 44-46:77–85. https://doi.org/10.1016/j.matbio.2015.01.013
14. Kelwick R, Desanlis I, Wheeler GN et al (2015) The ADAMTS (A Disintegrin and Metalloproteinase with Thrombospondin motifs) family. Genome Biol 16:113. https://doi.org/10.1186/s13059-015-0676-3
15. Esselens C, Malapeira J, Colome N et al (2010) The cleavage of semaphorin 3C induced by ADAMTS1 promotes cell migration. J Biol Chem 285(4):2463–2473. https://doi.org/10.1074/jbc.M109.055129
16. Rodriguez-Manzaneque JC, Carpizo D, Plaza-Calonge Mdel C et al (2009) Cleavage of syndecan-4 by ADAMTS1 provokes defects in adhesion. Int J Biochem Cell Biol 41(4):800–810. https://doi.org/10.1016/j.biocel.2008.08.014
17. Fontanil T, Rua S, Llamazares M et al (2014) Interaction between the ADAMTS-12 metalloprotease and fibulin-2 induces tumor-suppressive effects in breast cancer cells. Oncotarget 5(5):1253–1264. 10.18632/oncotarget.1690
18. Kramer N, Walzl A, Unger C et al (2013) In vitro cell migration and invasion assays. Mutat Res 752(1):10–24. https://doi.org/10.1016/j.mrrev.2012.08.001
19. Sun M, Zaman MH (2017) Modeling, signaling and cytoskeleton dynamics: integrated modeling-experimental frameworks in cell migration. Wiley Interdiscip Rev Syst Biol Med 9(1). https://doi.org/10.1002/wsbm.1365
20. Yarrow JC, Perlman ZE, Westwood NJ et al (2004) A high-throughput cell migration assay using scratch wound healing, a comparison of image-based readout methods. BMC Biotechnol 4:21. https://doi.org/10.1186/1472-6750-4-21
21. Zorn ML, Marel AK, Segerer FJ et al (2015) Phenomenological approaches to collective behavior in epithelial cell migration. Biochim Biophys Acta 1853(11 Pt B):3143–3152. https://doi.org/10.1016/j.bbamcr.2015.05.021
22. Van Horssen R, ten Hagen TL (2011) Crossing barriers: the new dimension of 2D cell migration assays. J Cell Physiol 226(1):288–290. https://doi.org/10.1002/jcp.22330

23. Kroening S, Goppelt-Struebe M (2010) Analysis of matrix-dependent cell migration with a barrier migration assay. Sci Signal 3(126):pl1. https://doi.org/10.1126/scisignal.3126pl1
24. Ashby WJ, Zijlstra A (2012) Established and novel methods of interrogating two-dimensional cell migration. Integr Biol (Camb) 4(11):1338–1350. https://doi.org/10.1039/c2ib20154b
25. Lobastova L, Kraus D, Glassmann A et al (2017) Collective cell migration of thyroid carcinoma cells: a beneficial ability to override unfavourable substrates. Cell Oncol (Dordr) 40(1):63–76. https://doi.org/10.1007/s13402-016-0305-5
26. Schindelin J, Arganda-Carreras I, Frise E et al (2012) Fiji: an open-source platform for biological-image analysis. Nat Methods 9(7):676–682. https://doi.org/10.1038/nmeth.2019
27. Strober W (2015) Trypan blue exclusion test of cell viability. Curr Protoc Immunol 111:A3.B.1–A3.B.3. https://doi.org/10.1002/0471142735.ima03bs111

Chapter 14

Analysis of Invasive Activity of CAF Spheroids into Three Dimensional (3D) Collagen Matrices

María Ángeles Villaronga, Saúl Álvarez Teijeiro, Francisco Hermida-Prado, Marta Garzón-Arango, Victoria Sanz-Moreno, and Juana María García-Pedrero

Abstract

Tumor growth and progression is the result of a complex process controlled not only by malignant cancer cells but also by the surrounding tumor microenvironment (TME). Cancer associated fibroblasts (CAFs), the most abundant cellular component of TME, play an active role in tumor invasion and metastasis by promoting cancer cell invasion through cell-cell interactions and secretion of pro-invasive factors such as extracellular matrix (ECM)-degrading proteases. Due to their tumor-promoting activities, there is an emerging interest in investigating CAFs biology and its potential as drug targets for cancer therapies. Here we describe an easy and highly reproducible quantitative method to analyze CAF invasive activity by forming multicellular spheroids embedded into a three-dimensional (3D) matrix that mimics in vivo ECM. Subsequently, invasion is monitored over time using a time-lapse microscope. We also provide an automated image analysis system that enables the rapid quantification of the spheroid area increase (invasive area) over time. The use of a 96-well plate format with one CAF spheroid *per* well and the automated analysis provides a method suitable for drug screening test, such as protease inhibitors.

Key words Cancer associated fibroblasts, Spheroids, Invasive activity, Extracellular matrix, Collagen, Proteases

1 Introduction

Emerging evidences indicate that tumors are highly complex heterogeneous structures in which growth is supported not only by the cancer cells themselves but also the surrounding microenvironment. Hence, cancer must be considered and consequently studied as a systemic disease. Therefore, an in-depth understanding of the tumor progression involves knowledge of the role of both tumor cells and infiltrating stroma. The tumor stroma is constructed by

María Ángeles Villaronga and Saúl Álvarez Teijeiro contributed equally to this work.

Santiago Cal and Alvaro J. Obaya (eds.), *Proteases and Cancer: Methods and Protocols*, Methods in Molecular Biology, vol. 1731, https://doi.org/10.1007/978-1-4939-7595-2_14, © Springer Science+Business Media, LLC 2018

various types of mesenchymal cells together with the extracellular matrix (ECM), collectively constituting the so-called tumor microenvironment (TME) [1].

A predominant component of TME is the cancer associated fibroblast (CAF) subpopulation. Mounting evidence over the last years shows that CAFs actively contribute to activate pro-tumorigenic functions, such as tumor growth, invasion, and metastasis. In addition, high CAF density has been associated with poor prognosis in various cancer types. CAFs promote the invasion of carcinoma cells that retain epithelial features and have a limited ability to degrade the ECM, through cell-cell interactions and secretion of pro-invasive factors, such as proteases. It has been shown that CAFs generate tracks to guide cancer cell migration by the action of matrix metalloproteinases (MMPs) [2, 3]. CAFs are genetically stable and present a pathologically activated state, responsible for their pro-tumorigenic functions, clearly distinct to normal fibroblasts. Hence, there is an increasing interest in studying the pro-tumorigenic functions of CAFs, and to evaluate their potential application as therapeutic targets to fight cancer. Further characterization of the mutual cross talk between cancer cells and CAFs and the underlying tumor-promoting mechanisms may ultimately contribute to identify potential novel therapeutic targets [4].

The herein-described method is a variation of the so frequently used 3D tumor spheroid invasion assay [5–7], adapted for analysis of CAF invasive properties. CAF spheroids are formed by the hanging drop method (gravity drives cell aggregation at the bottom of the drop) [8] and subsequently embedded into a 3D matrix that closely mimics the in vivo ECM. There are various gels with different composition commercially available in liquid form, which are chemically or physically solidified to form 3D matrices [9]. Depending on the research question, for CAF invasion analysis, we can either use collagen I matrices that mimic the interstitial ECM or a basement membrane-like matrix (Matrigel) composed of collagen IV, laminin, nidogen/entactin, and heparan sulfate proteoglycan. Herein, we provide a detailed protocol for 3D CAF invasion assays into collagen matrices. After matrix polymerization, the embedded CAF spheroids are overlaid with medium with or without any drug of interest.

Invasion is monitored at intervals of 30 min for a period of 20 h by using a time-lapse system, and images were analyzed using the ImageJ software with an automated macro adapted from one previously created [10]. This is a simple and highly reproducible method to measure CAF invasive activity. The use of a 96-well plate format monitoring one spheroid *per* well, coupled with the automated analysis, allows rapid testing of a high number of conditions simultaneously, thus representing a suitable and applicable system for drug screening.

This technique can be applied to study the contribution of different proteases to CAF invasiveness by using specific systems of protease overexpression/knockdown or pharmacological inhibitors. It is important to take into consideration the ECM substrates for the protease targeted in order to select the most appropriate matrix for the 3D invasion assay. Several families of proteases contribute to ECM degradation by direct cleavage of ECM proteins or indirectly activating other proteases that also lead to growth factor activation as well as cytoskeletal regulation and modification of downstream signaling pathways [11]. It is well recognized that CAFs represent one of the main sources of MMPs, thereby expressing and secreting different types, which vary greatly depending on the tumor type and stage. Accordingly, this context-dependent function of MMPs must be thoroughly characterized. In addition, it has been shown that CAFs also express other proteases, such as some ADAMs (A Disintegrin And Metalloproteinase), ADAMTSs (A Disintegrin And Metalloproteinase with ThromboSpondin motifs), cathepsins, and the serine protease urokinase-type plasminogen activator (u-PA) [12]; however, their function has not yet been elucidated.

2 Materials

2.1 Tissue Culture

1. Cells: Primary cancer-associated fibroblasts (CAFs) were isolated and cultured from a head and neck squamous cell carcinoma (HNSCC) resected at the Hospital Universitario Central de Asturias (HUCA), and the human FaDu cell line (from a hypopharyngeal carcinoma) was purchased from the American Type Culture Collection (ATCC®-HTB-43).
2. Culture medium: Dulbecco's modified Eagle's medium (DMEM) high glucose supplemented with 10% fetal bovine serum (FBS), with 2 mM L-glutamine and with MEM nonessential amino acids. Store at 4 °C. Warm up in a water bath at 37 °C before use.
3. Dulbecco's phosphate-buffered saline (PBS) without calcium and without magnesium. Warm up in a water bath at 37 °C before use.
4. Trypsin-EDTA 10×. Store at 4 °C. Warm up in a water bath at 37 °C before use.
5. Production of HNSCC conditioned medium (CM): HNSCC-derived cell lines are grown in serum-free DMEM for 72 h. Next, CM is collected, filtered through a 0.45 μm to remove cellular debris, aliquoted, and frozen at −80 °C until use.
6. Conical centrifuge tubes (15 and 50 mL).

2.2 CAF Spheroid Formation

1. Methyl cellulose solution: Weight out 3 g of methyl cellulose low viscosity in a 500 mL glass bottle with a magnetic stirring bar inside, and autoclave with cap loose for 20 min. Add 125 mL of warm medium (DMEM) to the autoclaved methyl cellulose, and incubate 15 min at 60 °C (shake the bottle to destroy clumps). Stir on a magnetic stirrer for 20 min, then add 120 mL of DMEM, and keep on the magnetic stirrer ~ 4 h at room temperature. Keep the bottle overnight at 4 °C. Add 5 mL of penicillin/streptomycin (10,000 U/mL) and stir thoroughly. Aliquot the methyl cellulose solution to 50 mL conical centrifuge tubes, centrifuge 20 min at 4 °C and 3200 × *g*, and carry the supernatant into 50 mL conical centrifuge tubes.
2. CAF culture medium.
3. Sterile phosphate-buffered saline, PBS buffer.
4. Sterile 100 mm or 150 mm tissue culture dishes (size depends on the number of CAF spheroids needed).

2.3 3D CAF Spheroid Invasion Assay into a Collagen I Matrix

1. Type I bovine collagen solution, 3 mg/mL.
2. 10× MEM culture medium. Store at 4 °C.
3. 10× reconstitution buffer: For a 50 mL solution, add 14.7 mL of sodium bicarbonate 7.5%, 10.1 mL of 1 M Hepes, and 25.2 mL of sterile water. Filter the solution through a 0.22 μm vacuum filter. Store at 4 °C.
4. 1 M sodium hydroxide (NaOH): Dissolve 2 g of NaOH in 50 mL of sterile water, and filter the solution through a 0.22 μm vacuum filter. Store at 4 °C.

2.4 Image Acquisition and Analysis

1. Zeiss Cell Observer Live Imaging microscope (Zeiss, Thornwood, NY) coupled with a CO_2 and temperature maintenance system.
2. Image analysis software (ImageJ).

3 Methods

The protocol described below is for a 3D CAF spheroid invasion assay on a 96-well plate format with one spheroid *per* well. To exemplify an application of this method, Fig. 1 shows data from a representative experiment monitoring CAF spheroid invasion upon treatment with GM 6001, a potent broad-spectrum inhibitor of MMPs and some ADAMs. We observed that GM 6001 potently inhibited CAF invasion, thus indicating the involvement of some of the targeted proteases in CAF invasive activity.

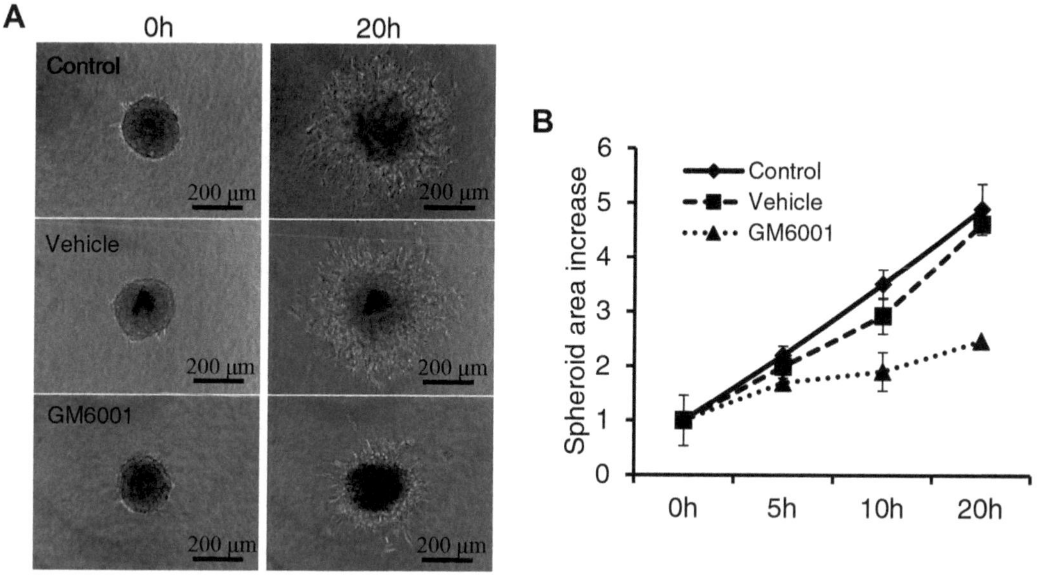

Fig. 1 Effect of the protease inhibitor GM6001 on CAF spheroid invasion into a 3D collagen I matrix. (**a**) Representative images of CAF spheroids treated for 20 h with FaDu-conditioned medium alone (control) or with vehicle (DMSO) or 10 μM GM6001. (**b**) Quantification of the spheroid area increase (invasive area) monitored at different time points. Data were normalized to the initial time point area ($t = 0$). The graph represents the mean ± SD of quadruplicates from each condition

3.1 CAF Spheroid Formation

CAFs are aggregated as spheroids after being cultured for 18 h in hanging drops of 25 μL of medium containing 20% of the methyl cellulose solution.

1. Trypsinize CAFs from a monolayer to a single cell suspension by adding trypsin EDTA-10× (0.5 mL for a 25 cm^2 or 1 mL for a 75 cm^2 flask). After incubation for 1 min at 37 °C, neutralize trypsin with culture medium, and centrifuge cell suspension at 244 × *g* for 5 min. Resuspend the pellet in culture medium and count cells.
2. Calculate the needed number of CAF spheroids to be assayed for invasion in the 96-well plate, considering at least four replicates *per* condition (*see* **Note 1**).
3. Calculate the volume of cell suspension required to form the total number of CAF spheroids needed, considering that each spheroid will be formed in a final volume of 25 μL (e.g., 1 mL for 40 spheroids). To facilitate manipulation, it is recommended to prepare a minimum volume of 500 μL (*see* **Note 2**).
4. Prepare a cell suspension of 80,000 cells/mL (considering 2000 cells/spheroid) in culture medium containing 20% of the methyl cellulose solution and 80% of culture medium. For 1 mL solution, transfer 80,000 cells into a 1.5 mL Eppendorf tube, add culture medium to 800 μL, and homogenize by soft

pipetting. Add 200 μL of methyl cellulose, and mix by inversion six to eight times (*see* **Notes 3** and **4**).

5. Pipette drops of 25 μL into the lid of the 100 mm tissue dish. Make sure that drops are placed sufficiently spaced to avoid fusion of spheroids. As estimation, it is possible to place at least 40 drops *per* dish. Fill the dish with 10 mL of sterile PBS and invert the lid very gently.
6. Place the plate in a humidified atmosphere at 37 °C and 5% CO_2 for 18 h (the cells in suspension will form hanging drops).

3.2 3D CAF Spheroid Invasion Assay into a Collagen I Matrix

The 96-well plate used for invasion assay must be first coated with a layer of collagen I gel (40 μL/well) and after polymerization for 1 h filled with another layer of collagen (70 μL/well). Then, one spheroid *per* well will be transferred on top, so that during the polymerization time of this second collagen layer, the spheroid will result completely embedded into the gel matrix. After solidification, each well will be filled with culture medium with or without any drug of interest to be tested. Here we describe the preparation protocol for bovine collagen matrix; however, it could be replaced with other matrices following appropriate gel polymerization protocol (*see* **Note 5**).

All the components for gel mix preparation must be kept on ice. The table below summarizes the list of reagents for 1 mL of 2.3 mg/mL collagen matrix, adapted from that described by VV. Artym et al. [13]. The total volume of gel needs to be scaled up according to the number of wells to be assayed. It is advisable to prepare an excess volume of 20% to account for pipetting difficulties/losses due to the high viscosity of collagen.

2.3 mg/mL collagen matrix	1 mL
Collagen (3.1 mg/mL stock)	750 μL
10× MEM	100 μL
Reconstitution buffer	150 μL
NaOH (1 M)	25 μL

1. Prechill all components for the gel mix preparation on ice.
2. Pipette the required amount of stock collagen, 10× MEM, reconstitution buffer, and NaOH, and mix slowly and gently by pipetting to homogenize and neutralize the collagen solution.
3. Incubate the neutralized collagen solution on ice for 3–5 min to allow the pH to equilibrate.
4. Centrifuge at 12,000 × *g* for 5 min at 4 °C to get rid of air bubbles.

5. Keep the tube with collagen solution on ice until use.
6. Gently dispense 40 μL of collagen solution into each well from the 96-well plate kept on ice.
7. Centrifuge the plate at 3000 × *g* for 30 s at 4 °C to ensure that the solution is uniformly distributed on the bottom of the well.
8. Incubate the plate at 37 °C and 5% CO_2 for 1 h.
9. After collagen polymerization, cool and keep the plate on ice.
10. Gently dispense 70 μL of collagen solution into each well and repeat **step** 7.
11. Transfer one CAF spheroid *per* well. Use a 2–20 μL micropipette setting the volume of liquid aspirated to 3 μL. Cut the tip to minimize disturbance of the spheroids, angle the tip toward the spheroid in each drop, and aspirate. Check that each spheroid is transferred and placed in the center of each well softly touching the collagen matrix with the tip and release the volume. Use a new tip when changing the cell type to avoid cross-contamination.
12. Using a microscope, check visually that all the wells contain one spheroid, as sometimes it could be kept in the tip or placed near the wall. Mark the empty wells, and repeat CAF spheroid transfer to them.
13. Use a sterile needle to remove the bubbles formed by spheroid transferring, if present.
14. Incubate the plate at 37 °C and 5% CO_2 to allow gel polymerization.
15. After 90 min, gently add 100 μL/well of HNSCC-CM alone or with any drug of interest, at 2× of the final concentration desired (*see* **Note 6**).
16. Fill with sterile PBS the empty wells to reduce evaporation.

3.3 Image Acquisition

1. Switch on the time-lapse microscopy and set the incubation parameters, 37 °C and 5% of CO_2. Allow to equilibrate for 1 h before placing the plate inside the stage incubation chamber (*see* **Note 7**).
2. Under acquisition tab, select phase-contrast channel with automatic exposure and time series of 30 min for 24 h.
3. Choose absolute fixed Z position as focus strategy.
4. By using the 10× objective, center and focus the spheroid in the field of view and set the position. This will keep all the fixed positions (coordinates *X*, *Y*, *Z*) during the whole acquisition.
5. After setting all the positions, click on "start scan."

3.4 Image Analysis

An ImageJ macro previously created [10] was adapted to be used with images acquired with the Zeiss Cell Observer Live Imaging microscope. This macro processes whole folders of images, records a file with spheroid measurements from each analyzed image (area, Ferret max, Ferret min, etc.), and draws a blue outline to delineate each spheroid area. First, the macro converts the images to black and white, by enhancing the contrast and then using the Otsu thresholding algorithm. Next, it proceeds to clean any artifacts from the image, fills gaps in the spheroid, removes debris, and determines the spheroid area.

The area increase (invasion) is calculated by dividing the area measured at each time point by the area measured at initial point. Results are represented as the mean area increase of four replicate spheroids plus the standard deviation.

4 Notes

1. For time-lapse image acquisition is recommended to use only the 60 central wells due to the high level of plate evaporation observed at the edge during long incubation times. Therefore, it is possible to test a maximum of 15 different conditions performed in quadruplicate.
2. Consider an excess volume of at least 25%, since sometimes when transferring the spheroids to the 96-well plate, they could be kept in the pipette or placed in the wall or well edge.
3. When assaying different subpopulations of fibroblasts (CAFs or normal fibroblasts) or cancer cells (with different size), spheroid concentration may need to be adjusted up or down in the range 20,000–120,000 cells/mL (500–3000 cells/spheroid) to ensure an adequate spheroid size. It should be visible to be transferred to the 96-well plate, although not too big to avoid that each spheroid exceeds the microscope field with 10× objective at the end point of the experiment.
4. If volumes higher than 1 mL of cell suspension are required, use a 2 mL Eppendorf tube or 15 mL conical centrifuge tube to ensure a good homogenization by inversion after methyl cellulose addition.
5. For preparing a basement membrane-like matrix, the growth factor-reduced Matrigel (BD Biosciences) may be used. Matrigel® is a viscous substance at 4 °C that solidifies at room temperature; hence, it must be always thawed and kept on ice and manipulated with prechilled tips. After thawing the 10 mL bottle, store in sterile 1 mL aliquots at −80 °C, and thaw the

amount required for an experiment to avoid repeating freeze-thaw cycles. Note the concentration of each particular batch in order to calculate volumes for preparing gels always at the same concentration and to get reproducible results. Gel neutralization is not necessary for basement membrane-like matrix solidification. Prechill the tubes and tips and dilute Matrigel in cold serum-free medium (DMEM) at a ratio 1:1. Afterward, proceed in the same way as described for a collagen matrix.

6. Conditioned media obtained from other cancer cell lines might be used. Thus, we have previously described the effect of CM from the human breast cancer cell line MCF-7 on the invasive activity of mammary fibroblasts [14].
7. If a time-lapse system is not available, take pictures of each spheroid both at the starting time point ($t = 0$) and at the end point of the invasion assay (e.g. 20 h), using a camera coupled to an inverted bright-field microscope (4–10× objective).

Acknowledgments

This study was supported by the Instituto de Salud Carlos III-FEDER (Funding Program from the European Union) (PI13/00259 and PI16/00280 to J.M.G.P. and CD13/00157 to M.A.V.), Consorcio CIBERONC (CB16/12/00390 to J.M.G.P.), and the Cancer Research UK (C.R.U.K.) (C33043/A12065 to V.S.M.).

References

1. Kalluri R (2016) The biology and function of fibroblasts in cancer. Nat Rev Cancer 16(9):582–598
2. Gaggioli C, Hooper S, Hidalgo-Carcedo C et al (2007) Fibroblast-led collective invasion of carcinoma cells with differing roles for RhoGTPases in leading and following cells. Nat Cell Biol 9(12):1392–1400
3. Labernadie A, Kato T, Brugués A et al (2017) A mechanically active heterotypic E-cadherin/N-cadherin adhesion enables fibroblasts to drive cancer cell invasion. Nat Cell Biol 19(3):224–237
4. Xing F, Saidou J, Watabe K (2011) Cancer associated fibroblasts in tumour microenvironment. Front Biosci 15:166–179
5. Vinci M, Box C, Eccles SA (2015) Three-dimensional (3D) tumour spheroid invasion assay. J Vis Exp 99:e52686
6. Vinci M, Gowan S, Boxall F et al (2012) Advances in establishment and analysis of three-dimensional tumour spheroid-based functional assays for target validation and drug evaluation. BMC Biol 10:29
7. Kramer N, Walzl A, Unger C et al (2013) In vitro cell migration and invasion assays. Mutat Res 752(1):10–24
8. Timmins NE, Nielsen LK (2007) Generation of multicellular tumour spheroid. Methods Mol Med 140:141–151
9. Katt ME, Placone AL, Wong AD et al (2016) *In Vitro* tumour models: advantages, disadvantages, variables, and selecting the right platform. Front Bioeng Biotechnol 4:12
10. Ivanov DP, Parker TL, Walker DA et al (2014) Multiplexing spheroid volume, Resazurin and acid phosphatase viability assays for high-throughput screening of tumour spher-

oids and stem cell neurospheres. PLoS One 9(8):e103817
11. Bonnans C, Chou J, Werb Z (2014) Remodelling the extracellular matrix in development and disease. Nat Rev Mol Cell Biol 15(12):786–801
12. Miles FL, Sikes RA (2014) Insidious changes in stromal matrix fuel cancer progression. Mol Cancer Res 12(3):297–312
13. Artym VV, Matsumoto K (2010) Imaging cells in three-dimensional collagen matrix. Curr Protoc Cell Biol Chapter 10:Unit 10.18.1–20
14. Fontanil T, Álvarez-Teijeiro S, Villaronga MA et al (2017) Cleavage of Fibulin-2 by the aggrecanases ADAMTS-4 and ADAMTS-5 contributes to the tumorigenic potential of breast cancer cells. Oncotarget 8(8):13716–13729

Chapter 15

Beyond the Proteolytic Activity: Examining the Functional Relevance of the Ancillary Domains Using Tri-Dimensional (3D) Spheroid Invasion Assay

Erico Tosoni Costa and Anamaria Aranha Camargo

Abstract

In this chapter, we describe a straightforward protocol to generate multicellular tumor spheroids (MTSs) and evaluate the role of specific genes in regulating cell invasiveness in real-time and tridimensional (3D) matrices. This approach provides advantages over other conventional invasion assays by offering intimate cell–cell and cell–ECM contacts and by mimicking the pathophysiological characteristics observed in tumor microenvironments (e.g., microregional gradients in glucose and O_2 concentrations and metabolic and proliferative tumor heterogeneity). We also provide an original and semiautomated approach to quantify MTS invasion using the freely available ImageJ software and plugins.

Key words Tridimensional (3D) assay, Multicellular tumor spheroids, A Disintegrin And Metalloproteinase (ADAM) family, Hydrogel, Tumor cell invasion

1 Introduction

It has long been deliberated that tissue invasion and metastasis are not intrinsic abilities of malignant cells but are strongly dependent on how tumor cells interact and respond to the "context" in which they are inserted. Indeed, bidirectional communication between subpopulations of tumor cells within a primary tumor and their microenvironment establishes a "dynamic reciprocity" that is critical for tumor initiation and progression and can influence therapeutic response and patient prognosis [1–5].

In particular, molecules capable of remodeling the microenvironment, as well as of releasing biologically active molecules, are powerful modulators of this reciprocity and can exacerbate malignant progression by altering the extracellular matrix (ECM) structure and composition [6].

The A Disintegrin And Metalloproteinase (ADAM) family members are good examples of this type of molecule. They belong to the metzincin superfamily of zinc-dependent endoproteases and

Santiago Cal and Alvaro J. Obaya (eds.), *Proteases and Cancer: Methods and Protocols*, Methods in Molecular Biology, vol. 1731,
https://doi.org/10.1007/978-1-4939-7595-2_15,

to the subfamily of adamalysins, which, in mammals, includes the ADAMs and the ADAMTSs (ADAMs with thrombospondin motifs) family members [7–9].

The ADAMs are multidomain proteins with a conserved and complex core structure containing pro-, metalloprotease-like, disintegrin-like, cysteine-rich, epidermal growth factor-like, transmembrane, and cytoplasmic domains [7]. The ADAMs are unique among type I transmembrane proteins in possessing both a disintegrin and a metalloprotease domain adjacent to each other.

Phylogenetically, the ADAMs evolved from a common ancestor gene with snake venom metalloproteases (SVMPs) [8, 10]. Their protease domain contains a conserved zinc-binding motif (HEXXHXXGXXH) that is indispensable for the catalytic activity of the adamalysins [8, 10–13]. Proteolytically active ADAMs act as ectodomain sheddases, releasing extracellular regions of membrane-bound proteins (e.g., adhesion molecules, growth factors, cytokines, chemokines, and receptors).

However, although all ADAM family members contain a metalloproteinase domain, nearly half of the 20 known human ADAM family members are predicted to be proteolytic inactive. Non-catalytic ADAMs present one or more amino acid substitutions in the conserved zinc-binding motif within the active site of the metalloprotease domain. Despite lacking the hallmark catalytic activity, non-catalytic ADAMs exhibit important adhesive and regulatory functions associated with the disintegrin and cysteine-rich ancillary domains.

This is the case of the non-catalytically active ADAM23 family member (also known as MDC3), which lacks the conserved catalytic motif within the metalloprotease-like domain [14] but exhibits important functions in normal brain development [15, 16] and cancer [4, 17, 18]. Through its disintegrin-like domain, ADAM23 binds $\alpha_v\beta_3$-integrin and mediates cell adhesion in neuroblastoma and melanoma cell lines, controlling tumor progression through cell–cell-mediated interactions [17, 18].

In addition, our recent studies demonstrated a pleiotropic effect of ADAM23 during tumor progression by promoting tumor cell proliferation while restraining cell migration, invasion, and metastasis. Using a tridimensional (3D) spheroid invasion assay, we demonstrated that mosaic clusters of tumor cells expressing different levels of ADAM23 act cooperatively during tissue invasion. In these mosaic clusters, ADAM23-negative cells promote tumor growth and metastasis by enhancing the proliferation and invasion of adjacent ADAM23-positive cells [4].

In this chapter, we provide a step-by-step description of the tridimensional (3D) spheroid invasion assay used to dissect the functional role of ADAM23 during tumor progression. The advantages of this 3D assay over other conventional invasion assays include (1) the simplicity of the analysis allowing the visualization of specific patterns of invasion (e.g., amoeboid or mesenchymal types) and monitoring individual invading cells in real time using an inverted microscope and (2) the particular spatial distribution of the cells within the spheroids which offers intimate cell–cell and cell–ECM contacts that better represent the pathophysiological characteristics observed in tumors (e.g., microregional gradients in glucose and O_2 concentrations and metabolic and proliferative tumor heterogeneity). All of these features interfere with gene and protein expression as well as with cell functionalities (e.g., cell polarization, differentiation), recapitulating an in vivo-like avascular condition (for a more detailed characterization of 3D culture systems, *see* refs. 19–24). Finally, in more complex protocols, the use of spheroids and the 3D invasion assays allows the co-culture of two (or more) different cell populations to elucidate the role of intratumoral heterogeneity and tumor cell cooperation in determining the invasive tumor phenotype [4].

2 Materials

2.1 Generation of Multicellular Tumor Spheroids (MTSs)

1. Single-cell suspension of tumor cells in complete culture medium.
2. 35-mm tissue culture dishes for protocol (A) or ultralow attachment (ULA) round bottom multi-well dishes (24-well, 48-well, or 96-well formats) for protocol (B) (*see* **Note 1**).
3. Sterile complete culture medium (CCM). The composition of the CCM depends on the cell type used in the assay (e.g., Leibovitz's L-15 medium with 10% heat-inactivated fetal bovine serum [FBS], 0.01 mg/mL bovine insulin, and 1% L-glutamine for MDA-MB-435 cells).
4. Sterile phosphate-buffered saline (PBS) solution.
5. Trypsin/EDTA solution: sterile 0.05% w/v trypsin and 0.02% w/v ethylenediaminetetraacetic acid (EDTA) solution.
6. 15 mL sterile conical tubes.
7. Neubauer chamber or hemocytometer.
8. 0.25% w/v trypan blue solution in PBS.

2.2 Preparation of 3D Matrices (Matrigel and Collagen Type I)

1. Reconstituted extracellular matrix from Engelbreth-Holm-Swarm (EHS) sarcoma, commercially available as Matrigel.
2. Acid collagen type I in 0.02 *N* hydrochloric acid.
3. Sterile serum-free medium (SFM) and SFM concentrated tenfold (SFM 10×). The composition of the SFM and SFM 10× depends on the cell type used in the assay (e.g., Leibovitz's L-15 medium or similar) (*see* **Note 2**).

4. Sterile reconstitution buffer solution concentrated tenfold (RB 10×): 2.2 g of $NaHCO_3$ and 4.8 g of HEPES diluted in 100 mL of distilled water (*see* **Note 2**).
5. Ultralow attachment (ULA) round bottom multi-well dishes (48-well or 96-well formats).
6. Sterile 3% w/v soft agar in PBS.
7. Sterile scalpel.

2.3 Image Analysis

1. Inverted microscope equipped with a 10× objective, bright-field optics and high-resolution capture camera.
2. ImageJ software v.1.50c or latter (Bethesda, MD, USA) and CLAHE (Contrast Limited Adaptive Histogram Equalization) plugin for enhancing the local contrast of MTSs automatically. ImageJ is freely available at https://imagej.nih.gov/ij/ and provides a wide range of analysis approaches via accessible plugins.

3 Methods

3.1 Generation of the Multicellular Tumor Spheroids (MTSs) by Cell Aggregation

There are many different strategies to generate MTSs (e.g., rotating-wall vessel culture, magnetic cell levitation, hang-drop assay, etc.) [21, 25]. In this section we describe two simple, easy-handling, and efficient protocols that do not require additional equipment other than those usually available in a regular tissue culture room: (A) the hang-drop protocol and (B) the multi-well-mediated aggregation protocol. We use protocol A for small MTSs up to 500 μm in diameter and protocol B for larger MTSs between 0.5 and 2 mm in diameter (*see* **Note 3** and Fig. 1).

In both cases, start by washing and detaching confluent monolayers of cells from culture dishes with trypsin/EDTA solution and resuspend the cells in sterile CCM to have ~10^5 viable cells/mL (*see* **Notes 4** and **5**):

1. Option (A): Hang-drop protocol. Plate 10 μL of cell suspension (i.e., 1000 cells) as a drop-like on the bottom of the lid of a 35-mm tissue culture dish. Make sure drops are placed sufficiently apart to not touch each other. Place 5 mL of sterile PBS in the dish to reduce evaporation of the drops, and place the lid in the PBS-filled dish (Fig. 1a). Incubate dishes using standard culture conditions for 48–72 h.
2. Option (B): Multi-well-based aggregation protocol. Plate 100–200 mL of cell suspension (1–2 × 10^4 cells/well) in 96-well ULA round bottom dish (*see* **Note 1**). Adjust the final volume to 0.5 mL/well with standard cell culture medium (Fig. 1b). Incubate dishes using standard culture conditions for 72–120 h.

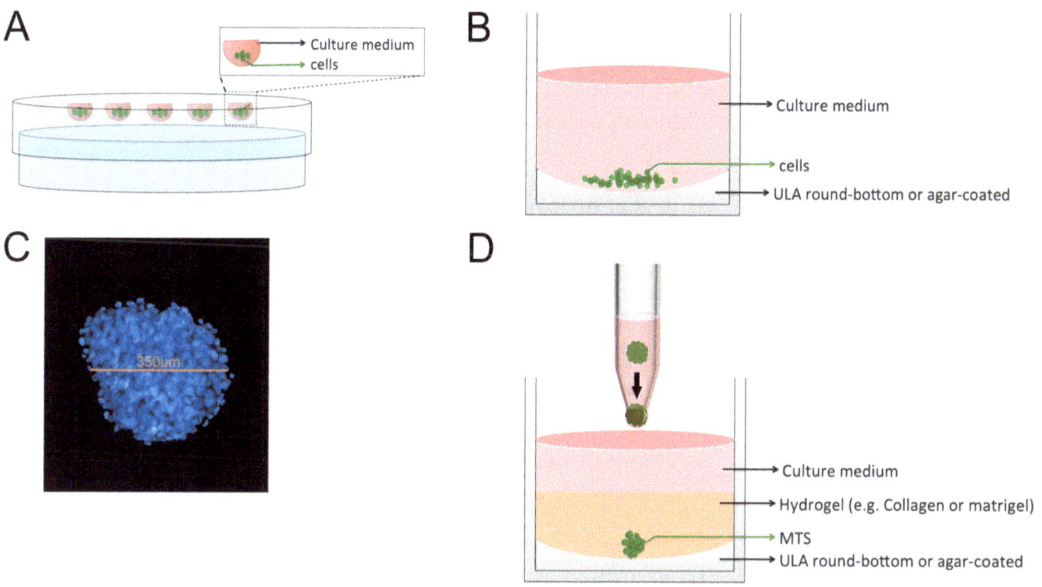

Fig. 1 Generation of MTSs by cell aggregation. (**a**) In the "hanging drop" method, cell aggregation is promoted by gravity at the liquid–air interface. (**b**) In multi-well-mediated aggregation, larger MTSs can be obtained by cell clustering at the center of a round-bottom 96-well or agar-coated well. In both methods, one MTS is generated per drop or well. (**c**) Immunofluorescent image of a small (diameter ~350 μm) and dense U87MG glioblastoma spheroid stained with DAPI. (**d**) Diagram illustrating how MTSs should be handled and individually transferred to multi-well plates containing 3D hydrogel matrices. The P200 pipette cut tip must be held vertically for 10–20 s to ensure that MTS move down into the tip and reach the first drop at the tip point

Monitor MTS formation daily for 4–7 days using an inverted microscopy.

3.2 Preparation of 3D Hydrogel Matrices

The matrix should provide a semisolid scaffold in which tumor cells interact, invade, and spread out from the MTS. The exact composition and concentration of the matrix will determine the invasive behavior (i.e., invasive pattern, speed, and persistence of cell invasion and cell morphology) (*see* **Note 6**).

In this section we will describe the preparation of two natural hydrogel matrices commonly used to assess tumor cell invasion in vitro: purified type I collagen and Matrigel. Alternative types of matrices, such as the commercially available synthetic hydrogel-based matrices (e.g., polyethylene) or natural composite matrices (mixtures of naturally occurring polymers, like hyaluronan and heparin), can also be used as scaffolds to recreate essential features of specific tissues (for additional information, see a recent review on hydrogels in reference 26).

Matrigel is a preparation rich in ECM proteins, such as laminin and type IV collagen, in addition to growth factors and enzymes [27], and it is much simpler to handle in the laboratory than collagen matrices. Once diluted to a working concentration (0.3–1.2 mg/mL) in PBS or SFM, Matrigel will rapidly self-assemble into a hydrogel at 22–35 °C (*see* **Note 6**).

Collagens have a pH-based gelling mechanism, so acid-soluble type I collagen must be reconstituted and the acidity neutralized to allow fibrillogenesis and gelification by adjusting the pH of the collagen stock solution to 7.0–7.4 as described below (*see* **Note 7**):

1. Before starting, prechill all dishes, sterile tips, pipettes, and conical centrifuge tubes at −20 °C for a few minutes.
2. Defrost aliquots of 10× SFM and 10× RB on melting ice.
3. Calculate the volume of the final collagen solution that is needed for the experiment, taking into account the desired final collagen concentration (e.g., 2–6 mg/mL) and well size (we recommend 300 μL for 48-well and 150 μL for 96-well). Prepare up to 30% more collagen solution than needed due to pipetting difficulties caused by collagen viscosity.
4. Pipette the required amount of collagen stock solution into a prechilled tube (e.g., 0.7 mL of a 6 mg/mL stock solution).
5. To neutralize the pH, add a seventh part of the volume of the collagen stock solution of SFM 10× (e.g., 0.1 mL), and mix slowly and gently by inverting the tube to avoid the introduction of air bubbles.
6. Add a seventh part of the volume of collagen stock solution of RB 10× (e.g., 0.1 mL), and mix gently by inverting the tube to avoid the introduction of air bubbles.
7. Dilute the reconstituted collagen to the desired final concentration using CCM (e.g., 1.2 mL to a final concentration of 2 mg/mL) (*see* **Note 6**).
8. Incubate the reconstituted collagen for 5 min on melting ice and measure the pH of the neutralized collagen with a pH paper strip (pH must be in the range of 7.0–7.4).
9. Spin collagen solution at 1600 × *g* in a prechilled microcentrifuge to eliminate air bubbles.

3.3 Embedding MTSs on 3D Matrices

Once MTS formation is macroscopically confirmed, MTSs can be easily handled and individually transferred to 48-well (for larger MTSs) or 96-well (for smaller MTSs) plates containing 3D matrices (Fig. 1d). Before embedding MTSs into 3D matrices, it is very important to keep all the components of the system (i.e., matrices, pipettes, multi-well plates, etc.) at 2–4 °C:

1. Pre-coat all wells with a thin layer (1–2 mm, called layer 1) of reconstituted hydrogel (100 μL/48-well or 50 μL/96-well) to prevent MTS dish contact. After coating, allow layer 1 to polymerize at 37 °C for 20 min.
2. Confirm layer 1 polymerization using a phase microscope (you should see an opaque matrix), and place the dish at room temperature for 10 min.

3. Add an additional layer of ice-cold reconstituted hydrogel on top of layer 1 (200 μL/48-well or 100 μL/96-well). This second layer will support the MTS, while layer one will prevent undesirable MTS dish contact (*see* **Note 8**). Due to fast jellification rates at room temperature, it is not recommended to prepare several secondary layers at the same time.
4. MTSs must be carefully captured using a P200 cut pipette tip and transferred immediately to the center of well using a minimum amount of culture medium (*see* **Note 9**, Fig. 1d).
5. After transferring all MTSs to the coated wells, allow the hydrogel to polymerize at 37 °C for 20 min.
6. Overlay layer 2 with standard culture medium. Capture and save images for each MTS using an inverted microscope ($t = 0$ days).
7. Incubate dishes at 37 °C. MTSs cultures will require periodic medium changes. Intervals between medium changes and image captures will vary depending on the cell line used for the assays.

3.4 Image Acquisition and Analysis

As mentioned before, one of the advantages of this 3D invasive assay is that the invasive cells can be easily visualized using an inverted microscope. When properly embedded in permissive and homogeneous matrices, invasive cells spread out from MTS in a "starburst" format. The evolution and dynamic of this spreading pattern is, however, strongly dependent on the invasive mode, MTS size, and matrix composition and concentration (Fig. 2).

Therefore, parameters for image acquisition, like time intervals, magnification, and experimental endpoints, must be adjusted for each condition. For instance, 4× objectives are usually appropriated for whole MTS visualization (*see* Fig. 4a), while 10× or 20× objectives are needed for monitoring changes in cell morphology or invasive modes (*see* Fig. 4b). Acquired images must be of high quality, well focused, well contrasted, and captured in grayscale without any special preprocessing (*see* **Note 10**).

In this section we will describe a simple and original approach for MTS invasion analysis using the freely available ImageJ software and plugins.

During the spreading process, invasive cells can remain linked (e.g., in groups or aligned in "Indian file") or can detach from the MTS and spread as isolated cells (Fig. 2—in detail). In terms of image analysis, detached isolated cells can be visualized as non-contiguous pixels located within a defined range from the MTS. In order to better characterize MTS invasion, three concentric zones should be defined: two invasive zones, named leading edge (LE) and intermediate zone (I), and a noninvasive core (C). Detached isolated or small clusters of fast-invasive cells are usually detected at

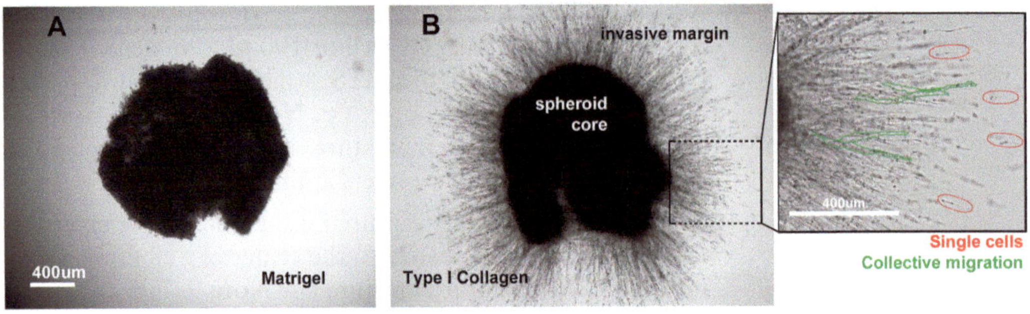

Fig. 2 Effects of matrix composition on the invasive phenotype. Phase-contrast images at day 10 of MDA-MB-435-derived melanoma spheroids embedded in 70% Matrigel (*left*) or 3 mg/mL type I collagen (*right*) (Courtesy of authors)

the "LE" zone, while the bulk of the invasive cells are detected in the "I" zone. The "C" zone is a noninvasive zone named spheroid core (Fig. 3).

The pipeline below describes the steps necessary to quantify invasion, using representative images of the MDA-MB-435 spheroids, which we have previously used to address the functional impact of ADAM23 gene silencing in the tumor cell invasion phenotype [4]:

1. Open the raw image obtained at $t = 0$ days of the invasive assay using ImageJ (version 1.50c). The image should be in grayscale (8-bit) and should be representative of the spheroid core (C). The MTS image at this time point should be very well contrasted (Fig. 4a).
2. Before start working, it is important to calibrate the scale to allow reliable measurements. To set the scale go to *Analyze* > *Set scale*.
3. Adjust *brightness* and *contrast* automatically.
4. To improve image analysis go to *Edit* > *Options* > *Profile Plot options* > "check" *sub-pixel resolution* to activate subpixel accuracy.
5. Select the *Wand tool* and click at the center of the MTS. Next, double-click on the wand tool icon to open the configuration dialog box. Select the "8-connected" mode and adjust tolerance value manually to visualize the borders of the MTS (e.g., Fig. 4a, $t = 0$ h for the core or $t = 240$ h for intermediate zone).
6. Improve the quality of the selected image by using the *Edit* > *Selection* > *Interpolate* > "check" *Smooth* (we set interval to 2 pixels).
7. Open ROI (region of interest) manager (Analyze > tools > ROI manager) and save this selected area by clicking "add." Rename it accordingly (e.g., "core area").

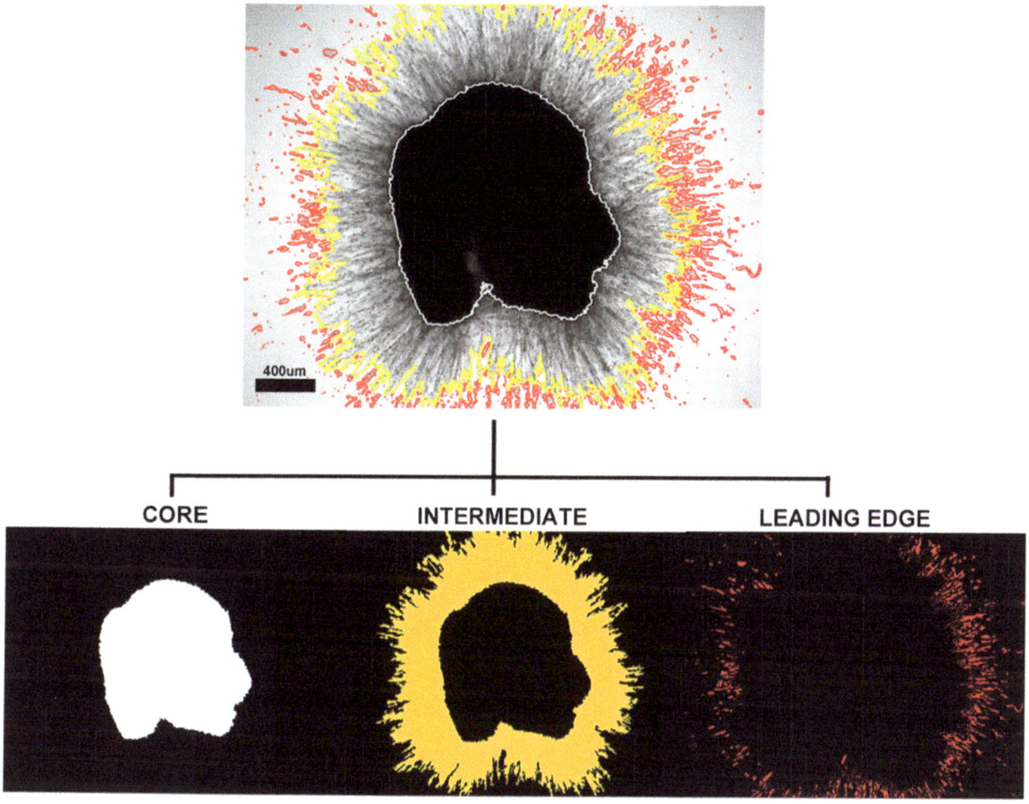

Fig. 3 Image of invasive MDA-MB-435 spheroid embedded in type I collagen (3 mg/mL, $t = 240$ h) and their corresponding segmented images: a noninvasive core zone (core) and two invasive zones, Intermediate invasive cells (yellow) and leading edge invasive cells (red) (Courtesy of authors)

8. Calculate area of the selected region using *Plugins* > *Analyze* > *Measure and set label.* Set area name accordingly and click "ok" (save image).

   Next, open the raw image captured at the end of invasive assay (e.g., at day 10) (Fig. 3b). To calculate intermediate layer (I) repeat **steps 1–8** as described above. At **step 5**, increase tolerance value manually to include the invasive zone in the selected area. Note that the "I" zone also includes the spheroid core (C) and that not all invasive cells can be selected due to non-contiguous pixels corresponding to detached invasive cells (Fig. 4a, center).

9. To calculate the leading edge (LE) layer, reopen the image obtained at the end of the invasive assay and repeat **steps 2–4** as described above.

10. To correct uneven illuminated background, apply subtract background: Processes > Subtract Background. We chose the *sliding paraboloid* and light background options with the *rolling ball* radius set to 15 pixels.

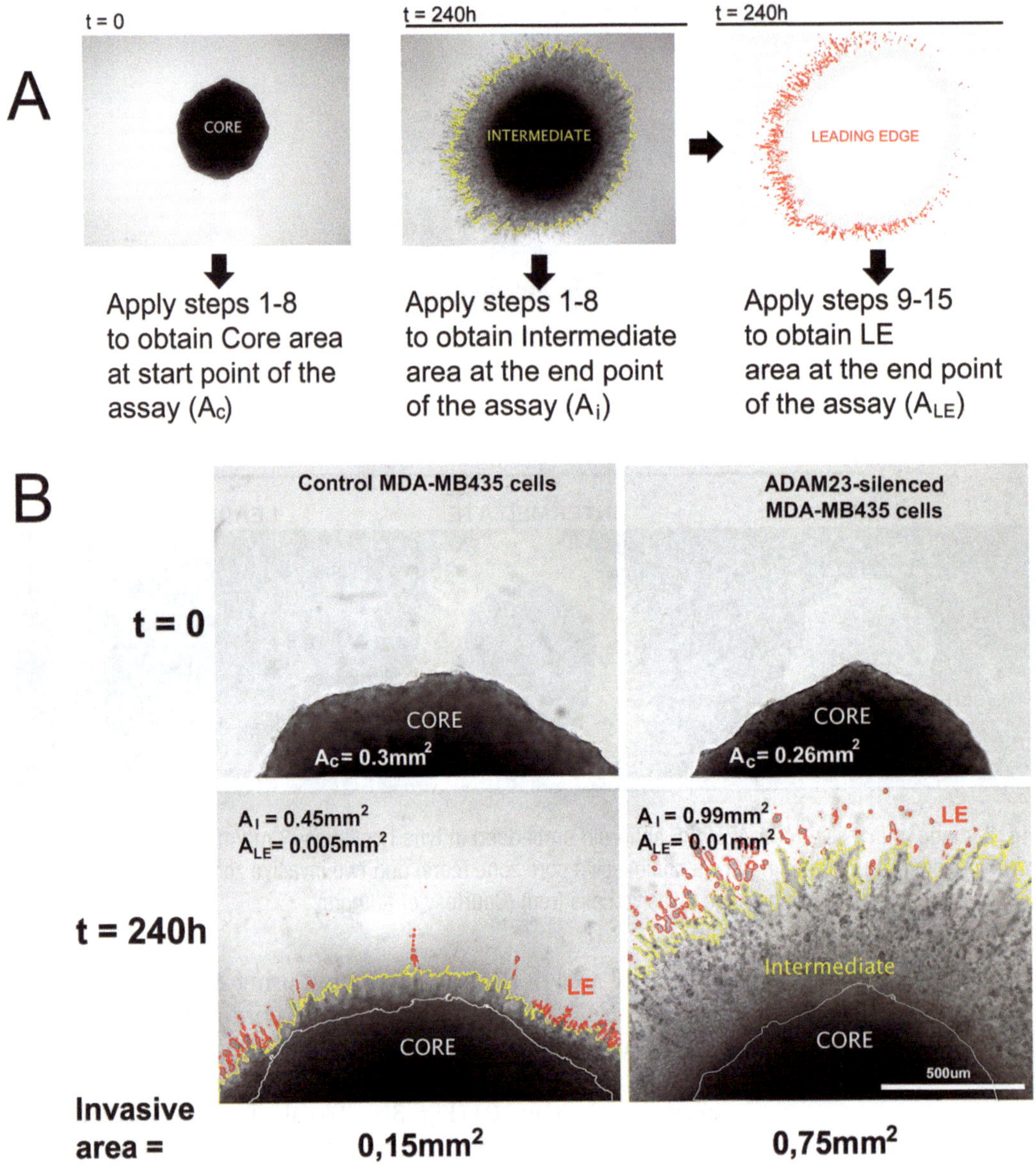

Fig. 4 Representative images of MDA-MB-435 cell line MTS embedded in type I collagen (3 mg/mL). MTSs can be imaged over time using bright-field microscopy to quantify the invasive behavior based on the distance traveled by invasive cells from the spheroid core. (**a**) Diagrams of MTS segmentation in three concentric zones using ImageJ software (4× objective); (**b**) invasive behavior and quantification of the invasive area of spheroids formed by MDA-MB-435 ADAM23-positive cells (left) versus their highly invasive ADAM23-negative cells (ADAM23-shRNA silenced cells, (right) (10× objective) (for a full description of the role of ADAM23 gene in cell invasion, *see* Ref. 4) (Courtesy of authors)

11. In the ROI manager window, click on preselected area representative "I" zone and fill it with white color: *Edit > Fill.*
12. Enhance the local contrast of the image by running the CLAHE (Contrast Limited Adaptive Histogram Equalization) plugin. The plugin CLAHE uses three critical parameters, we recommend the following values: block size = 127, histogram bins = 256, and maximum slope = 3.
13. Run the *threshold* command: *Image > Adjust > Threshold.* Set the threshold levels manually to include all remaining invasive cells. Here we used the default method (*see* Fig. 4a, right).
14. To create the LE area: *Edit > Selection > Create Selection.* Store the LE selection to the list of ROI manager. Rename it as LE.
15. Calculate area of the selected region in: *Plugins > Analyze > Measure And Set Label*

Finally, export measurements of different parameters (area, perimeter, diameter, etc.) to a worksheet. The invasive area can be calculated as: (*I* area + *LE* area) – *C* area (*see* comparative examples in the Fig. 4b).

4 Notes

1. Alternatively to the use of non-adherent dishes in protocol (B), flat-bottom multi-well dishes coated with 1% soft agar can be used to prevent cell dish adhesion. Dishes can be coated with soft agar by pipetting 100–300 μL/96-well of 1% soft agar (1–2 mm coating) diluted in preheated SFM (55 °C) and allowing to solidify at room temperature. Take care to cover the surface completely, and respect the indicated temperature to fill the wells homogeneously. The use of multi-well dishes larger than 24-well format can result in the formation of multiple spheroids per well with variables diameters.
2. All buffers should be filtered using 0.45 μm sterile filters before use.
3. Depending on the cell line, MTS aggregation dynamics, sizes, and volumes may vary, so cell concentration and aggregations periods should be adjusted accordingly. MTSs may also aggregate in non-spherical shapes due to different types of cell–cell interactions. In some models, the inability to aggregate may also be an intrinsic characteristic of the cell line. In terms of microregional heterogeneity, small spheroids are more homogeneous than larger spheroids. The latter ones can exhibit central hypoxia and, eventually, develop a central necrosis.

4. Be careful not to over digest with trypsin to avoid cell damage. If possible, detach cells using PBS and EDTA plus mechanical scraping to preserve cell–cell adhesion molecules at cell surface. Obtaining single-cell suspensions is not strictly necessary. If PBS and EDTA is used, cell suspension can still present cell clumps when examined microscopically, and as far as these clumps do not interfere with cell counting, they do not represent a significant problem.
5. Optimal cell density needs to be determined for each cell line in order to obtain MTSs with desirable diameters. Usually 4 days after seeding is sufficient to visually confirm MTS formation. MTSs can be maintained in culture for several weeks upon adequate medium changes.
6. Optimal hydrogel concentration should be empirically determined for each cell type: lower concentrations may not provide a significant impediment to segregate invasive from noninvasive cells, whereas higher concentrations may completely prevent cell invasion.
7. Natural hydrogels usually start gelling when kept at room temperature. Use the indicated temperature (4–10 °C) for all solutions and materials to avoid heterogeneous jellification. Always pipette the hydrogel solutions slowly and gently to avoid introducing air bubbles. Harsh pipetting can cause precipitation and form clumps. Collagens must be reconstituted on ice immediately before use. Differently from reconstituted collagen keep at 4 °C, polymerized collagen forms a turbid and opaque matrix.
8. It is important to note that invasive cells usually tend to take paths of least resistance in the surrounding matrix. Despite the relative homogeneity of 3D matrices, invasive cells also find preferable routes to spread in vitro. Easier migratory routes could be artificially generated by improper polymerization of the matrices, and this may represent a relevant experimental bias.
9. To avoid diluting layer 2, after capturing the MTS, the cut P200 pipette tip must be held vertically for 10–20 s to ensure that the MTS move down the tip. Do not dispense the full volume of the pipette tip, only the first drop containing the MTS.
10. To study invasion kinetics, time-lapse videos can be used. Invasive cells will gradually come in and out of focus when they enter or exit the optical.

Acknowledgment

This work was supported by grants from FAPESP (16/07463-4), Hospital Sírio-Libanês and Ludwig Institute for Cancer Research (LICR), São Paulo, Brazil.

References

1. Fidler IJ (1978) Tumor heterogeneity and the biology of cancer invasion and metastasis. Cancer Res 38(9):2651–2660
2. Bissell MJ, Hall HG, Parry G (1982) How does the extracellular matrix direct gene expression? J Theor Biol 99(1):31–68
3. Quail DF, Joyce JA (2014) Microenvironmental regulation of tumor progression and metastasis. Nat Med 19(11):1423–1437
4. Costa ET, Barnabé GF, Li M et al (2015) Intratumoral heterogeneity of ADAM23 promotes tumor growth and metastasis through LGI4 and nitric oxide signals. Oncogene 34:1270–1279
5. Klemm F, Joyce JA (2015) Microenvironmental regulation of therapeutic response in cancer. Trends Cell Biol 25(4):4198–4213
6. Bonnans C, Chou J, Werb Z (2014) Remodelling the extracellular matrix in development and disease. Nat Rev Mol Cell Biol 15:786–801
7. White JM (2003) ADAMs: modulators of cell–cell and cell–matrix interactions. Curr Opin Cell Biol 15(5):598–606
8. Takeda S, Takeya H, Iwanaga S (2012) Snake venom metalloproteinases: structure, function and relevance to the mammalian adam/adamts family proteins. Biochim Biophys Acta 1824(1):164–176
9. Kelwick R, Desanlis I, Wheelter GN et al (2015) The ADAMTS (A Disintegrin and Metalloproteinase with Thrombospondin motifs) family. Genome Biol 16:113
10. Bode W, Gomis-Ruth F-X, Stockler W (1993) Astacins, serralysins, snake venom and matrix metalloproteinases exhibit identical zinc-binding environments (HEXXHXXGXXH and met- turn) and topologies and should be grouped into a common family, the metzincins. FEBS Lett 331(1–2):134–140
11. Black RA, Rauch CT, Kozlosky CJ et al (1997) A metalloproteinase disintegrin that releases tumour-necrosis factor-alpha from cells. Nature 385(6618):729–733
12. Black RA, White JM (1998) ADAMs: focus on the protease domain. Curr Opin Cell Biol 10(5):654–659
13. Schlondorff J, Blobel CP (1999) Metalloprotease-disintegrins: modular proteins capable of promoting cell-cell interactions and triggering signals by protein-ectodomain shedding. J Cell Sci 112(Pt21):3603–3617
14. Sagane K, Ohya Y, Hasegawa Y et al (1998) Metalloproteinase-like, disintegrin-like, cysteine-rich proteins MDC2 and MDC3: novel human cellular disintegrins highly expressed in the brain. Biochem J 334(Pt1):93–98
15. Mitchell KJ, Pinson KI, Kelly OG et al (2001) Functional analysis of secreted and transmembrane proteins critical to mouse development. Nat Genet 28(3):241–249
16. Leighton PA, Mitchell KJ, Goodrich LV et al (2001) Defining brain wiring patterns and mechanisms through gene trapping in mice. Nature 410(6825):174–179
17. Cal S, Freije JM, Lopez JM et al (2000) ADAM23/MDC3, a human disintegrin that promotes cell adhesion via interaction with the alphavbeta3 integrin through an RGD-independent mechanism. Mol Biol Cell 11(4):1457–1469
18. Verbisck NV, Costa ET, Costa FF et al (2009) ADAM23 negatively modulates alpha(v) beta(3) integrin activation during metastasis. Cancer Res 69:5546–5552
19. Vinci M, Gowan S, Boxan F et al (2012) Advances in establishment and analysis of three-dimensional tumor spheroid-based functional assays for target validation and drug evaluation. BMC Biol 10:29
20. Kunz-Schughart LA (1999) Multicellular tumor spheroids: intermediates between monolayer culture and in vivo tumor. Cell Biol Int 23(3):157–161
21. Antoni D, Burckel H, Josset E et al (2015) Three-dimensional cell culture: a breakthrough in vivo. Int J Mol Sci 16(3):5517–5527

22. Sutherland RM (1988) Cell and environment interactions in tumor microregions: the multicell spheroid model. Science 240(4849): 177–184
23. Cukierman E, Pankov R, Stevens DR et al (2001) Taking cell-matrix adhesions to the third dimension. Science 294(5547):1708–1712
24. Pampaloni F, Reynaud EG, Stelzer EHK (2007) The third dimension bridges the gap between cell culture and live tissue. Nat Rev Mol Cell Biol 8(10):839–845
25. Souza GR, Molina JR, Raphael RM et al (2010) Three-dimensional tissue culture based on magnetic cell levitation. Nat Nanotechnol 5(4):291–296
26. Caliari SR, Burdick JA (2016) A practical guide to hydrogels for cell culture. Nat Methods 13:405–414
27. Hughes CS, Postovit LM, Lajoie GA (2010) Matrigel: a complex protein mixture required for optimal growth of cell culture. Proteomics 10(9):1886–1890

Chapter 16

Analyzing the Type II Transmembrane Serine Protease Hepsin-Dependent Basement Membrane Remodeling in 3D Cell Culture

Shishir M. Pant, Denis Belitskin, Hanna Ala-Hongisto, Juha Klefström, and Topi A. Tervonen

Abstract

Breakdown of the basement membrane is a key step that precedes tumor invasion, and accumulating evidence suggests a key role for the type II transmembrane proteases (TTSPs) in that process. Overexpression of a TTSP hepsin characterizes many solid cancers, including prostate, breast, and ovarian cancer, and in experimental tumor models, the elevated proteolytic activity of hepsin simultaneously activates several growth factors and cleaves basement membrane protein laminin-332, which is an essential component of the cell-basement membrane junction hemidesmosome. These hepsin-dependent molecular events associate with dramatic loss of basement membrane integrity in mouse tumor models and in three-dimensional (3D) epithelial culture. In particular, the 3D culture systems offer unprecedented possibilities to clarify the mechanistic basis of destructive interactions between out-of-control serine protease activity and the basement membrane structure. Here, we describe how to establish 3D mammary epithelial culture in an exogenous basement membrane-free egg white matrix and provide a protocol for quantitative analysis of the impact of hepsin on laminin-332 and its hemidesmosomal receptor α6-integrin by means of confocal microscopy imaging. These protocols were established to facilitate studies aiming to decipher the exact role of oncogenic proteases in tumor invasion processes and to identify novel therapeutic agents able to intervene these cancer critical processes.

Key words Hepsin, 3D culture, Basement membrane, Hemidesmosome, Laminin-332, α6-Integrin, Immunofluorescence confocal microscopy

1 Introduction

Type II transmembrane serine proteases (TTSPs) are a small family of proteases involved in diverse physiological functions such as tissue homeostasis, iron metabolism, blood pressure regulation and blood coagulation, neural tube closure, hearing, and epithelial differentiation [1, 2]. TTSPs are predominantly transported and integrated into plasma membrane as inactive zymogens (proenzymes)

Santiago Cal and Alvaro J. Obaya (eds.), *Proteases and Cancer: Methods and Protocols*, Methods in Molecular Biology, vol. 1731, https://doi.org/10.1007/978-1-4939-7595-2_16,

followed by irreversible activation by auto- or trans-proteolytic processing of the conserved activation domain [1, 3]. The enzymatic activity of processed TTSPs is thereafter dynamically controlled by numerous cell surface and soluble cognate inhibitors [2].

In human cancers, many TTSPs show altered protein expression and activity [4, 5]. Specifically, hepsin is one of the most frequently overexpressed TTSPs in prostate, ovarian, endometrial, and breast cancer [6–11]. The oncogenic role of hepsin in primary tumor growth, invasion, and metastasis has been demonstrated in several mouse models of prostate and breast cancer [7, 8, 11–13].

Accumulating evidence suggest that the oncogenic action of hepsin involves degradatory effects on the basement membrane (BM). BM is a specialized form of the extracellular matrix, which normally separates epithelial cells from the surrounding stroma. Interestingly, degradation of BM is a defining feature of all advanced solid cancers, which supports the notion that loss of BM components provides a permissive microenvironment for invasiveness phenotype of cancer [14, 15]. In the normal adult resting breast epithelial structures, the expression of hepsin is restricted to the mammary epithelial cells, and the strongest staining localizes to the basement membranes (BM) [8]. Further studies in three-dimensional epithelial organoid cultures have pinpointed the expression of hepsin to hemidesmosomal cell-BM and desmosomal cell-cell junctions [7, 8]. The first findings linking hepsin to degradation or remodeling of BM were made by Klezovitch et al., demonstrating that ectopic probasin promoter-driven hepsin overexpression alters the immunostaining pattern of laminin-332 (formerly known as laminin-5) and β4-integrin in mouse prostate. When these components of BM are stained in normal prostate, they form continuous ringlike BM structures around the epithelial structures, but overexpression of hepsin resulted in discontinuities and gaps in the immunostaining. These changes suggested some level of degradation or remodeling of the BM structure [12]. The damaging interaction between overexpressed hepsin and the BM structure has been corroborated in breast cancer models harboring either endogenously or ectopically overexpressed hepsin. For example, in a transgenic mouse model of MYC-driven breast cancer, overexpression MYC together with loss of a tumor suppressor LKB1 in the mammary epithelial cells leads to overexpression of the endogenous hepsin and concomitant breakdown of BM. In the ex vivo explants, which were grown in three-dimensional (3D) BM gels and engineered to express the same oncogenic lesions, the observed BM defects were rescued by shRNA-mediated hepsin inhibition [7]. Furthermore, an acute doxycycline-induced hepsin overexpression in 3D cultures of human mammary epithelial cells leads to a loss of laminin-332 and α6-integrin immunofluorescent staining, which defects can be rescued with an investigational drug targeting the cell surface serine protease activity [8]. It has been demonstrated that hepsin can proteolytically cleave the β3-chain of laminin-332. Such proteolytic event could compromise the ability of laminin-332 to bind its hemidesmosomal receptor β4-integrin, which together with α6-integrin forms a cellular part of the hemidesmosome junction [16, 17].

The mammary epithelial structures formed in reconstituted 3D BM matrices closely resemble mammary alveolar (acinar) structures with hollow cavities (lumen) and sometimes with capacity to secrete milk proteins [18, 19]. The cells forming these structures are apicobasally polarized, enabling the formation of blanket-like BM on the basal surface of the cells and correctly localized apical cell-cell junctions. These fundamental functional and structural characters of organized epithelial structures are lacking in monolayer cell culture as the plastic-attached epithelial cells are typically not polarized. The correct biological context provided by polarized 3D epithelial structures for a protein function is exemplified in the case of hepsin. In 2D cultures of mammary epithelial cells, hepsin localizes to desmosomal cell-cell junctions, which is likely not an artifact either as hepsin is basolaterally localized also in tissue sections of human breast [8]. However, only in 3D cultures, hepsin colocalizes with BM and the hemidesmosomal components α6-integrin and laminin [7, 8]. Hence, 3D cultures offer unique possibilities to study interactions between tumorigenesis relevant cell surface proteases and BM components as well as the functional consequences of BM degradation or remodeling.

There are number of commercially available reconstituted basement membrane-based matrices which support formation of polarized 3D structures, for example, Engelbreth-Holm-Swarm (EHS) mouse sarcoma-derived Matrigel™ [20]. However, reconstituted BM matrices occasionally pose problems for experimentalists as they contain growth factors and exogenous BM proteins derived from the tumor. One way to circumvent these problems is to use synthetic or natural hydrogels [21]. In our laboratory, we have successfully adapted egg white hydrogels to culture various mammary epithelial cells and tumor breast tumor cell lines in 3D [22]. Non-transformed human mammary epithelial MCF10A cells form polarized and lumen-containing acinar structures in egg white with basement membrane forming on the basal side of the structures [8]. The egg white 3D cultures offer many unique possibilities to explore epithelial cell secreted BM components and the remodeling actions of hepsin on BM.

Here, we describe a method to culture human mammary epithelial MCF10A cells in 3D egg white, fixation and immunostaining procedures of the structures, digital imaging of the immunostained acinar structures with confocal microscope, and analysis of the basement membrane degradation by hepsin. The described methods are not only applicable to hepsin but can be adapted to study the role of different transmembrane serine proteases on BM remodeling and degradation in various cancer relevant contexts.

2 Material

2.1 Hepsin Expression Validation

1. MCF10A-hepsin^{IND20} cells as described in [8].
2. Complete medium: mammary epithelial basal medium (MCDB 170) supplemented with 70 μg/mL bovine pituitary extract (BPE), 5 ng/mL epithelial growth factor (EGF), 5 μg/mL transferrin, 10^{-5} M isoproterenol, 0.5 μg/mL hydrocortisone, 5 μg/mL insulin, 50 μg/mL amphotericin B, and 50 μg/mL gentamicin.
3. Polybrene.
4. G418 disulfate salt solution.
5. Phosphate-buffered saline (PBS).
6. Lysis buffer (1% Triton X-100 in PBS supplemented with complete Mini, EDTA-free Protease Inhibitor Cocktail and PhosSTOP both from Roche) 1 tablet each for 10 mL lysis buffer.
7. Doxycycline hyclate.

2.2 3D Culture, Fixation, and Staining

1. Organic eggs.
2. Büchner funnel 2 mm.
3. 8-chamber slides.
4. Microscope coverslips.
5. Trypsin–EDTA (10× solution).
6. Paraformaldehyde phosphate buffer (PFA) (used as diluted to 2% in PBS).
7. Methanol.
8. Immunofluorescence (IF) buffer (7.7 mM NaN_3, 0.1% bovine serum albumin, 0.2% Triton X-100, and 0.5% Tween-20 in PBS).
9. Blocking buffer—IF buffer supplemented with 10% normal goat serum.
10. Hoechst 33258.
11. Antibodies:
    (a) Hepsin (rabbit polyclonal antibody) (Cayman Chemicals).
    (b) α6-Integrin (mouse monoclonal antibody) (Millipore).
    (c) Alexa Fluor 546, goat anti-mouse IgG.
    (d) Alexa Fluor 488, goat anti-rabbit IgG.

(e) Microscope coverslips.

(f) Immu-Mount reagent (Thermo Fisher Scientific).

2.3 Imaging

1. Confocal microscope Leica TCS SP8.
2. Lasers: argon (488), helium-neon (543 and 633), and diode (405) lasers.
3. Objective 40× DIC.
4. Two descanned high sensitivity hybrid GaAsp detectors (HyD) and one photomultiplier tube (PMT) detector.

3 Methods

3.1 Validation of Ectopic Hepsin Expression (2D Culture and Validation)

1. Culture MCF10A-hepsin^{IND20} cells in complete medium at 37 °C and 5% CO_2, and add G418 disulfate salt solution (1:125) to select the positive cells.
2. To check hepsin expression levels, seed approximately 3–4 × 10^5 MCF10A-hepsin^{IND20} cells/well in a 6-well plate with 2 mL of complete medium.
3. Once the cells are 80% confluent, add 100 ng/mL of doxycycline to the cells to induce hepsin expression (*see* **Note 1**).
4. After 48 h incubation, lyse the cells with 100 μL lysis buffer.
5. Validate hepsin protein expression by Western blot analysis.

3.2 Setting Up 3D Egg White Culture

1. Purchase organic eggs from grocery store and clean the egg shell with 70% ethanol. Separate the egg white from the yolk and filter it through Büchner funnel (*see* **Note 2**).
2. Aliquot and store at −80 °C.
3. Thaw egg white in room temperature before use (*see* **Note 3**).
4. Coat each chamber of 8-chamber slide with 50 μL egg white. Spread the egg white in the chamber with a pipette to avoid monolayer cell growth (*see* **Note 4**).
5. Add 20 μL egg white at the center of the slide to avoid any gaps, thus making the final volume of egg white 70 μL (*see* **Note 5**).
6. Incubate the egg white-coated slides at 60 °C for 50–60 min, until egg white becomes semisolid (*see* **Note 6**).
7. While the egg white is incubating, trypsinize MCF10A-hepsin^{IND20} cells with 1× trypsin–EDTA and resuspend in complete medium.
8. Wash the chambers with 400 μL MCDB media, to wash out any loose egg white (*see* **Note 7**).

9. Seed 2,000 viable cells per chamber in 400 μL MCDB media on top of the egg white (*see* **Note 8**).
10. Change media on the 4th day of culture after carefully aspirating the old media. Add 900 ng/mL doxycycline to the medium on the 4th day to induce hepsin expression, Milli-Q water was used as vehicle (*see* **Note 9**), culture the cells until day 7 (*see* **Note 10**).

3.3 Fixing 3D Culture

1. Remove the medium and wash the cells twice with 400 μL PBS, 20 min each wash (*see* **Note 11**).
2. Fix the cells with 200 μL of 2% PFA at room temperature for 20 min.
3. After fixation, wash the cells twice with 400 μL PBS, 20 min each wash (*see* **Note 12**).

3.4 Immunostaining of the 3D Culture

1. Permeabilize the fixed 3D culture cells 200 μL of ice-cold 100% methanol (*see* **Note 13**).
2. Wash three times with PBS, 10 min each wash.
3. Incubate the cells with 200 μL blocking buffer at room temperature for 1.5 h.
4. After blocking, incubate the cells in primary antibodies diluted in 150 μL of blocking buffer overnight at 4 °C (antibody concentration ranges from 1:250 to 1:500; *see* **Note 14**).
5. Wash cells three times with 400 μL of IF buffer at room temperature (20 min each wash on a rocker (*see* **Note 15**)).
6. Incubate the cells with appropriate Alexa Fluor-conjugated secondary antibody diluted in 150 μL of blocking solution (*see* **Note 16**) (antibody concentration ranges from 1:300 to 1:500; *see* **Note 14**) at room temperature for 45 min.
7. Wash the 3D cultures twice with 400 μL of IF buffer at room temperature.
8. Counterstain the nuclei with 150 μL of Hoechst 33258 (1:10,000 in PBS) for 15 min at room temperature. Wash once with PBS.
9. After the immunostaining, carefully detach the chamber from the slide, dip the slide into conical centrifuge tube with water, carefully dry the excess water from the slide, and mount the full-length coverslip using few drops of Immu-Mount reagent (*see* **Note 17**).

3.5 Imaging

Images for the basement membrane integrity (α6-integrin) were acquired using confocal microscope Leica TCS SP8 equipped with argon (488), helium-neon (543 and 633), and diode (405) lasers and 40× DIC objective. Fluorescence signal was detected using two descanned high sensitivity hybrid GaAsp detectors (HyD) and one conventional PMT detectors.

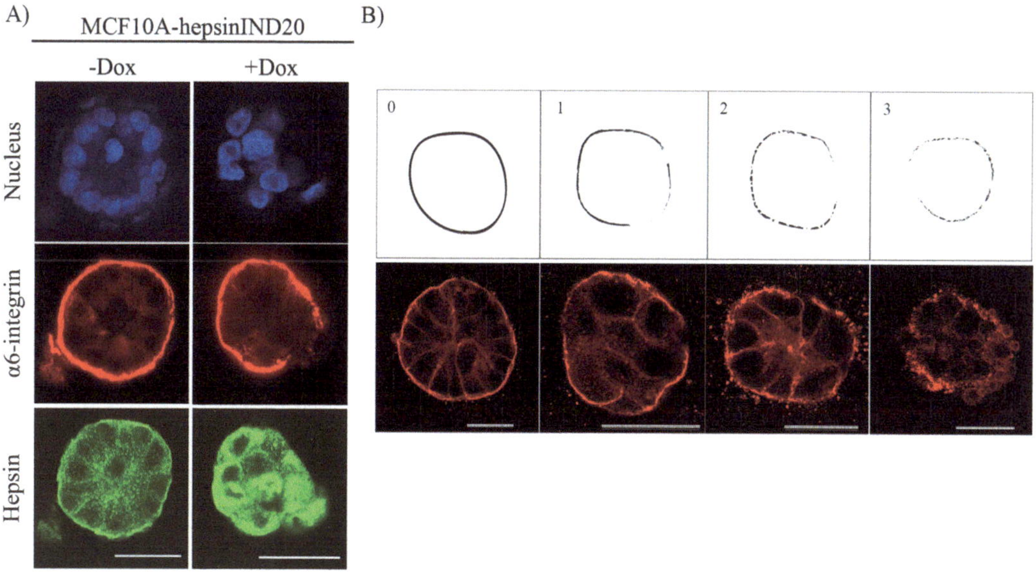

Fig. 1 Hepsin overexpression disrupts basement membrane in 3D culture. (**a**) Representative image of MCF10A-hepsinIND20 organoids cultured on egg white showing deterioration of basal α6-integrin immunoreactivity. MCF10A-hepsinIND20 organoids were grown for 4 days followed by addition of 900 ng/mL doxycycline or carrier (H_2O). The organoids were further grown for 3 more days before immunostaining. (**b**) Schematic representation of different categories of basement membrane degradation highlighting the loss of α6-integrin immunoreactivity upon hepsin induction. Scale bar = 25 μm

3.6 Analysis of the Basement Membrane Degradation

Images were then analyzed manually using Photoshop software. The organoids were divided into four different categories based on the level of damage to the basement membrane which appear as discontinuous staining of the basement membrane (α6-integrin). The MCF10A organoids (without hepsin overexpression) with intact basement membrane were used as control and scored (0). Hepsin overexpressing organoids were further divided into low (score 1), moderate (score 2), and high (score 3) level of damage caused to the basement membrane (Fig. 1a and b). The results were derived by quantitating organoids from ten field of views per experiment, from three biological replicates.

4 Notes

1. Hepsin induction should be tested with increasing concentration of doxycycline both in monolayer and 3D culture system. The concentrations provided may vary depending on the transduction efficacy and amount of viral transgene integrations.
2. Egg white should be separated carefully without mixing the yolk and filtered through 2 mm Büchner funnel without using

the filter paper. Since egg white is viscous, it might be desirable to cut the tip of the pipette tips. If the egg white forms clumps, it should be discarded.

3. In case of stored egg white, it is necessary to check the consistency after thawing as long-term storage may lead to increased clump formation and the egg white may not spread evenly around the chamber.
4. While coating the 8-well chamber with egg white, it is necessary to spread the egg white at the bottom of the chamber avoiding any gaps. Since the presence of small gap may lead to cell monolayer formation.
5. After coating the chamber with 50 μL egg white, it is desirable to add 20 μL egg white at the center of the well, as the egg white in contact with the sidewalls of the chamber may stick and rise on the sidewalls because of the capillary actions. This may lead to uneven distribution of the egg white at the center of the well.
6. After heating the egg white, it is important to check that the egg white is semisolid and has turned slightly opaque. However, it is important not to let the egg white dry out. The time period provided is a guideline and might need to be optimized.
7. It is necessary to wash the egg white with the media before seeding the cells to get rid of any loose egg white at the top. The presence of loose egg white leads to loss of organoids during the following washing steps.
8. It is desirable to optimize the number of cells seeded on the egg white depending upon the readout. Higher number of cell or longer growth period might result in fusion of the organoids or formation of cell monolayer.
9. An important consideration while optimizing hepsin induction in 3D culture is that it might require up to tenfold increase in doxycycline concentration compared to the monolayer culture.
10. Depending on the hepsin expression levels and the desired readout, the time period for hepsin induction should be optimized.
11. Special care should be given during the washes to avoid loss of egg white and the organoids. Wash steps can be shortened or even omitted to maximize the acinus yield.
12. If the immunofluorescent staining is not started on the same day, store the cells at 4 °C in the last PBS wash buffer.
13. Methanol at −20 °C was used to permeabilize the cells.

14. Both primary and secondary antibody concentrations might require further optimization as the concentrations provided in this protocol are only guidelines.
15. Wash time can be shorter (15 min) depending on the antibody.
16. Antibody solution volume can be reduced to save antibody, however, the egg white should not dry out during the incubation.
17. Excess water can be sucked out carefully by suction system mounted with pipette tip.

Acknowledgments

We would like to acknowledge all the members of the Klefström laboratory for their critical input in developing this protocol. Special thanks to Tiina Raatikainen and Tarja Välimäki for technical assistance. Biomedicum Imaging Unit and Biomedicum Functional Genomics Unit are acknowledged for core services and technical support. This study was supported by funding from the Academy of Finland, TEKES, Finnish Cancer Organizations, Doctoral Program in Biomedicine, and University of Helsinki.

References

1. Szabo R, Bugge TH (2011) Membrane-anchored serine proteases in vertebrate cell and developmental biology. Annu Rev Cell Dev Biol 27:213–235. https://doi.org/10.1146/annurev-cellbio-092910-154247
2. Antalis TM, Buzza MS, Hodge KM et al (2010) The cutting edge: membrane-anchored serine protease activities in the pericellular microenvironment. Biochem J 428(3):325–346. https://doi.org/10.1042/BJ20100046
3. Hedstrom L (2002) Serine protease mechanism and specificity. Chem Rev 102(12):4501–4524
4. Murray AS, Varela FA, List K (2016) Type II transmembrane serine proteases as potential targets for cancer therapy. Biol Chem 397(9):815–826. https://doi.org/10.1515/hsz-2016-0131
5. Tanabe LM, List K (2016) The role of type II transmembrane serine protease-mediated signaling in cancer. FEBS J. https://doi.org/10.1111/febs.13971
6. Dhanasekaran SM, Barrette TR, Ghosh D et al (2001) Delineation of prognostic biomarkers in prostate cancer. Nature 412(6849):822–826. https://doi.org/10.1038/35090585
7. Partanen JI, Tervonen TA, Myllynen M et al (2012) Tumor suppressor function of liver kinase B1 (Lkb1) is linked to regulation of epithelial integrity. Proc Natl Acad Sci U S A 109(7):E388–E397. https://doi.org/10.1073/pnas.1120421109
8. Tervonen TA, Belitskin D, Pant SM et al (2016) Deregulated hepsin protease activity confers oncogenicity by concomitantly augmenting HGF/MET signalling and disrupting epithelial cohesion. Oncogene 35(14):1832–1846. https://doi.org/10.1038/onc.2015.248
9. Xing P, Li JG, Jin F et al (2011) Clinical and biological significance of hepsin overexpression in breast cancer. J Investig Med 59(5):803–810. https://doi.org/10.2310/JIM.0b013e31821451a1
10. Matsuo T, Nakamura K, Takamoto N et al (2008) Expression of the serine protease hepsin and clinical outcome of human endometrial cancer. Anticancer Res 28(1A):159–164
11. Miao J, Mu D, Ergel B et al (2008) Hepsin colocalizes with desmosomes and induces progression of ovarian cancer in a mouse model. Int J Cancer 123(9):2041–2047. https://doi.org/10.1002/ijc.23726

12. Klezovitch O, Chevillet J, Mirosevich J et al (2004) Hepsin promotes prostate cancer progression and metastasis. Cancer Cell 6(2):185–195. https://doi.org/10.1016/j.ccr.2004.07.008
13. Li W, Wang BE, Moran P et al (2009) Pegylated kunitz domain inhibitor suppresses hepsin-mediated invasive tumor growth and metastasis. Cancer Res 69(21):8395–8402. https://doi.org/10.1158/0008-5472.CAN-09-1995
14. Pantel K, Brakenhoff RH (2004) Dissecting the metastatic cascade. Nat Rev Cancer 4(6):448–456. https://doi.org/10.1038/nrc1370
15. Guan X (2015) Cancer metastases: challenges and opportunities. Acta Pharm Sin B 5(5): 402–418. https://doi.org/10.1016/j.apsb.2015.07.005
16. Tripathi M, Nandana S, Yamashita H et al (2008) Laminin-332 is a substrate for hepsin, a protease associated with prostate cancer progression. J Biol Chem 283(45):30576–30584. https://doi.org/10.1074/jbc.M802312200
17. Walko G, Castanon MJ, Wiche G (2015) Molecular architecture and function of the hemidesmosome. Cell Tissue Res 360(3):529–544. https://doi.org/10.1007/s00441-015-2216-6
18. Bissell MJ, Rizki A, Mian IS (2003) Tissue architecture: the ultimate regulator of breast epithelial function. Curr Opin Cell Biol 15(6): 753–762
19. Debnath J, Brugge JS (2005) Modelling glandular epithelial cancers in three-dimensional cultures. Nat Rev Cancer 5(9):675–688. https://doi.org/10.1038/nrc1695
20. Debnath J, Muthuswamy SK, Brugge JS (2003) Morphogenesis and oncogenesis of MCF-10A mammary epithelial acini grown in three-dimensional basement membrane cultures. Methods 30(3):256–268
21. Hoffman AS (2002) Hydrogels for biomedical applications. Adv Drug Deliv Rev 54(1):3–12
22. Kaipparettu BA, Kuiatse I, Tak-Yee Chan B et al (2008) Novel egg white-based 3-D cell culture system. BioTechniques 45(2):165–168., 170-161. https://doi.org/10.2144/000112883

Chapter 17

Evaluation of Tumor Vasculature Using a Syngeneic Tumor Model in Wild-Type and Genetically Modified Mice

Francisco Javier Rodríguez-Baena, Silvia Redondo-García, María del Carmen Plaza-Calonge, Rubén Fernández-Rodríguez, and Juan Carlos Rodríguez-Manzaneque

Abstract

The relevance of tumor vasculature has been extensively recognized, and it is still the focus of numerous lines of research for basic, translational, and clinical scientists. Indeed, the knowledge of some of its regulatory mechanisms has provoked the generation of ongoing cancer therapies. Within the context of the tumor microenvironment, the information that the analysis of the vasculature provides is very valuable, and it might reveal not just its quality and the response against a specific therapy but also its close relationship with neighboring stromal and tumor players.

Studies during last decades already supported the contribution of extracellular proteases in neovascularization events, including ADAMTS. However, deeper analyses are still required to better understand the modulation of their proteolytic activity in the tumor microenvironment. Future studies will clearly benefit from existing and ongoing genetically modified mouse models.

Here we emphasize the use of syngeneic models to study the vasculature during tumor progression, supported by their intact immunocompetent capacities and also by the range of possibilities to play with engineered mice and with modified tumor cells. Although various high-tech and sophisticated approaches have already been reported to evaluate tumor neovascularization, here we describe a simple and easily reproduced methodology based in the immunofluorescence detection of vascular-specific molecules. A final in silico analysis guarantees an unbiased quantification of tumor vasculature under different conditions.

Key words Extracellular microenvironment, In silico analysis, Metalloproteinase, Tumor stroma, Vasculature

1 Introduction

A profound knowledge of tumor neovascularization has been pursued since last decades of the twentieth century, and it is still a main topic of research for numerous laboratories. The understanding of the regulatory mechanisms of vascularization has already allowed the design of new and ongoing cancer therapies, so its continuous

Santiago Cal and Alvaro J. Obaya (eds.), *Proteases and Cancer: Methods and Protocols*, Methods in Molecular Biology, vol. 1731, https://doi.org/10.1007/978-1-4939-7595-2_17, © Springer Science+Business Media, LLC 2018

evaluation appears as a requirement for basic and translational investigations [1]. More recent advances remarked the concept of tumor heterogeneity, supporting fundamental roles to distinct tumor subpopulations, like cancer stem and tumor-initiating cells, but also to non-tumor compartments such as the vascular niche, immune-related infiltrates, and cancer-associated fibroblasts [2]. Although a great body of techniques has been developed to study the tumor microenvironment, still the information that vasculature provides is unique regarding its functional characteristics such as permeability and leakage, distribution throughout the tumor, association to supportive cells, and relationship with molecular and cell players within the tumor scenario. Importantly, the literature attributes to the vascular niche a main role for the appearance of resistance episodes to chemotherapy but also to antiangiogenic agents [3].

In this setting, the impact of the vasculature on the communication between cancer cells and stroma constituents during distinct stages of tumor progression has been an inspiring field of investigation during the last decades. Among the multitude of factors within this intricate scenario, some extracellular proteases have been already a target of interest as modifiers of the tumor microenvironment. However, their inhibition with non-specific drugs was a total failure, unveiling at the same time their complexity [4]. The contribution of extracellular proteases during vascularization has been outlined previously [5]. Their participation during the degradation of the vascular basement membrane has been reported, facilitating angiogenic sprouting but also tumor invasion through modified extracellular matrices [6]. Indeed, bioactive proteolytic fragments from ECM have shown both angioinhibitory and proangiogenic properties [7]. As regards to ADAMTS proteases, studies about their contribution during vascularization revealed a multifaceted scenario that requires a deeper understanding of the extracellular microenvironment [8]. For example, the angiostatic properties of the first member ADAMTS1 have been described in distinct models [9–11], but other studies support a pro-metastatic and tumorigenic role [12–15]. In fact some of these reports suggest the necessity to discern if the protease is provided by tumor or stromal components, together with their overlapping with vascular-related substrates.

At this point, the tremendous importance of mouse models to study tumor biology does not require a thoughtful presentation. Their use forms part of a majority of studies in outstanding basic and clinical cancer research journals. Indeed the relevance of some of these models to investigate matrix metalloproteinases has been reviewed elsewhere [16]. Furthermore, the current development of new editing tools would expand the generation of genetically modified mice almost for unlimited purposes. The specific use of syngeneic models still allows to study tumor progression in an immunocompetent setting and also permits the use of compatible tumor cells that could be alternatively modified, independent of the host mouse itself. Here we described the use of B16F1 mouse melanoma cells, first isolated from lung metastases from the original B16F0 melanoma [17], and Lewis Lung Carcinoma (LLC) [18], both of them compatible with a C57BL/6 background and widely used to study tumor progression and metastasis. Significantly, while the overall or cell-specific expression levels of a protease, or any gene of interest, could be modified in a mouse model with consequences for the stroma constituents, the additional possibilities are remarkable to modify such expression in the tumor compartment, represented by the injected cell line. In this line, a recent study has been reported for ADAMTS1 [15]. Furthermore, the use of these animal models to accomplish intricate molecular and cellular determinations is easily suitable, as noted in this chapter, including the therapeutic treatment with novel drugs or combinations to translate to the clinic.

Finally, multiple assays have been developed to evaluate angiogenesis and vascularization, including the use of mouse tumor models [19]. Indeed, very sophisticated noninvasive and microscopy tools have been described [20, 21], but they are far from a routine basis. Here we described a simple immunofluorescence-based methodology that allows the visualization of tumor vasculature and an easy unbiased quantification by an in silico approach.

2 Materials

2.1 Equipment and Reagents for Cell Culture

1. Tissue culture hood/biological safety cabinet.
2. CO_2 incubator with humid atmosphere.
3. Light microscope.
4. Liquid handling pipettes and disposable sterile tips.
5. 1.5 mL conical tubes.
6. Tissue-culture grade plates.
7. Neubauer hemocytometer.
8. Dulbecco's Modified Eagle Medium (DMEM).
9. Penicillin/streptomycin (P/S).
10. Fetal bovine serum (FBS).
11. Phosphate buffered saline (PBS).
12. 0.05% trypsin.
13. Trypan blue cell culture solution.

14. Mouse melanoma B16F1 (and derived) and Lewis lung carcinoma (LLC) cells are suitable for these assays, according to their C57BL/6 strain background (*see* **Note 1**).

2.2 Equipment and Reagents for Tumor Induction, Monitoring, and Dissection

1. 1 mL syringes with 25 G needle.
2. Caliper.
3. Anesthesia vaporizer and distributor.
4. Sterile scissors.
5. Sterile tweezers.
6. Sterile surgical scalpel.
7. Pins or small needles to fasten mice.
8. Precision scale.
9. 15 and 50 mL conical tubes.
10. Rack holders.
11. Digital camera.
12. Parafilm M.
13. Ruler.
14. Dry ice.
15. Isoflurane.
16. Two- to three-month-old C57BL/6 mice are used (*see* **Note 2**). All mice were kept and maintained under standard 12 h light-dark cycles, ad libitum, and with standard chow pellet diet.

2.3 Equipment and Reagents for Tumor Fixation and Block Preparation for Sectioning

1. Embedding cassettes.
2. Base molds.
3. Steel forceps.
4. Water bath.
5. Superfrost microscope slides.
6. Microtome.
7. 4% paraformaldehyde (PFA) or 10% neutral buffered formalin (NBF) in 1× PBS for tumor fixation.
8. Pure water (Elix® Millipore) (pH_2O).
9. Different ethanol solutions (100, 96, and 70% v/v pH_2O).
10. Xylene or substitute.
11. Paraffin wax.
12. PBS.

2.4 Equipment and Reagents for Immunofluorescence and Vasculature Detection

1. TPX staining holders and tray (microwave proof).
2. Histology staining set or nylon gaskets.
3. Microwave.
4. Epifluorescence microscope.

5. Humid chamber for antibody incubation.
6. Glass coverslips.
7. Xylene or substitute.
8. Different ethanol solutions (100, 96, and 70% v/v pH_2O).
9. PBS.
10. PAP pen (Cat. Z377821, Sigma).
11. 0.05% Tween 20 in 1× PBS (PBST) for tissue permeabilization and washes.
12. Blocking solution: 3% bovine serum albumin (BSA), 1% donkey serum, and 0.05% Tween 20, in 1× PBS.
13. Antibody incubation solution: 1% BSA, 1% donkey serum, and 0.05% Tween 20, in 1× PBS.
14. Antigen retrieval solutions: 10 mM Tris–HCl pH 7 for CD31 and endomucin antibodies. 10 mM sodium citrate pH 10 for endomucin antibody.
15. Primary antibodies: rabbit polyclonal to CD31 and rat monoclonal to endomucin (Cat. 65495, SCBT).
16. Secondary antibodies: For CD31, use anti-rabbit Alexa Fluor 488 and Alexa Fluor 555. For endomucin, use anti-rat Alexa Fluor 488 and Alexa Fluor 555.
17. 4′,6′-Diamino-2-phenylindole (DAPI).
18. Mowiol reagent microscopy grade for immunofluorescence.
19. 1,4-Diazabicyclo-[2.2.2]-octane (DABCO) as antifading agent to prevent photo bleaching. It needs to be previously prepared by adding it to warm Mowiol at a 2.5% final concentration. This solution last up to 1 month at 4 °C.

2.5 Software Analysis Requirements

1. ImageJ or Fiji software (NIH, USA).
2. Wimasis®, alternative non-free web-based software for the analysis of the vasculature (*see* **Note 3**).

3 Methods

3.1 Preparation of Tumor Cell Suspension for Injection

Cell lines are maintained under optimal growth conditions at 37 °C, 5% CO_2, and 95% humidity atmosphere. Tumor cells should be in culture at least 1 week after thawing to achieve standard growth rates.

1. Cells are passaged at least 24–48 h prior to cell suspension preparation (scheme in Fig. 1a).
2. A confluence of 80–90% is optimal for cell suspension preparation. Overconfluent cell cultures might compromise cell growth rate, so it should be avoided.

3. Prior to trypsinization, the culture media is removed followed by two gentle washes with sterile PBS.
4. For a 100 mm plate, add 1 mL of 0.05% trypsin. Place the plate for 5 min in the incubator, and check under a light microscope for cell detachment.
5. Add 2–3 mL of complete growth medium (DMEM, 10% FBS and 1% P/S), and pipette gently up and down until a single-cell suspension is obtained. Place the solution in a conical tube and spin the samples during 5 min, 300 × *g* at RT.
6. Discard the supernatant, add sterile PBS, and pipette up and down to rinse cells from media and serum debris. Spin again during 5 min, 300 × *g* at RT. Repeat this process twice.
7. Finally resuspend the cell pellet in sterile PBS, and check cell density and viability using trypan blue. Proper final dilutions are 1×10^6 cells/100 μL for B16F1 and 5×10^5/100 μL for LLC. For other cell lines, please follow recommendations provided by the bibliography.
8. Aliquot an excess of cells in 1.5 mL conical tubes, according to the number of mice to be injected (scheme in Fig. 1a). This excess is to prevent possible mistakes during the injection process. Tubes should be sealed with parafilm in order to avoid unexpected leakage and variations in the volume.
9. Proceed as soon as possible with the injection of the cell suspension to avoid cell death. It is recommended to put back in a culture plate the remaining cells after the injection, in order to evaluate cell death during all the injection process. Under normal circumstances cells remain viable during 2 h at least.

3.2 Tumor Induction and Monitorization

1. Mice are anesthetized in an isoflurane-based vaporizer chamber at least 10 min prior to tumor cell injection.
2. Prepare the syringe with the cell suspension, avoiding the presence of bubbles to inject the correct cell number. Do not forget to gently swirl the syringe right before the injection to avoid the deposition of cells.
3. Pinching the animal skin, perform a subcutaneous injection with the desired amount of cell suspension (100 μL is recommended) with a controlled release in the right flank of the animal (scheme in Fig. 1a) (*see* **Note 4**).
4. Place the injected animal into the housing cages, and observe its full recovery from the anesthesia.
5. Tumor growth is monitored every 2–3 days, up to day 21 or until the tumor reaches the desired or allowed volume (*see* **Note 5**). Use a caliper and take photographs for the record.
6. All animals are sacrificed using the proper animal welfare ethical guidelines.

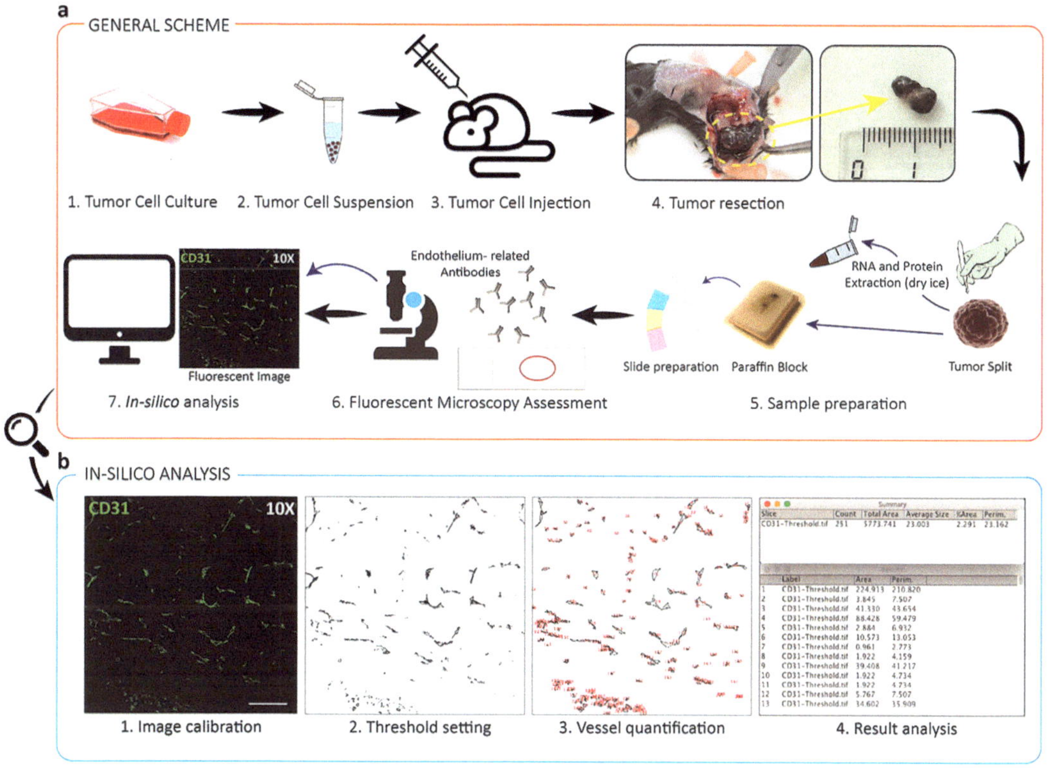

Fig. 1 (**a**) General scheme representing the procedures performed to obtain vasculature parameters from syngeneic tumors. (**b**) Main steps for in silico analysis of images

3.3 Tumor Resection, Paraffin Embedding, and Sectioning

1. Place the mice, recently sacrificed, over a proper surface for surgery procedures (e.g., cork surface with filter paper). This procedure needs to be fast, rigorous, and neat in order to prevent tumor damaging and degradation of the biological material. It is important to take all necessary measurements prior to the sample split for different purposes.
2. Fasten the animal facing the tumor using laboratory pins or small needles in every limb.
3. Spray the mouse surface with 70% EtOH.
4. Using forceps and scissors, pinch the animal skin and make a small incision in the surrounding tumor area. Keep cutting the skin around the tumor until a pocket is open.
5. Use a scalpel and a new blade to separate the skin from the tumor without altering the tumor structure (scheme in Fig. 1a).
6. Remove the tumor, place it in a piece of parafilm, and proceed with the macroscopic examination. A cold surface could be used to maintain the integrity of the tumor.

7. Weight the tumor, and measure three different dimensions with the caliper to obtain the tumor volume. Take a photograph of the tumor showing a ruler or scale (scheme in Fig. 1a).
8. Cut the tumor into pieces with a clean scalpel in order to split the sample for different experimental purposes (scheme in Fig. 1a). For RNA and protein extraction, a small representative piece can be frozen in dry ice (less or more than 30 mg, respectively, is recommended).
9. For fixation, a representative piece of the tumor is immersed in 10% NBF (or 4% PFA). The fixative volume should be about 20 times that of the tumor weight (e.g., 2 mL of fixative for 100 mg of tumor). Fixation should be carried for 24–48 h at RT.
10. If long storage of the fixed tissue is required, transfer the sample to a 70% EtOH solution after fixation (*see* **Note 6**).
11. Proceed with a standard paraffin-embedding protocol.
12. From paraffin tumor blocks, obtain the desired microtome sections (scheme in Fig. 1a). For vasculature analyses, section thickness should be between 5 and 10 μm.

3.4 Immunofluorescence of Vasculature with Specific Antibodies

1. Preheat the sample slides in an oven to 65 °C during 1 h or until the wax has melted down. Wait 1–2 min to cool down the slides before proceeding with further steps. Place the slides into xylene or substitute solution three times during 5 min each (*see* **Note 7**).
2. To rehydrate the sample, follow with two immersions into absolute EtOH during 5 min each.
3. Place the slides in 96% EtOH during 5 min, twice.
4. Place the slides in 70% EtOH during 5 min.
5. Place the slides in fresh pH_2O during 5 min.
6. Place the slides in fresh sterile PBS during 5 min.
7. For antigen retrieval, place the slides in a microwave-proof gasket immersed in the antigen retrieval solution, and incubate them during 10 min at 800 W. Alternative antigen retrieval protocols could be approached according to the manufacturer's antibody guidelines.
8. Let the samples cool down at least 20–30 min before continuing the procedure.
9. Wash twice the slides with PBST.
10. With the PAP pen, draw a circle surrounding the tumor sample without touching its edges and avoiding the sample to dry.

11. Place the slides in a humid chamber, and add 50–100 μL of blocking solution. Incubate during 1 h in darkness.
12. Wash twice with PBST.
13. Primary antibody incubation is performed in a dark and humid chamber, with 50–100 μL of antibody incubation solution, including antibodies at the following dilutions: 1:50 for CD31 antibody and 1:100 for endomucin antibody. Overnight incubation at 4 °C is recommended, although alternative conditions could be followed according to manufacturer's guidelines.
14. Wash twice with PBST.
15. Secondary antibody incubation is performed during 1 h at RT in a dark and humid chamber, with 50–100 μL of antibody incubation solution, including antibodies at 1:100 dilution.
16. Wash twice with PBST.
17. Add DAPI (1 μg/mL final concentration) in 1× PBS and incubate 5 min in darkness.
18. Wash three times with PBST.
19. Dry the slides using a soft tissue without damaging the tumor section. Then add 20–30 μL of Mowiol with antifading agent as mounting media.
20. Place a glass coverslip and let the samples dry at RT in darkness for 2 h and overnight at 4 °C. Then, samples are ready for analysis, or they can be stored at 4 °C.
21. Assess immunofluorescence using an epifluorescence microscope. In this case, an Axioimager A1 microscope (Zeiss) was used to obtain 10× magnification images of the samples (scheme in Fig. 1a).
22. The whole tumor section is imaged for further in silico analysis. Images obtained must be converted to 8-bit and should be stored as black and white and tiff extension (scheme in Fig. 1a).

3.5 In Silico Analysis of Tumor Vasculature

The following steps refer to the use of ImageJ (version 1.48v) or Fiji (version 2.0.0-rc-48/1.50i). It is an open access and can be downloaded from NIH secure server (https://imagej.nih.gov/ij/ or https://imagej.net/Fiji/Downloads). As previously stated, images to be analyzed should meet particular requirements. For a specific set of samples, at least one of the images needs to be saved with the scale. This scale will allow to determine the area and to calculate the vessel perimeter and additional parameters.

1. The image with the scale needs to be opened first to calibrate the program (Fig. 1b).
2. Using the "line tool," draw a line coinciding with the length of the scale. Use the zoom option to enlarge the scale and ease the task.
3. Select the known scale (100 μm generally) and calibrate: Analyse—Set Scale. Change "Known distance" to 100 μm and "Unit of length" to μm, and check "Global" to apply the same scale within the following images (*see* **Note 8**).
4. Open the image of interest: File—Open—Select image. A new window will pop up. Uncheck "Disable Global Calibration" to maintain the same calibration for all images, and check "Disable these Messages" to avoid this window to appear every time that a new image is open.
5. Delimitate area sample using rectangular, oval, polygon, or freehand selection tools, depending on area's shape. Using the command *Ctrl* (or *Cmd* in Mac OS) + *A*, or Edit—Selection—Select All, the total area of the picture can be selected.
6. Measure area using the command *Ctrl* (or *Cmd* in Mac OS) + *M* or Analyze—Measure. Copy area measurement in a spreadsheet.
7. To segment the image and measure the blood vessel area is necessary to select a threshold by selecting Image—Adjust—Threshold—Set—Ok. The threshold will be given depending on the images that have been taken (Fig. 1b). When users take different pictures, the threshold may change due to different microscopy settings (*see* **Note 9**).
8. Select which results are required (the most commonly used are vessel count, total area, average size, % area and perimeter): Analyse—Set Measurements.
9. To measure blood vessels, click Analyse—Analyse Particles. You need to select a particle size to discriminate from background signal or debris. For this, start selecting from 1 to infinity and also check the "display results" box and also "show" outlines. This would generate a new image in which every vessel is surrounded by a circle and numerated. Repeat this procedure changing the particle range until the user criteria is met (Fig. 1b).
10. In this section also check the boxes "Clear results" and "Summarize" to sum up the results and "Include holes" to count open blood vessels.
11. Click "OK" and the analyzed results and image will appear in a new window. Copy the results into a new spreadsheet. Follow with the rest of the images (Fig. 1b) (*see* **Note 10**).

4 Notes

1. Additional tumor cell lines can be used for this assay as long as they are compatible with the specific available mouse strain.
2. A wide set of genetically modified mice could be used in a similar manner to the syngeneic model described here. In addition, tumor progression can be challenged with distinct therapeutic regimes (according to the field of interest of the reader). Therefore, the vasculature would be analyzed at different time points, drug concentrations, combinatory therapies, etc. As an example, Fig. 2 shows a practical example of the evaluation of tumor vasculature in wild-type and *Adamts1* knockout mice [15].
3. Wimasis (https://www.wimasis.com/en/) is a web-based software with multifunctional tools for cell and histology analyses. The assessment of the vasculature is one of their functions, and the outcome is complete and reliable.
4. Depending on the tumor cell line or the experiment's purpose, the injection area can vary. For the procedures carried in this protocol, a subcutaneous right flank injection is preferred. Nevertheless, subcutaneous injections can be performed in the neck and other areas.
5. Prior to the animal sacrifice, additional procedures could be performed to obtain more information about the tumor vasculature. For example, the injection of fluorescent-labeled lectins provides a fluorescent detection of tumor and tissue vessels without further antibody incubation [22, 23]. Also, the injection of pimonidazole (Hypoxyprobe, Inc.) provides a helpful insight about hypoxic areas to study tumor vessel functionality [15].
6. The tumor size and volume should be measured prior to its fixation. If the piece is too large, the fixation would take a longer time. If the fixation is not enough, the tumor could shrink and crack the paraffin wax in the block. Regarding fixation reagent, NBF is preferred according to its longer lifespan.
7. The deparaffinization process is recommended to be carried under a gentle agitation, helping to the removal of wax from undesired areas and also to the penetration and replacement of fixative solution by water.
8. For test calibration, draw a line again in the known scale within the same first image. Click Analyze—Measure; the known line should be 100 μm. For every analysis, a single calibration with a single scale bar is necessary. Be aware that the scale calibration disappears when you close the program. Every analysis should be performed at once in order to obtain comparable results.

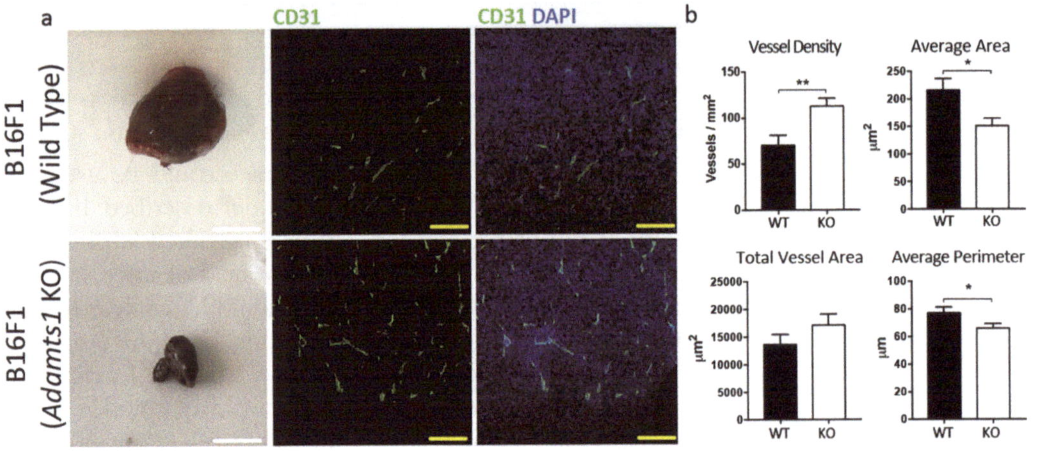

Fig. 2 Characterization of vasculature in B16F1-derived tumors in wild-type and *Adamts1* knockout mice. (**a**) Images of representative tumors obtained in wild-type and *Adamts1* knockout mice at day 18 postinjection (white scale bar = 5 mm) (left column) and fluorescence microscopy of representative sections showing CD31 and DAPI staining (yellow scale bar = 200 μm) (center and right columns). (**b**). Graphs representing results after in silico analyses of vasculature, including vessel density (vessels/mm^2), average vessel area (μm^2), total vessel area (μm^2), and average vessel perimeter. Bars show mean values ± SEM. Statistical analyses show unpaired t test. (*, $p < 0.05$; **, $p < 0.01$) (adapted from [15])

9. To set a correct threshold, it is necessary to discriminate between real vessels and unspecific noise. Adjusting these parameters, the image would turn into binary and the number of pixels would be counted. For this, a strict parameter set could lose information and non-well-adjusted could add wrong data to the results. Please note that the threshold may not be applied to all the images in the set; this depends on the user ability to obtain similar images from the fluorescence microscope.
10. Given the time-consuming task of this kind of analyses, the creation of a macro that automatizes the work is suggested. Official macros and plugins are available in the software website. These tools are intended as a collaborative work that researchers can share with each other to facilitate these tasks. Macros can be easily created with low levels of programming and software knowledge.

Acknowledgment

Work in the author's laboratory has been supported by grants from the Ministerio de Economía y Competitividad and Instituto de Salud Carlos III from Spain and cofinanced by FEDER (PI13/00168 and PI16/00345 to JCRM). SRG is supported by a contract from Garantía Juvenil (PEJ-2014-A-38416-MINECO-FSE).

For data shown, all mice were kept in the Centro de Investigaciones Biomédicas-UGR Animal Facility under pathogen-free conditions and according to institutional guidelines.

References

1. Carmeliet P, Jain RK (2011) Molecular mechanisms and clinical applications of angiogenesis. Nature 473(7347):298–307. https://doi.org/10.1038/nature10144
2. De Sousa E, Melo F, Vermeulen L et al (2013) Cancer heterogeneity – a multifaceted view. EMBO Rep 14(8):686–695. https://doi.org/10.1038/embor.2013.92
3. Jain RK (2014) Antiangiogenesis strategies revisited: from starving tumors to alleviating hypoxia. Cancer Cell 26:605–622. https://doi.org/10.1016/j.ccell.2014.10.006
4. Turk B (2006) Targeting proteases: successes, failures and future prospects. Nat Rev Drug Discov 5(9):785–799. https://doi.org/10.1038/nrd2092
5. Handsley MM, Edwards DR (2005) Metalloproteinases and their inhibitors in tumor angiogenesis. Int J Cancer 115(6):849–860. https://doi.org/10.1002/ijc.20945
6. Lu P, Takai K, Weaver VM et al (2011) Extracellular matrix degradation and remodeling in development and disease. Cold Spring Harb Perspect Biol 3:a005058. https://doi.org/10.1101/cshperspect.a005058
7. Bix G, Iozzo RV (2005) Matrix revolutions: "tails" of basement-membrane components with angiostatic functions. Trends Cell Biol 15:52–60. https://doi.org/10.1016/j.tcb.2004.11.008
8. Rodríguez-Manzaneque JC, Fernández-Rodríguez R, Rodríguez-Baena FJ et al (2015) ADAMTS proteases in vascular biology. Matrix Biol 44–46:38–45. https://doi.org/10.1016/j.matbio.2015.02.004
9. Reynolds LE, Watson AR, Baker M et al (2010) Tumour angiogenesis is reduced in the Tc1 mouse model of Down's syndrome. Nature 465(7299):813–817. https://doi.org/10.1038/nature09106
10. Martino-Echarri E, Fernández-Rodríguez R, Rodríguez-Baena FJ et al (2013) Contribution of ADAMTS1 as a tumor suppressor gene in human breast carcinoma. Linking its tumor inhibitory properties to its proteolytic activity on nidogen 1 and nidogen-2. Int J Cancer 133(10):2315–2324. https://doi.org/10.1002/ijc.28271
11. Casal C, Torres-Collado AX, Plaza-Calonge MCDC et al (2010) ADAMTS1 contributes to the acquisition of an endothelial-like phenotype in plastic tumor cells. Cancer Res 70(11):4676–4686. https://doi.org/10.1158/0008-5472.CAN-09-4197
12. Lu X, Wang Q, Hu G et al (2009) ADAMTS1 and MMP1 proteolytically engage EGF-like ligands in an osteolytic signaling cascade for bone metastasis. Genes Dev 23(16):1882–1894. https://doi.org/10.1101/gad.1824809
13. Ricciardelli C, Frewin KM, Tan IDA et al (2011) The ADAMTS1 protease gene is required for mammary tumor growth and metastasis. Am J Pathol 179(6):3075–3085. https://doi.org/10.1016/j.ajpath.2011.08.021
14. Rocks N, Paulissen G, Quesada-Calvo F et al (2008) ADAMTS-1 metalloproteinase promotes tumor development through the induction of a stromal reaction in vivo. Cancer Res 68(22):9541–9550. https://doi.org/10.1158/0008-5472.CAN-08-0548
15. Fernández-Rodríguez R, Rodríguez-Baena FJ, Martino-Echarri E et al (2016) Stroma-derived but not tumor ADAMTS1 is a main driver of tumor growth and metastasis. Oncotarget 7(23):34507–34519. 10.18632/oncotarget.8922
16. Wieczorek E, Jablonska E, Wasowicz W et al (2015) Matrix metalloproteinases and genetic mouse models in cancer research: a mini-review. Tumor Biol 36(1):163–175. https://doi.org/10.1007/s13277-014-2747-6
17. Poste G, Doll J, Hart IR et al (1980) In vitro selection of murine B16 melanoma variants with enhanced tissue-invasive properties. Cancer Res 40(5):1636–1644
18. Bertram JSJ, Janik PP (1980) Establishment of a cloned line of Lewis lung carcinoma cells adapted to cell culture. Cancer Lett 11(1):63–73. https://doi.org/10.1016/0304-3835(80)90130-5

19. Simons M, Alitalo K, Annex BH et al (2015) State-of-the-art methods for evaluation of angiogenesis and tissue vascularization: a scientific statement from the American Heart Association. Circ Res 116(11):e99–e132. https://doi.org/10.1161/RES.0000000000000054
20. Vakoc BJ, Lanning RM, Tyrrell JA et al (2009) Three-dimensional microscopy of the tumor microenvironment in vivo using optical frequency domain imaging. Nat Med 15(10): 1219–1223. https://doi.org/10.1038/nm.1971
21. Missbach-Guentner J, Hunia J, Alves F (2011) Tumor blood vessel visualization. Int J Dev Biol 55:535–546. https://doi.org/10.1387/ijdb.103229jm
22. Robertson RT, Levine ST, Haynes SM et al (2015) Use of labeled tomato lectin for imaging vasculature structures. Histochem Cell Biol 143(2):225–234. https://doi.org/10.1007/s00418-014-1301-3
23. Rodriguez-Manzaneque JC, Lane TF, Ortega MA et al (2001) Thrombospondin-1 suppresses spontaneous tumor growth and inhibits activation of matrix metalloproteinase-9 and mobilization of vascular endothelial growth factor. Proc Natl Acad Sci U S A 98(22):12485–12490. https://doi.org/10.1073/pnas.171460498

Chapter 18

3D Image Analysis of the Microvasculature in Healthy and Diseased Tissues

Álvaro Sahún-Español, Cristina Clemente, and Alicia G. Arroyo

Abstract

The vasculature ensures optimal delivery of nutrients and oxygen throughout the body. The ability to respond to changing tissue demands requires constant reshaping of the vascular network through modulation of its density, diameter, or patterning. These processes are especially prominent after tissue damage or in tumors. The matrix metalloproteinase (MMP) family of endopeptidases are key contributors to vascular remodeling, able to cleave all extracellular matrix components and also soluble factors and membrane receptors. Observations recorded over several decades have established that the vasculature changes in pathological contexts, and this has formed the basis for developing angiotherapies as a novel approach to treating disease. For example, inhibition of angiogenesis or normalization of the vasculature has been proposed as treatment for cancer and chronic inflammatory diseases. In contrast, boosting angiogenesis may be helpful in ischemic conditions such as myocardial infarction and in regenerative medicine. Classical histological methods for the analysis of tissue vasculature have relied on thin sections that do not capture the complex 3D structure of the vascular network. Given the importance of understanding disease-associated vascular changes for the development of rational angiotherapeutic interventions, we present a protocol for thick section-based 3D image analysis of vasculature structure and function.

Key words Vasculature, Thick section, Volumetric, Three-dimensional, Mouse, Confocal microscope, Quantification

1 Introduction

The vasculature must continually adapt to tissue demands in order to ensure optimal delivery of nutrients and oxygen throughout the body, particularly after tissue damage or in tumors. This adaptation requires constant reshaping of the vascular network by modulating its density, diameter, and/or complexity. Being aware of the vasculature changes in pathological contexts, researchers have proposed angiotherapies as a feasible treatment strategy.

When activated, the normally quiescent vasculature promotes the formation of new vessels from pre-existing ones in a process called angiogenesis. Angiogenic vascularization is a critical step in tumor growth, with tumors reportedly unable to grow in the

Santiago Cal and Alvaro J. Obaya (eds.), *Proteases and Cancer: Methods and Protocols*, Methods in Molecular Biology, vol. 1731, https://doi.org/10.1007/978-1-4939-7595-2_18, © Springer Science+Business Media, LLC 2018

absence of proper vascularization to more than 2–3 mm in diameter [1]. In addition, vascularization not only provides the tumor with nutrients but is also necessary for metastasis to occur [2, 3]. Because of this, some therapies are focused on abrogating tumor angiogenesis by depriving the tumor of oxygen and nutrients, causing a reduction in tumor growth. This therapeutic approach is very common for some types of cancer, such as breast cancer [4]. However, vascular architecture in the tumor is chaotic and tortuous, with vessels having irregular diameters and poor functionality due to improper lumen formation. Tumor vasculature also has defects in pericyte coverage and in endothelial cell junctions, making it highly permeable to nutrients and metastatic cells [5]. This extremely complex and abnormal vasculature has raised questions about drug delivery and efficacy of anti-angiogenic therapies [6]. An alternative approach is to normalize the aberrant vasculature to make the tumor more accessible to drugs, which has proved successful with some types of cancer [7]. In other cancers, such as pancreatic cancer, tumor growth and spread are reduced by strategies to increase vascular development [8]. These examples demonstrate the importance of a thorough understanding of the vascular plexus when deciding on the appropriate therapeutic approach.

Understanding the vascular architecture is essential not only for tumor angiotherapies but also for other pathological settings. A prominent example is regenerative medicine. An injured tissue needs to be revascularized in order to obtain oxygen and nutrients and to allow infiltration by effector immune cells for proper repair and regeneration [9]. Much of the attention in this area is focused on heart repair after myocardial infarction, and boosting angiogenesis after an ischemic event is considered one of the most promising approaches to improving cardiac repair and avoiding negative postinfarction effects [10, 11]. In the case of the injured heart, it is also important to understand the process of arteriogenesis, the growth of functional collateral arteries from pre-existing arterio-arteriolar anastomoses.

Angiotherapies are thus relevant to a broad spectrum of pathologies, including tumors and chronic inflammatory diseases that could benefit from angiogenesis inhibition or normalization of the aberrant vasculature. Ischemic disorders such as myocardial infarction by its part can benefit from boosting the vascularization as a promising strategy to promote tissue repair and regeneration. Angiotherapies have classically targeted angiogenic factors such as VEGFA and related receptors; however, other potential targets are the matrix metalloproteinases (MMPs), a family of proteolytic enzymes that make a varied contribution to angiogenesis and vasculature remodeling. MMPs are endopeptidases that play an important role in extracellular matrix (ECM) degradation and also modulate the bioactivity of soluble factors and membrane receptors. There are currently 25 metalloproteinases characterized in mammals [12–14]. MMPs such as MT1-MMP (MMP14) directly degrade the ECM, allowing ECs to migrate and form the vascular net in vitro and in vivo [15, 16]. In addition, the degradation of their substrates releases peptidic fragments that modulate angiogenesis. Examples include the proangiogenic C-terminal non-collagenous 1 domains produced by the degradation of collagen [17] and the VEGFA inhibitor endostatin, generated by the activity of MMP3, MMP9, MMP12, MMP13, and MMP20 [18]. MMPs can also process other proteins related to angiogenesis. For example, MMP9 can release VEGFA from the ECM, allowing its binding to VEGFR and thus promoting the angiogenic switch in tumors [19]. In addition, MMP9 and MMP14 (MT1-MMP) can both release and activate TGF-β [19, 20].

Quantitative assessment of the structure and function of the vasculature is thus of key importance (1) to increase knowledge about the basic mechanisms by which the vasculature contributes to tissue damage and repair and (2) for the implementation of rational angiotherapies adapted to specific pathophysiological contexts.

When studying the vasculature under pathological conditions, it is important to address parameters related to the abundance, function, and pattern of the vasculature. This is achieved by quantitating endothelial cell (EC) content, vascular volume fraction or density, vessel number and length, and also other parameters such as pattern and order (tortuosity, thickness), maturation (perivascular coverage), and functionality (vascular perfusion, vascular stability, and leakage). All these parameters are essential indicators of vasculature status [21], and a precise understanding should be considered together with the three-dimensional (3D) structure of the vascular network, a feature of the vascular architecture that has been often dismissed. Tissue vasculature is conventionally analyzed by histology and immunohistochemistry for specific markers on 5–10 μm sections. These approaches have yielded crucial information about the number and density of capillaries, EC content, and perivascular coverage. Moreover, analysis of sections from tissue perfused with antibodies or dextran has allowed partial functional analysis [22]. However, in recent years, the need to understand the vasculature as a connected network has prompted researchers to move from the use of thin sections that provide 2D information to thicker sections that allow 3D volumetric studies (Table 1). Some specific vascular plexus have a flattened structure, such as the superficial vascular plexus of the postnatal retina [23, 24]; however, many other vascular nets develop in 3D, with vessels sprouting in all directions [25]. Because of this, 3D image acquisition and analysis is becoming an essential requirement for vascular biology researchers [26]. To reconstruct the vascular tree and enable reliable data quantification, we and others [26] specifically recommend the use of 40- to 50-μm-thick sections or whole-mount

Table 1
Pros and cons of 2D vs 3D imaging

Method	Advantages	Limitations
2D	Low sample requirements	Loss of structural network
	Quick (staining protocol, image acquisition, quantification)	Only able to quantify vascular area or endothelial cell number
	Low tool requirements (standard fluorescence microscope, widely used analysis software)	Difficult to visualize rare events (tip cells or intussusception)
		Loss of tissue integrity even in serial slicing, you can lose some material because of the cut
3D	Visualization of structural network	More sample requirements
	Visualization of rare events (tip cells or intussusception)	Time consuming (staining protocol, image acquisition, quantification)
	Possibility to quantify parameters such as branching points or tortuosity	Specific tool requirements (mandatory use of confocal microscope and 3D analysis software)
	Maintenance of tissue integrity	Depth limitation for antibody penetration
	Parameters with direct biological meaning (true vessel length)	

samples of thin tissues (such as skin or gut); this task may be facilitated by new optimized clearing protocols [27].

New or improved protocols for the study of the vascular network in tissues are of great interest to scientists working in fields from oncology to regenerative medicine. Here we present a protocol for 3D analysis of the vascular plexus architecture and its functionality. This protocol can be used for the in-depth study of changes to the vasculature in pathologies such as cancer and myocardial infarction among others as well as the impact of specific molecular pathways or angiotherapies.

2 Materials

2.1 Mouse Injection for Functional In Vivo Analysis

1. Homemade restraining device. For IV injection, the mouse must be immobilized. This restraining accessory, made by 3D printing, allows the researcher to restrict mouse movement, leaving the tail exposed in the correct position for IV injection. Both ends of the device are open, one to allow the mouse to breathe and the other to leave the tail exposed. If this device is unavailable, a conical centrifuge tube open at both ends can be used instead.
2. Warming chamber.
3. 70% ethanol.
4. 1 mL syringe.
5. 25 G needles.
6. Dextran tetramethylrhodamine 70,000 MW (dextran-TRITC).
7. *Griffonia simplicifolia* lectin I/isolectin B4 (IB4).
8. Anesthesia: Medeson 1 mL (medetomidine/Domtor), Zoletil 100 mg (tiletamine + zolazepam).
9. Dextran-TRITC preparation: Dissolve lyophilized dextran-TRITC in PBS at 71.5 μM (5 mg/mL), aliquot, and store at −20 °C in the dark.
10. Anesthesia preparation: To prepare Zoletil, add 5 mL of solvent liquid to the lyophilized reagent and mix, and then add 20 mL of saline solution and mix. To prepare Domtor, add 9 mL of saline solution to 1 mL of reagent and mix. For anesthesia, mix the Zoletil and Domtor preparations 1:1, prepare 1 mL aliquots, and store at −20 °C until use.

2.2 Tissue Dissection and Processing

1. CO_2 chamber.
2. Dissection material: Forceps, scissors.
3. Phosphate-buffered saline (PBS): Dissolve 8 g of NaCl (final 137 mM), 1.78 g Na_2HPO_4 dihydrate (final 10 mM), 0.2 g KCl (final 2.7 mM), and 0.24 g KH_2PO_4 (final 1.8 mM) in 500 mL Milli-Q water. Sterilize at 121 °C for 20 min and adjust to pH 7.4. Store at room temperature.
4. 10 mL syringe.
5. 30 G needles.
6. Paraformaldehyde powder (PFA): Warm 400 mL PBS to 60 °C. Next, add 16 g of PFA (highly toxic! Use a biohazard hood and prepare in the dark). When dissolved, filter with a 0.22 μm filter and adjust to pH 7.4. Store in the dark at 4 °C for up to a week; for longer periods, store 10–13 mL aliquots at −20 °C.

7. Sucrose.
8. Intermediate Cryomold.
9. Optimal cutting temperature compound (OCT, Tissue-Tek O.C.T. Compound).
10. Sucrose solution preparation: 0.44 and 0.88 M (15% and 30%, respectively) sucrose solutions are prepared by dissolving 1.5 or 3 g of sucrose in 10 mL PBS. Stir until sucrose is totally dissolved. Solutions are best prepared fresh for every experiment but can be stored for short periods at 4 °C.

2.3 Tissue Cutting

1. Cryostat.
2. Cutting material: Blades, forceps.
3. 48-well flat-bottom cell culture plates.

2.4 Staining

1. Methanol.
2. Hydrogen peroxide, 30% w/v.
3. Triton X-100.
4. Normal goat serum (NGS). Dissolve the vial in Milli-Q water, aliquot, and store at −20 °C.
5. Rocker.
6. Blocking solution: 0.3% Triton X-100 + 2% NGS in PBS. Store at 4 °C.
7. Washing solution: 0.15% Triton X-100 in PBS.
8. Primary antibodies: Anti-CD31, anti-Erg, and anti-smooth muscle actin (anti-SMA) (Table 2).
9. Secondary antibodies: Alexa-647-conjugated goat anti-hamster, Alexa-488-conjugated goat anti-rabbit, Alexa-488-conjugated streptavidin (Table 2).
10. Hoechst 33342, trihydrochloride, trihydrate (Table 2).

2.5 Mounting

1. Paintbrush.
2. Petri dish.
3. Superfrost slides.
4. Coverslips.
5. Mounting medium (Fluoromount-G).

2.6 Image Acquisition

1. Confocal microscopy: For reliable 3D image acquisition, confocal microscopy with an automatized plate should be available, as well as the possibility for intensity adjustment through Z stacks during acquisition. In addition, a set of at least four wavelength channels is required: an ultraviolet laser (excitation ~352 nm, for Hoechst), a blue laser (excitation ~490 nm,

Table 2
List of antibodies and reagents used in this protocol

Marker	Supplier	Ref.	Dilution/ concentration	Staining	Comments
CD31	Millipore	MAB1398Z	1/200 2.5 μg/mL	ECs from blood and lymphatic vessels (membrane)	–
Erg	Abcam	ab92513	1/100 5 μg/mL	ECs (nuclear)	–
SMA	Sigma	C6198	1/300 5 μg/mL	VSMCs (cytoplasmatic)	Cy3 directly labeled
Dextran-TRITC	Invitrogen	D1819	100 μL of 5 mg/mL	Permeability	i.v. injection
Isolectin B4 (IB4)	Vector	B-1205	100 μL of 0.5 mg/mL	Perfusion	i.v. injection
2.4G2 (CD16/CD32)	BD Pharmingen	553142	1/100 5 μg/mL	Fc receptors	Blocking antibody
Alexa Fluor 647 goat α-hamster	Jackson ImmunoResearch	127-605-160	1/500 1 μg/mL	--	CD31 secondary antibody
Alexa Fluor 488 goat α-rabbit	Life Technologies	A11034	1/500 4 μg/mL	--	Erg secondary antibody
Alexa Fluor 488 streptavidin	Life Technologies	S32354	1/500 4 μg/mL	--	IB4 secondary antibody
Hoechst 33342	Invitrogen	H1399	1/5.000 2 μg/mL	Nuclei	--

for FITC and Alexa-488), a green laser (excitation ~556 nm, for dextran-TRITC and Cy3), and an infrared laser (excitation ~649 nm, for Alexa-647). We acquire images using a Nikon A1R confocal microscope with NIS-Elements software.

2.7 Image Quantification

1. Image analysis requires dedicated 3D software tools. Although 3D data can be processed with standard programs such as ImageJ with the use of specific plugins, we recommend the use of specialized software. Most of these programs use the voxel as the basic unit instead of the pixel (the homologous basic unit in two-dimensional images). They are generally able to perform analyses such as delimitation of a volumetric region, masking fluorescence in order to generate an individual mask containing the specific fluorescent signal of the raw channel, and 3D co-localization assays to detect structures that share the same location or are in close apposition. Volocity, Amira, or Bioimage 3D are all examples. Vaa3D, although more suitable for larger volumes (SPIM data), may be another option. Furthermore, computer programming in MATLAB can be used to generate specific plugins for these programs for improved 3D analysis. Here, analysis and semiautomatic quantifications are performed using Imaris 7.7.2 (Bitplane).

3 Methods

3.1 Mouse Procedures (Only for In Vivo Staining)

For in vivo staining, we use C57BL6 adult mice (15 weeks old):

1. Warm the mice to 39 °C in a warming chamber for 5–10 min to dilate the tail vein and flush with 70% ethanol (*see* **Note 1**).
2. Using a 25 G needle, inject 100 μL of 71.5 μM (5 mg/mL) of dextran-TRITC (70 kDa) intravenously 30 min previous to the sacrifice.
3. Using a 25 G needle, intravenously inject 100 μL of IB4 20 min before sacrifice (*see* **Note 2**).

3.2 Sample Collection

3.2.1 For In Vivo Staining

1. After dextran-TRITC and IB4 administration, mice were anesthetized by intraperitoneal injection with 200 μL of Zoletil/Domtor (Z/D).
2. Check the anesthesia with the plantar reflex.
3. Flush the animal with 70% ethanol and open the thoracic cavity without cutting large vessels.
4. Remove the lungs.
5. Perfuse the animal with 20 mL of 1% PFA by direct injection through the aorta (*see* **Note 3**).
6. Extract the tissue and place it in cold PBS.

7. Postfix the tissue with 4% PFA 2 h at 4 °C.
8. Place the samples in 30% (w/v) sucrose in PBS at 4 °C overnight (o/n).

3.2.2 For Ex Vivo Staining

1. Sacrifice mice in a CO_2 chamber.
2. Using a 10 mL syringe with a 30 G needle, perfuse the mice through the aorta with cold PBS until all blood is washed out.
3. Dissect the organ/tissue of interest and place it in 4% PFA o/n at 4 °C (*see* **Note 4**).
4. Wash the organ three times with PBS for 10 min each (*see* **Note 5**).
5. In order to preserve tissue structure when freezing, the sample must be embedded in sucrose. Place the sample in 15% (w/v) sucrose in PBS until it sinks at 4 °C. Then transfer it to 30% (w/v) sucrose in PBS again until it sinks at 4 °C.

3.3 Tissue Freezing and Sectioning

1. Put some drops of OCT in the Cryomold. Then, dry the sample gently with a piece of paper, and place it over the OCT drops in the correct orientation. Then fill the Cryomold with OCT and freeze and store the sample at −80 °C.
2. Take the OCT block from the Cryomold, and use a drop of OCT to attach it to the cryostat adapter in the desired orientation.
3. Take a 48-well plate and fill as many wells as staining panels you have with 300 μL PBS.
4. For 3D analysis, cut sections at around 40–50 μm thick. At this thickness, cutting along the OCT block produces a roll of OCT. This roll contains the thick tissue section and so must be gently collected using tweezers and placed in the well containing PBS. We recommend adding two to three sections per well in order to have technical replicates for each staining.

3.4 Immunostaining

1. Replace the PBS, and agitate the samples for 5 min at room temperature (RT) to eliminate residual OCT (*see* **Note 6**).
2. Add blocking solution to the wells and incubate for 1 h at RT (*see* **Note 7**).
3. Prepare the primary antibodies in fresh blocking solution. Each well requires 100 μL final volume to cover the sections. We recommend the following dilutions, although antibodies should be correctly titrated: 1/200 for CD31 (used for in vivo and ex vivo staining) and 1/100 for Erg (used for ex vivo staining).
4. Add the diluted primary antibodies to the sections and incubate at 4 °C o/n with gentle agitation.

5. The next day, wash the sections three times for 30 minutes in washing solution followed by a further wash for 1 h.
6. To the washed sections, add directly labeled anti-SMA antibody (used in ex vivo staining) at 1/300 in blocking solution and also add the secondary-labeled antibodies diluted 1/500. We recommend goat anti-hamster 647 for CD31 and goat anti-rabbit 546 for Erg. For in vivo IB4 staining, add Alexa-488-conjugated streptavidin at 1/500. Finally, add also Hoechst for nuclear staining at 1/5000 (*see* **Note 8**).
7. Incubate secondary antibodies o/n at 4 °C with gentle agitation (*see* **Note 9**).
8. The next day, wash the sections four times in washing solution for 30 min each. Finally, wash the sections for 1 h in PBS without detergent.
9. Mount the sections on slides. Remove the sections from the wells using a paintbrush, and place them in a PBS-filled petri dish. Using the paintbrush, pick sections up one at a time and place them on the slide.
10. Once the sections are attached to the slide, remove the PBS and dry the surface thoroughly. Fluoromount-G or other mounting medium can then be added and a coverslip placed over the sections.

3.5 Image Acquisition

1. Place the slide on the confocal microscope stage and use the 10× objective to find the tissue section of interest. Change the objective depending on the requirements (for general visualization of the vascular plexus, 10× should be enough; when studying cells, 20× is recommended). Finally, adjust the focus to examine the sample.
2. Once a representative area for analysis has been located, acquire confocal sections every 1 μm through the entire sample depth. If possible, maintain a constant temperature in order to avoid loss of focus, and try to adjust the intensity along Z stack acquisition. If tile scanning, set up the overlay at 10%. Laser parameters should be adjusted according to the staining performance; however, the intensity should be set at 20–30% of the total laser intensity for all markers except for Hoechst (nuclear signal) and the anti-SMA and anti-CD31 antibodies, whose bright signal will require 12–15% laser intensity. Offset should not exceed −15, and gain should be set at around 110–130, except for anti-SMA and anti-CD31, for which gain should be no more than 100. We recommend a resolution of 1024 × 1024. With these settings, a four laser 3 × 3 tile scan with 45 stacks (45 images) will require approximately 1 h of acquisition (*see* **Note 10**).

3. A stack of sequential images will be obtained covering the full thickness of the sample. Maximal intensity projection (MIP) generates a consensus image to present the volumetric information in 2D. Nevertheless, MIP may overestimate some parameters such as vessel density [21] (*see* **Note 11**). In the current protocol, we therefore propose analysis and quantification of the 3D composition provided by the image stack without a preprocessing step that eliminates 3D properties.

As an example, we show representative images of CD31 staining obtained in thick sections (xenograft tumor) and whole mount (skin wound healing) (Fig. 1a). The same figure shows representative images of cardiac injury (neonatal cryoinjury and adult permanent ligation of the left anterior descending [LAD] artery) obtained with different antibodies (Fig. 1b, ex vivo, and Fig. 1c, in vivo).

3.6 Image Quantification

3.6.1 Generation of Volumes of Interest (VOI)

When the image contains healthy and injured areas (Figs. 1 and 2) or any regions of specific interest, these areas should be selected and isolated so that they can be analyzed separately. The first step is thus to extract 3D regions containing the information you want to quantify:

1. To generate the volume of interest (VOI), a region of interest (ROI) is drawn in a section in the middle of the stack. The same ROI is then copied to the other images in the stack (*see* **Note 12**).
2. The 3D software will connect these ROIs to create a 3D mask. This mask is a volumetric selection containing the whole volume of interest. This volume can be analyzed independently, allowing injured and healthy regions to be analyzed separately.

The mask contains the fluorescence channels of every antibody used, enabling analysis of different parameters. For a first screening, the structural parameters of the vascular plexus can be analyzed, including the number of endothelial cells, perivascular coverage, general vascular density, and even volumetric parameters specifically related to capillary structure or to the presence of arterioles. A functional analysis can then be used to calculate number of perfused (functional) vessels or dextran extravasation (vascular leakage). Other analysis options include calculation of arteriolar thickness or further analysis of the leakiness of the vascular net. We use cardiac injury (both cryoinjury and LAD ligation) as a model for all these analyses because it provides a vascular plexus containing capillary and arteriolar structures and showing impaired function.

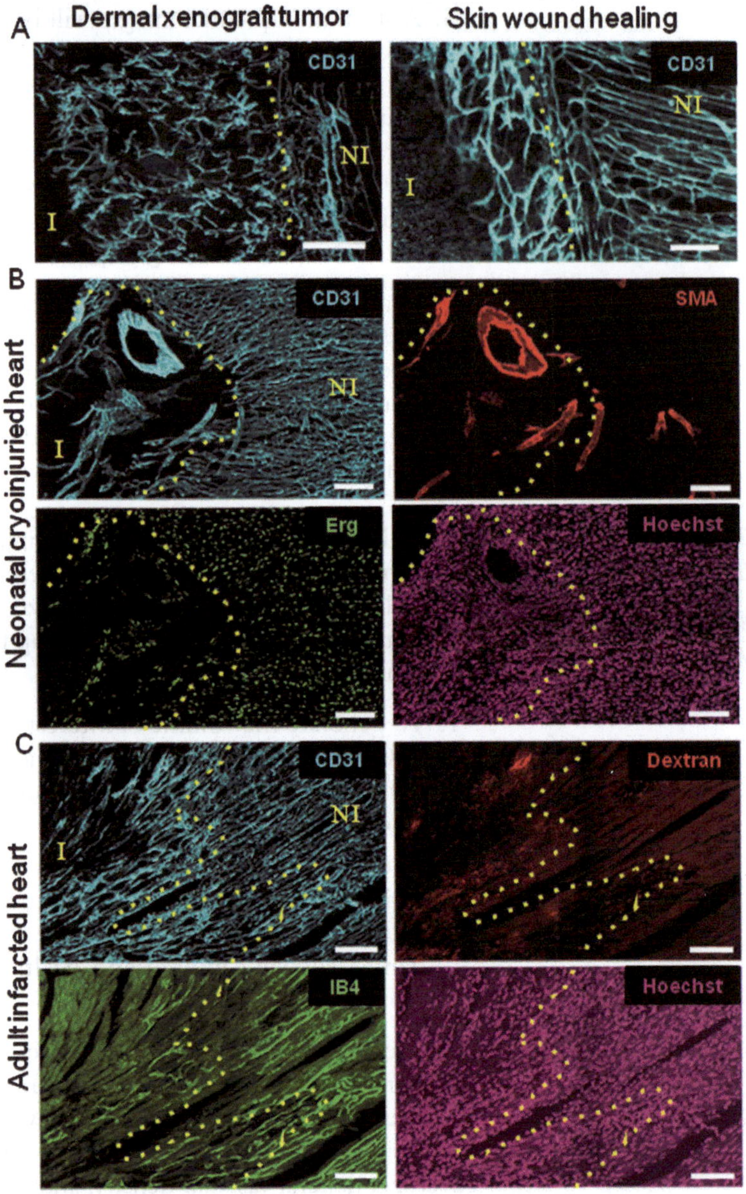

Fig. 1 Examples of immunostaining in thick sections (50 μm). (**a**) CD31 staining in a thick section of a dermal xenograft tumor (left) and a whole mount of wounded skin on day 6 post wound (right). (**b**) Sections of neonatal heart cryoinjured (CI) at P1, dissected at 14 days post-CI and stained for Hoechst, Erg, CD31, and SMA. (**c**) Sections of adult heart infarcted by left anterior descending (LAD) artery ligation, dissected 3 days post-injury and stained for Hoechst, isolectin B4, CD31, and dextran (70 kDa). Dotted lines separate the healthy region (right) from the injured area (left). *I* injured, *NI* noninjured; Scale bar: 200 μm in **a** left and 100 μm in **a** right, **b** and **c**

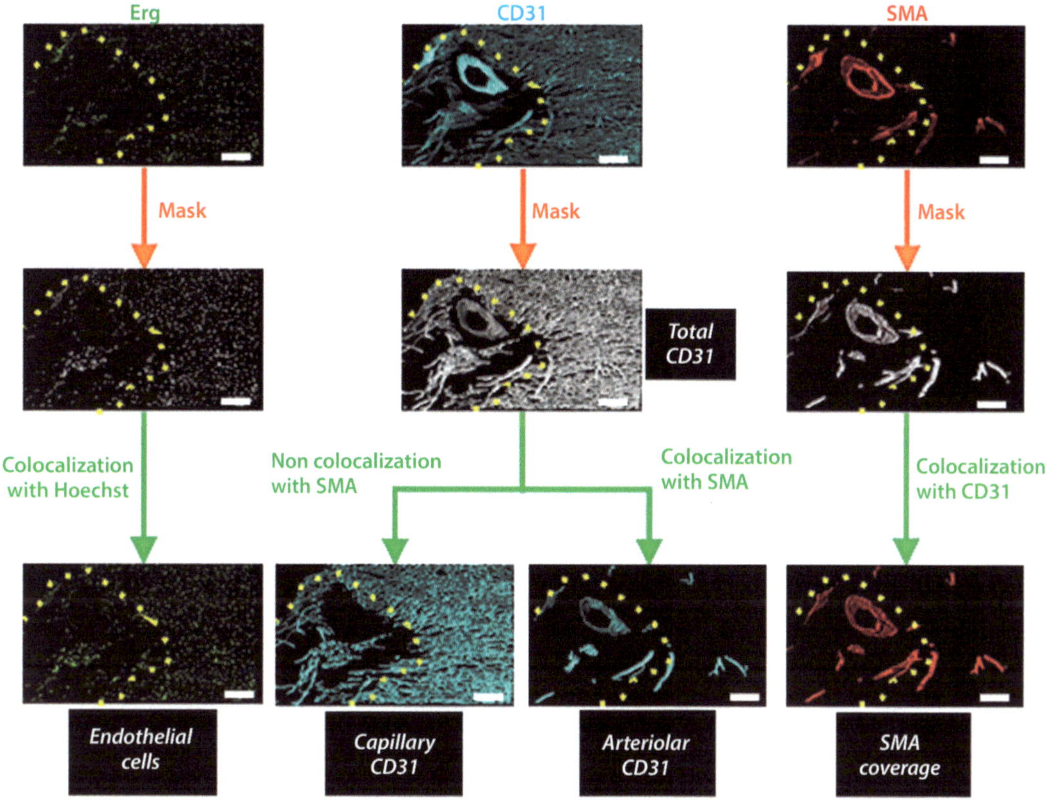

Fig. 2 3D image quantification workflow: vascular architecture quantification. From the masks for CD31, SMA, and Erg, we obtain volumetric three-dimensional information about the endothelial arteriolar and capillary structures as well as about SMA coverage and endothelial cell number. Scale bar: 100 μm

3.6.2 Structural Parameters (Fig. 2)

Here we provide guidelines for analyzing vasculature-associated cellular components as well as the basic structural parameters related to volumetric quantitation of the vasculature and its coverage by SMA^{+} perivascular cells. As an example, we use the cryoinjury model in a P1 postnatal heart 14 days after cryoinjury.

1. One of the most important components of the vascular plexus is the population of endothelial cells (ECs) forming the vascular net. Before extracting volumetric information about the vascular plexus, EC content can be measured by generating a mask from the Erg^{+} fluorescence channel. This mask identifies each of the Erg^{+} nuclei, and dedicated 3D software quantifies the number of Erg^{+} nuclei.
2. A more precise measure of EC number requires a refining step. Since Erg is a nuclear marker, the Erg signal should colocalize with Hoechst (nuclei). Therefore, after generating the Erg mask (**step 1**), a Hoechst co-localization assay should be performed and only cells doubly positive for Erg and Hoechst

considered as ECs. In the co-localization analysis, the 3D software takes each positive Erg unit and checks if the associated voxels (volumetric information homologous to the pixels in 2D images) are also positive for the Hoechst fluorescence signal. If voxels for a cell in the Erg mask also show an intense Hoechst signal, the software will mark the double-positive cell as a genuine EC.

3. The 3D analysis software will provide an absolute number of ECs present in the tissue, and this number can be normalized to the total number of cells, determined as the total number of Hoechst-positive elements (Table 3).
4. Another important parameter is the volume that the vascular net occupies within the tissue; and to obtain a precise picture of the state of the vascular plexus, information about EC number must be combined with volumetric data. General vascular volume is quantified by generating a volumetric mask from the fluorescence channel corresponding to the $CD31^+$ vascular signal. This mask will be a volumetric net containing all $CD31^+$ fluorescent signals. Dedicated 3D software quantifies the number of positive voxels inside the mask, thereby obtaining a volumetric measure of the CD31 signal. This $CD31^+$ volume can then be normalized to the total region volume, thus yielding the vascular volume density, which can also be expressed as a percentage (Table 3).
5. Vascular smooth muscle cells (VSMCs) are perivascular cells that surround the endothelial layer, providing contractility to large arterioles and arteries and mechanical stability to some capillaries of the microvasculature. VSMC coverage of the endothelium provides crucial information about the arteriolar plexus. VSMCs can be specifically identified from the expression of SMA. A mask of the SMA fluorescent signal provides volumetric information about VSMC coverage.
6. Injured tissue can contain SMA-positive nonvascular elements (e.g., myofibroblasts within infarcted regions) [22], and this can lead to these structures being erroneously identified as VSMCs. Non-VSMC SMA^+ cells can be eliminated from the mask by considering only SMA^+ structures in close apposition to the $CD31^+$ EC signal. The co-localization assay checks which SMA^+ structures (**step 5**) are in close apposition to $CD31^+$ voxels, and only these structures are retained as genuine VSMCs (*see* **Notes 13** and **14**).
7. The 3D software then calculates the number of voxels inside this refined SMA^+ volumetric mask, providing the volume associated with the VSMC signal. Normalizing to the total region volume gives a measure of the presence of arterioles and the percentage of SMA^+ volume (Table 3).

Table 3
Quantification of vascular structural parameters in neonatal cryoinjured heart

	Infarcted region	Non-infarcted region
CD31 volume (%)	7.3	13.8
SMA volume (%)	3.5	0.8
Arteriolar volume (%)	37.1	2.9
Capillary volume (%)	62.8	97.0
Number of ECs (%)	13.9	36.4

Images shown in Fig. 1b were quantified according to the protocol and pipeline described in Fig. 2

8. Phenotypic analysis may require separation of the capillary plexus from arterioles. Again, this is achieved by co-localization analysis. In this case, from the $CD31^+$ volumetric mask (**step 4**), you retain only those $CD31^+$ structures in close apposition with the SMA^+ fluorescence channel. The selected $CD31^+$ vessels will correspond to VSMC-covered $CD31^+$ endothelium, classified as arteriolar endothelium (*see* **Note 15**). Again, using the 3D analysis software to quantify voxels inside the generated mask, we can provide volumetric information about this specific endothelium. We recommend normalization to the total $CD31^+$ volume (**step 4**) to obtain the final percentage of arteriolar endothelium in the analyzed vasculature (Table 3).
9. The same analysis will yield a mask of $CD31^+$ structures that are not in close apposition to SMA, corresponding to the capillary endothelium. The specific volumetric mask will give a 3D measure that can be normalized to the total vascular $CD31^+$ volume to determine the capillary plexus as a percentage of the total vasculature (Table 3).

3.6.3 Functional Parameters (Fig. 3)

Analyzing the performance of vascular structures in vivo is a crucial part of 3D vasculature analysis. Staining for functional parameters can provide information about the vasculature perfusion (identifying lumenized vessels that are receiving blood flow) and also about the leakage of the vascular plexus (an index of the stability of the vascular net). For this analysis, we show an example of artery ligation in adult mice at 3 days post infarction.

1. First, generate a volumetric mask from the fluorescence channel for the $IB4^+$ vascular signal. This mask will reveal the volumetric net of perfused vessels. These vessels, which have taken

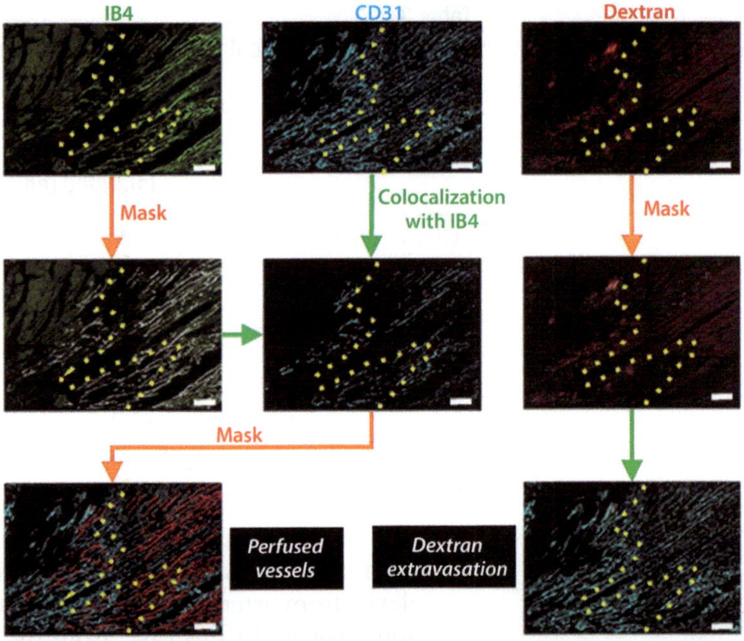

Fig. 3 3D image quantification workflow: functional quantification. From the Isolectin B4, CD31, and dextran masks, we can obtain information about the perfusion and leakage of the vascular net. Scale bar: 100 μm

up the IV-injected IB4 and are thus competent for blood flow, should be considered functional.

2. Select the $CD31^+$ fluorescence signal from within the IB4 mask (**step 1**). Rather than positively selecting that part of a fluorescence channel showing co-localization, as in previous examples (Subheading 3.6.2 **step 2**, **6**, and **8**), here the procedure involves elimination of $CD31^+$ fluorescence that is not inside the mask voxels, thus leaving only the fluorescent signal associated with the mask. In this specific case, CD31 fluorescence that does not co-localize with the voxels in the IB4 mask (**step 2**) is eliminated, yielding a CD31 fluorescence channel of double-positive ($CD31^+$ and $IB4^+$) vessels.
3. Using the 3D software, a volumetric mask can then be generated over the IB4-co-localized $CD31^+$ fluorescence signal, enabling determination of the volume of correctly perfused vasculature.
4. The perfused vasculature (**step 3**) can be normalized to the whole vascular plexus, obtained from the general mask of the $CD31^+$ vascular signal (Subheading 3.6.2 **step 4**) (*see* Table 4).
5. Following the same principle, a volumetric mask can be generated of the dextran surface and normalized to the vascular

Table 4
Quantification of vascular functional parameters in adult infarcted heart

	Infarcted region	Non-infarcted region
CD31 volume (%)	9.9	11.4
Perfused vessel volume (%)	11.2	47.6
Extravasated dextran volume	1.5	0.1

Images shown in Fig. 1c were quantified according to the protocol and pipeline described in Fig. 3

plexus volume. This reveals the volume of extravasated dextran, giving a measure of the stability and leakage of the vascular plexus (Table 4).

These masking and co-localization functions are integral to all 3D programs; however, individual programs can also include specific tools that allow a more detailed analysis. For example, Imaris 7.7.2 includes the distance transformation map, which can substitute the co-localization assays and determine structures by simply checking the distance between them. There are also customized algorithms (MATLAB programming) that allow quantification of other structural parameters such as number of segments, vessel radius, branching nodes, etc. (*see* **Note 16**).

4 Notes

1. Tail vein dilatation is crucial when working with dark strains (such as C57BL6), in which the tail is darker and the vein difficult to see. For white strains (such as BALB/c), this is less important because the vein is clearly visible.
2. The first tail injection should be distal to the second. Alternatively inject each component in different veins.
3. From here on, samples are maintained and manipulated in the dark to prevent loss of dextran fluorescence.
4. Some antibodies may require a milder fixation, and PFA concentrations from 0.4% to 2% can be used.
5. For whole-mount staining, go directly to the step 3.4 (immunostaining). Whole-mount samples can be stored for up to a month in PBS at 4 °C.
6. During staining, liquids should be removed with care, using a p200 pipette. Avoid suction to prevent sample damage.

7. Anti-CD16/CD32 antibodies should be included when staining samples with high numbers of inflammatory cells in order to avoid the possible non-specific reactions of their FcR receptors.
8. DAPI (4′,6-diamidino-2-phenylindole, dihydrochloride) or Hoechst can be added for nuclear staining indistinctly.
9. From here on, samples are maintained and manipulated in the dark to preserve the fluorescence signal.
10. For the 3D acquisition of full structures, such as tumors or hearts, a 512 × 512 pixel resolution should be enough for quantification of vessel density, perfusion, and extravasation, making it possible to reduce microscopy acquisition time, obtain smaller files, and thus speed up analysis. Acquisition time can also be reduced by acquiring optical sections in the Z stacks at 1.5–2 μm intervals.
11. Maximal intensity projections are useful for rapid visualization of the sample, giving an initial idea of the parameters that may be of interest for 3D quantification.
12. The region of interest in damaged tissue can be delineated by selecting the aberrant $CD31^+$ vasculature; however, other markers such as the macrophage marker CD68 can also be used.
13. The endothelial cells and VSMC layers are closely apposed but do not coincide exactly. Co-localization analysis can be used to specifically select VSMCs because the endothelial and perivascular cell fluorescence signals are superimposed. However, some 3D analysis programs (e.g., Imaris version 7.7.2) can perform distance transformation maps that examine the inter-signal distance instead of co-localization. This tool, although not included in every 3D software package, can be more specific, and we encourage its use when available.
14. Any remaining anomalous SMA structure should be eliminated manually.
15. In the heart model, most SMA^+-covered vessels correspond to arterioles. However, in other contexts such as tumors, SMA^+-covered vessels may not correspond to arterioles but to more mature or stabilized vessels; the immature vessels will be those with less or no SMA coverage.
16. With this kind of 3D images, it is possible to analyze other structural parameters, such as tortuosity and number of branch points, providing information about how the vessel network is structured. This kind of analysis can be done with programs like Imaris (the one that we use here) and also with customized software implemented in MATLAB, for example [28].

Acknowledgments

We thank Simon Bartlett for English editing. This work was supported by grant SAF2014-52050R from the Spanish Ministry of Economy and Competitiveness. A.S-E. is funded by a fellowship from Obra Social "La Caixa." The CNIC is supported by the Ministry of Economy, Industry and Competitiveness and the Pro-CNIC Foundation and is a Severo Ochoa Center of Excellence (SEV-2015-0505).

References

1. Greenblatt M, Shubi P (1968) Tumor angiogenesis: transfilter diffusion studies in the hamster by the transparent chamber technique. J Natl Cancer Inst 41(1):111–124
2. Parangi S, O'Reilly M, Christofori G et al (1996) Antiangiogenic therapy of transgenic mice impairs de novo tumor growth. Proc Natl Acad Sci U S A 93(5):2002–2007
3. Folkman J (2002) Role of angiogenesis in tumor growth and metastasis. Semin Oncol 29(6 Suppl 16):15–18. https://doi.org/10.1053/sonc.2002.37263
4. Fakhrejahani E, Toi M (2014) Antiangiogenesis therapy for breast cancer: an update and perspectives from clinical trials. Jpn J Clin Oncol 44(3):197–207. https://doi.org/10.1093/jjco/hyt201
5. Weis SM, Cheresh DA (2005) Pathophysiological consequences of VEGF-induced vascular permeability. Nature 437(7058):497–504. https://doi.org/10.1038/nature03987
6. Bae YH, Park K (2011) Targeted drug delivery to tumors: myths, reality and possibility. J Control Release 153(3):198–205. https://doi.org/10.1016/j.jconrel.2011.06.001
7. Carmeliet P, Jain RK (2011) Principles and mechanisms of vessel normalization for cancer and other angiogenic diseases. Nat Rev Drug Discov 10(6):417–427. https://doi.org/10.1038/nrd3455
8. Wong PP, Demircioglu F, Ghazaly E et al (2015) Dual-action combination therapy enhances angiogenesis while reducing tumor growth and spread. Cancer Cell 27(1):123–137. https://doi.org/10.1016/j.ccell.2014.10.015
9. Madeddu P (2005) Therapeutic angiogenesis and vasculogenesis for tissue regeneration. Exp Physiol 90(3):315–326. https://doi.org/10.1113/expphysiol.2004.028571
10. Zhang H, van Olden C, Sweeney D et al (2014) Blood vessel repair and regeneration in the ischaemic heart. Open Heart 1(1):e000016. https://doi.org/10.1136/openhrt-2013-000016
11. Porrello ER, Olson EN (2014) A neonatal blueprint for cardiac regeneration Stem Cell Res 13 (3 Pt B):556-570. doi:https://doi.org/10.1016/j.scr.2014.06.003
12. Rundhaug JE (2005) Matrix metalloproteinases and angiogenesis. J Cell Mol Med 9(2):267–285
13. Siefert SA, Sarkar R (2012) Matrix metalloproteinases in vascular physiology and disease. Vascular 20(4):210–216. https://doi.org/10.1258/vasc.2011.201202
14. Zhou Z, Apte SS, Soininen R et al (2000) Impaired endochondral ossification and angiogenesis in mice deficient in membrane-type matrix metalloproteinase I. Proc Natl Acad Sci U S A 97(8):4052–4057. https://doi.org/10.1073/pnas.060037197
15. Galvez BG, Genis L, Matias-Roman S et al (2005) Membrane type 1-matrix metalloproteinase is regulated by chemokines monocyte-chemoattractant protein-1/ccl2 and interleukin-8/CXCL8 in endothelial cells during angiogenesis. J Biol Chem 280(2):1292–1298. https://doi.org/10.1074/jbc.M408673200
16. Galvez BG, Matias-Roman S, Albar JP et al (2001) Membrane type 1-matrix metalloproteinase is activated during migration of human endothelial cells and modulates endothelial motility and matrix remodeling. J Biol Chem 276(40):37491–37500. https://doi.org/10.1074/jbc.M104094200
17. Koziol A, Gonzalo P, Mota A et al (2012) The protease MT1-MMP drives a combinatorial proteolytic program in activated endothelial cells. FASEB J 26(11):4481–4494. https://doi.org/10.1096/fj.12-205906
18. Sudhakar A, Sugimoto H, Yang C et al (2003) Human tumstatin and human endostatin exhibit distinct antiangiogenic activities mediated by alpha v beta 3 and alpha 5 beta 1 integrins.

Proc Natl Acad Sci U S A 100(8):4766–4771. https://doi.org/10.1073/pnas.0730882100

19. Bergers G, Brekken R, McMahon G et al (2000) Matrix metalloproteinase-9 triggers the angiogenic switch during carcinogenesis. Nat Cell Biol 2(10):737–744. https://doi.org/10.1038/35036374
20. Mu D, Cambier S, Fjellbirkeland L et al (2002) The integrin alpha(v)beta8 mediates epithelial homeostasis through MT1-MMP-dependent activation of TGF-beta1. J Cell Biol 157(3):493–507. https://doi.org/10.1083/jcb.200109100
21. Walchli T, Mateos JM, Weinman O et al (2015) Quantitative assessment of angiogenesis, perfused blood vessels and endothelial tip cells in the postnatal mouse brain. Nat Protoc 10(1):53–74. https://doi.org/10.1038/nprot.2015.002
22. Cunha SI, Pardali E, Thorikay M et al (2010) Genetic and pharmacological targeting of activin receptor-like kinase 1 impairs tumor growth and angiogenesis. J Exp Med 207(1):85–100. https://doi.org/10.1084/jem.20091309
23. Pitulescu ME, Schmidt I, Benedito R et al (2010) Inducible gene targeting in the neonatal vasculature and analysis of retinal angiogenesis in mice. Nat Protoc 5(9):1518–1534. https://doi.org/10.1038/nprot.2010.113
24. Tual-Chalot S, Allinson KR, Fruttiger M et al (2013) Whole mount immunofluorescent staining of the neonatal mouse retina to investigate angiogenesis in vivo. J Vis Exp 77:e50546. https://doi.org/10.3791/50546
25. Walls JR, Coultas L, Rossant J et al (2008) Three-dimensional analysis of vascular development in the mouse embryo. PLoS One 3(8):e2853. https://doi.org/10.1371/journal.pone.0002853
26. Jester JV, Ho-Chang J (2003) Modulation of cultured corneal keratocyte phenotype by growth factors/cytokines control in vitro contractility and extracellular matrix contraction. Exp Eye Res 77(5):581–592
27. Richardson DS, Lichtman JW (2015) Clarifying tissue clearing. Cell 162(2):246–257. https://doi.org/10.1016/j.cell.2015.06.067
28. Gkontra P, Żak MM, Norton K-A et al (2015) A 3D fractal-based approach towards understanding changes in the infarcted heart microvasculature. Springer 9351:173–180. https://doi.org/10.1007/978-3-319-24574-4_21

Chapter 19

Human Tumor Tissue-Based 3D In Vitro Invasion Assays

Pirjo Åström, Ritva Heljasvaara, Pia Nyberg, Ahmed Al-Samadi, and Tuula Salo

Abstract

Here we describe a protocol to utilize human benign leiomyoma tissue in in vitro 3D model that enables an assessment of cell invasion. The chapter also describes detailed instructions for image analysis to quantify the results. Leiomyoma is a benign tumor of the uterus which mimics authentic components of the tumor microenvironment including fibroblasts, vessels, collagen fibers, and extracellular protein composition. The leiomyoma invasion model represents a superior 3D model for cell invasion studies compared to the other non-human organotypic models.

Key words 3D in vitro model, Invasion, Human tissue, Leiomyoma, Extracellular matrix, Tumor microenvironment, Immunohistochemistry, Image analysis, Cancer cells, Co-culture

1 Introduction

Extracellular matrix (ECM) protein mixtures of non-human origin, such as Matrigel from Engelbreth-Holm-Swarm (EHS) mouse sarcoma cells, are the prevailing substrates in the majority of in vitro cell invasion studies [1]. We have recently described a novel protein extract made of human uterus leiomyoma tissue and demonstrated that it is superior to Matrigel in in vitro cancer and angiogenesis studies [2]. However, such protein mixtures lack the complex 3D architecture which also influences proteolytic actions during cell invasion [3]. The described organotypic leiomyoma 3D solid disc model utilizes human tissue material with authentic components of the tumor microenvironment (TME) such as fibroblasts, insoluble and soluble ECM components, and a complex tumor tissue architecture including nerves and vessels [3–5]. Although cells in the myoma discs are not viable, their presence is important as they simulate the in vitro tumor cellular environment [6]. Additionally, myoma discs are hypoxic providing natural surroundings for cancer cells in vitro [3]. Hence, in this human 3D organotypic model,

Santiago Cal and Alvaro J. Obaya (eds.), *Proteases and Cancer: Methods and Protocols*, Methods in Molecular Biology, vol. 1731, https://doi.org/10.1007/978-1-4939-7595-2_19, © Springer Science+Business Media, LLC 2018

tumor progression and cell invasion can be investigated in vitro in an environment that closely mimics the in vivo situation.

2 Materials

Human uterine leiomyoma tissue can be obtained from routine surgical operations after the informed consent of the donors and kept frozen. Their use should be approved by ethical guidelines and regulations that follow international, national and institutional standards in each country, with the strictest legal and ethical standards.

Like all human tissues, the human leiomyoma specimens are potentially biohazardous material, and thus they should only be handled by trained personnel. Processing of the myoma samples must be performed in dedicated areas, in a laminar hood with biosafety level 2. A full risk assessment should be performed on all steps of the protocol. Human samples should be stored in designated areas, and their disposal should comply with institutional guidelines.

This model is suitable for several malignant and stromal cell lines. Cell line-specific media and reagents used for growing the cells should be applied in this model. The procedure needs the following materials:

1. Human uterine leiomyoma tissue.
2. Cultured tumor and other stromal cells.
3. Cell culture reagents (depending on the cell type).
4. Transwell chambers (sterile 6.5 mm Transwell polycarbonate membrane inserts with an 8.0 μm pore size).
5. Slicing device or a sterile knife.
6. 8 mm biopsy punch.
7. 24- and 12-well plates.
8. Sterile tweezers (blunt and sharp).
9. CryoTubes.
10. Custom-made sterile metal grids.
11. DMSO (dimethyl sulfoxide).
12. Microscope equipped with camera.
13. Standard histology reagents for embedding and staining [(a) 4% formaldehyde in phosphate-buffered saline, (b) ethanol, (c) Tissue-Clear (xylene substitute), (d) paraffin blocks, (e) microtome, (f) slides, (g) hematoxylin-eosin, (h) xylene, (i) mounting medium].

3 Methods

The myoma invasion assay takes 10–14 days:

Day 0: Transfer myoma pieces to Transwell inserts, seed cells on top of the myoma.

Day 1: Transfer myomas onto the metal grids.

Days 3–13: Change the media according to the culture protocol of your cells.

Days 10–14: Collect the myomas for analyses, and continue to further sample processing and analyses.

3.1 Preparing the Myoma Discs for Organotypic Culture

1. Cut the leiomyoma tissue into 4 mm thick slices using a slicing device or a large knife in a sterile fashion (Fig. 1a, b, *see* **Note 1**).
2. In a cell culture laminar hood, make cylinder-shaped discs from the 4 mm leiomyoma slices using an 8 mm biopsy punch (Fig. 1c).
3. Store the discs at −70 °C or in liquid nitrogen in CryoTubes filled with 1000 μL of the desired culture medium with 10% DMSO (*see* **Note 2**). Alternatively, the myoma discs can also be lyophilized (*see* **Note 3**).

3.2 Invasion Assay (Day 0)

1. Remove myoma discs from the freezer or liquid nitrogen, thaw them, and immerse the discs into the desired culture medium in a 50 mL conical tube (eight discs in 30–40 mL of medium). Rinse overnight at room temperature (or if the tissue is bloody, for up to 3 days at 4 °C). Prepare at least three parallel myoma discs per experimental condition.
2. Use sterile blunt tweezers to transfer myoma discs gently into Transwell inserts placed in a 24-well plate avoiding tissue damage (Fig. 1d, *see* **Note 4**).
3. Immediately after the transfer, add 0.5 mL of culture medium to the lower chamber. Put the plate into cell culture incubator while preparing the cells.
4. Trypsinize the cells according to the protocol used for your cells.
5. Resuspend the cells and count cell number. Suspend the cells in an appropriate volume of cell culture medium (e.g., for HSC-3 oral squamous cell carcinoma cells, approximately 1.4×10^7 cells per mL is a good cell density). For co-culture experiments *see* **Note 5**.
6. Add tumor cells on top of the myoma in 50 μL of their normal culture medium (*see* **Note 6**). The appropriate number of the cells depends on the cell line used, e.g., for HSC-3 cells, 700,000 cells per myoma disc is recommended. Also include myomas without cancer cell seeding in the study (control).
7. Culture at the appropriate conditions overnight.

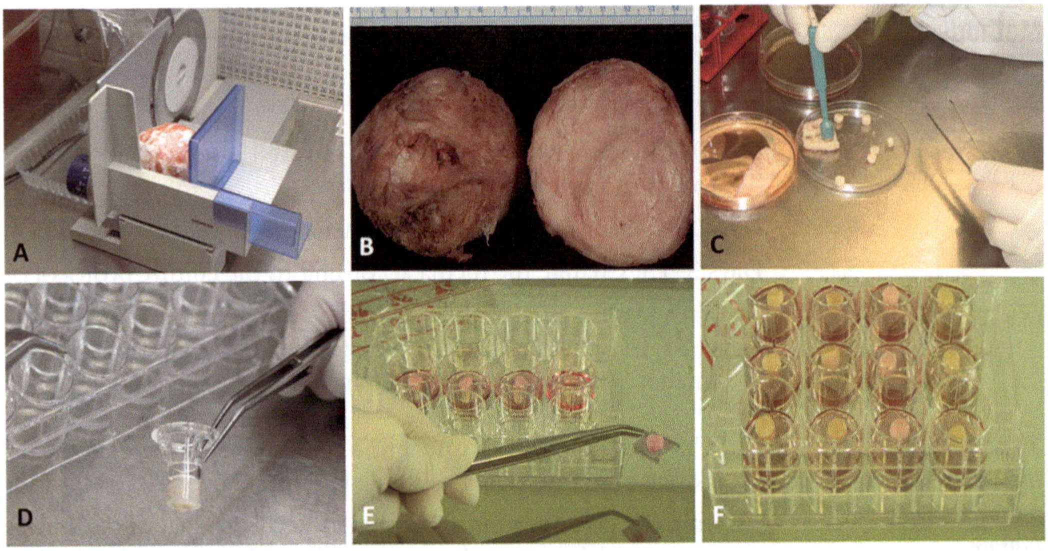

Fig. 1 Selected steps for preparation of the myoma disc for invasion assay. (**a**) Cut the myoma tissue into 4 mm slices using a slicing device. (**b**) Myoma slices after cutting. (**c**) Cut myoma discs using 8 mm biopsy punch. (**d**) Insert the disc inside the Transwell chamber. (**e**) Transfer the disc from the Transwell chamber onto a metal grid. (**f**) Culture the myoma discs on the grids in a 12-well plate

3.3 Transfer the Myomas onto the Steel Grids (Day 1) and Culturing (Until Days 10–14)

1. Place sterile metal grids in the wells of a 12-well plate.
2. Add 1 mL of culture medium (with or without test substance, e.g., cancer drugs) to the wells.
3. Take myoma discs from the Transwell inserts and place them on the grids (Fig. 1e). Make sure that the cells are on the upper side of the myoma disc.
4. Culture at suitable conditions for up to 2 weeks, changing the media (1 mL) at desired intervals depending on the cell line (Fig. 1f; *see* **Note 7**).

3.4 Processing of the Discs for Analyses (Days 10–14)

1. Prepare the tissues for histology.
   (a) Paraffin processing: Remove the myoma discs from the metal grids, and place them in plastic cassettes of a suitable size (*see* **Note 8**). Immerse tissues in 4% formaldehyde in phosphate-buffered saline (pH 7.2–7.4) fixative for a maximum of 24 h; longer incubation can destroy antigens. Use gentle agitation, e.g., a small magnetic stirrer placed in a plastic cassette that will enhance penetration of fixative to tissues. The volume of the fixative solution should be approximately 50-fold the volume of the tissue.
   (b) Frozen sample preparation: Slice the myomas into two halves and freeze the myoma tissue quickly in liquid nitrogen

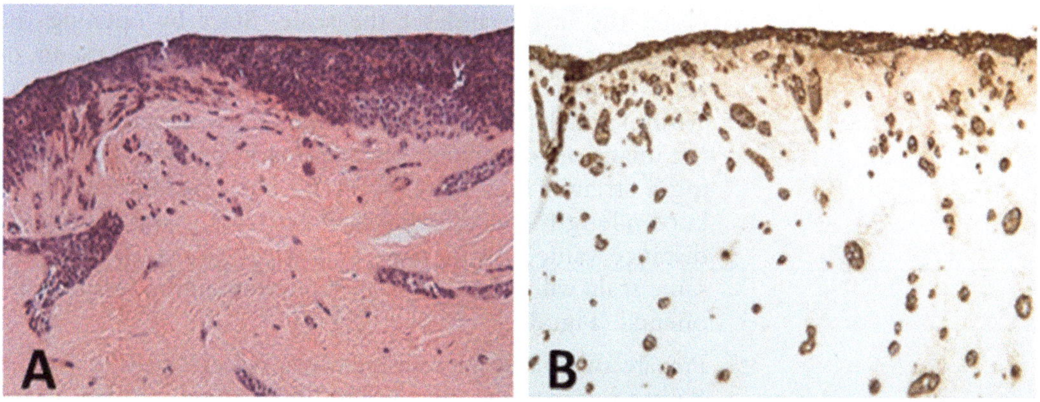

Fig. 2 Histological sections of myoma discs with carcinoma cells after 10 days in culture. (**a**) Hematoxylin and eosin staining. (**b**) Pan-cytokeratin AEI/AE3 immunohistochemical staining

or place the disc in a plastic Cryomold (in the correct orientation for cutting) and cover with optimal cutting temperature compound (OCT) and rapidly freeze on an aluminum plate on the dry ice.

2. Place the cassettes under running tap water for 4 h. Dehydrate the tissue in stepwise ethanol concentration: (a) 40% for at least 4 h, (b) 50% for overnight, (c) 70% for 1 h, (d) 95% for 2 h, and (e) 100% for 2 h. All steps should be done under gentle agitation.
3. To remove all ethanol, immerse the tissue in Tissue-Clear for 30 min under agitation.
4. Cut the myoma disc in two halves, orientate each halve in the cassette, embed it in paraffin, and place the cassette on a cold plate to solidify.
5. Cut 5–6 μm myoma sections and stain, for example, with hematoxylin and eosin for tissue morphology (Fig. 2a). Immunohistochemical staining, e.g., anti-pan-cytokeratin antibody AEI/AE3, can be used to stain the carcinoma cells (Fig. 2b).

3.5 Analyzing the Invasion

The invasion area and invasion depth can be examined using image analysis software. Here we describe the use of Fiji software for analyzing the invasion area and depth. However, there are also several other ways to apply Fiji software in image analyses [7].

1. Acquire three to five images of the whole invasion area (5× objective), or scan the area with a whole slide imaging scanner. Avoid the areas right next to the myoma edges during the image analysis (*see* **Note 9**).

2. Open the image and set the scale. Start by opening the Imagej.jar- file. Open the image from *File* ➔ *Open* menu, or take the picture from a folder, and drag it on the ImageJ symbol which will open the image. You can set the size of the image once you have opened it: Choose a tool for drawing a straight line from the menu bar, and draw a line of known length. Select *Analyze* ➔ *Set Scale*, insert the known distance value and its unit, and select *Global*, so that the same scale will be used also in the following images that are opened (Fig. 3a).
3. Prepare the image for measurements. Select *Image* ➔ *Type* ➔ *8-bit*, to change the picture into an 8-bit gray-shaded image. Select *Image* ➔ *Adjust* ➔ *Threshold*, and use the mouse to adjust the scroll bars so that the regions to be studied are colored red (Fig. 3b).
4. Define the epithelium and invasive regions. Select the Wand (tracing) tool with which you can define a uniform area. Click on the epithelium to draw/create a yellow line around the selected region. Select *Analyze* ➔ *Analyze Particles.* You can select the minimum and maximum size of the particles to be measured on the part *Size (μm*2)*. Select *OK* to measure the surface area of the selected regions (Fig. 3c). Select *Edit* ➔ *Clear*, to remove the already measured region from the image (Fig. 3d). Continue by drawing a line around the invasive region, or you can also select *Edit* ➔ *Selection* ➔ *Select all*, if the scale bar has been removed from the image. Select *Analyze* ➔ *Analyze Particles* ➔ *OK*, to measure the surface area of the selected regions/particles. Now the surface areas and number of particles within the area are shown in the *Summary* window (Fig. 3e).
5. Measuring the depth of invasion: Adjust the settings for the measurements *Analyze* ➔ *Set Measurement*; from here you only select *Limit Threshold* and *Display Label.* Select the *Straight* tool from the menu, and draw a vertical line starting from the lower threshold of the epithelium and ending at the particle that invaded the deepest/furthest (Fig. 3f). Select *Analyze* ➔ *Measure* to obtain the result of the measurement in the *Results* window. Measure the invasion depths for three separate invasive particles with the deepest/furthest invasion.
6. Handling the results: The results can be copied from the *Summary* and *Results* windows straight into an Excel file. The average of invasion depth is calculated based on the measurements taken from three separate invasion particles.

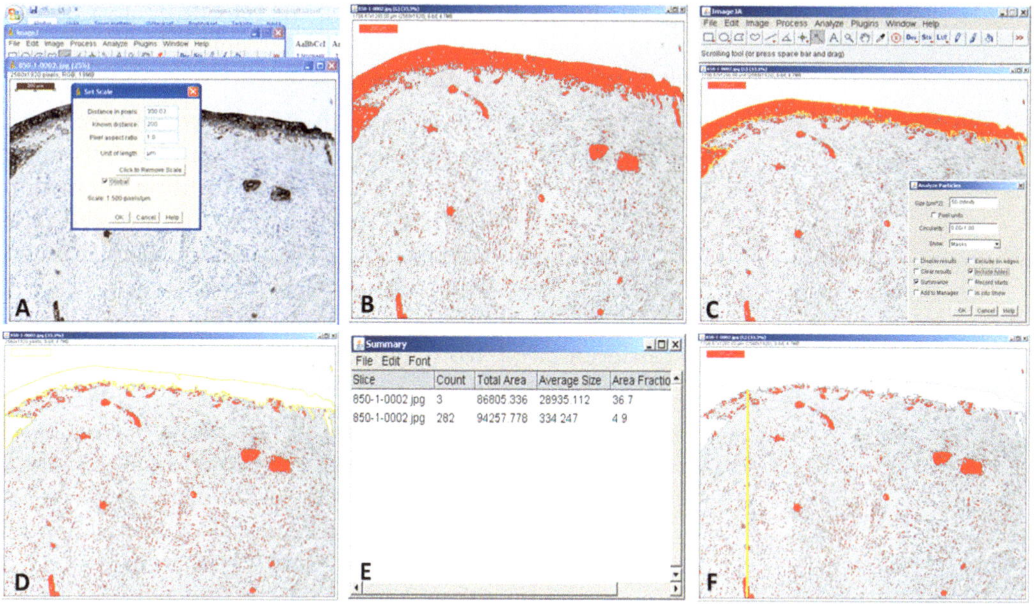

Fig. 3 Selected steps for measuring the invasion area and invasion depth. (**a**) Open the desired image and set the scale. (**b**) Change the image to 8-bit depth, and then adjust the threshold to get the stained area red in color. (**c**) Use the tracing tool to select the area of non-invaded cancer cells. (**d**) Remove the non-invaded cancer cells and the scale bar from the image. (**e**) Summary of the results. (**f**) Measure the invasion depth by drawing a straight line from the bottom of the non-invaded cancer cells to the deepest point of the invaded cancer cells

4 Notes

1. In each individual experiment, use tissue discs from the same leiomyoma specimen. Special care should be taken when working with human tissues. All steps should be carried out in cell culture.
2. You can put up to eight myoma discs in each CryoTube.
3. To lyophilize the myoma discs, first put them onto 24- or 48-well plates, one disc per well, cover with Parafilm, and freeze at −70 °C. Pierce the Parafilm and lyophilize the discs for 72 h using a Heto Drywinner DW3. After lyophilization, place the discs in an exicator. The discs are rehydrated by rinsing them at 4 °C in the desired culture medium overnight. After rehydration, the discs can be used in the same manner as non-lyophilized native discs.
4. Myoma disc and the membrane should be packed tightly without any empty space between them to allow capillary flow of media into the myoma. If the disc is too high, cut it carefully to fit into the insert.

5. The myoma in vitro 3D invasion model can be also used to co-culture cancer cells with other adherent and non-adherent cells within the tumor microenvironment:
   (a) Adherent cells. Cancer cells can be co-cultured with fibroblasts, macrophages, stem cells, and other adherent cells by mixing the cells before adding them onto the myoma discs. The ratio between different cell types can be decided depending on the aim of the experiment and type of the cells. If needed, cells can be transfected with green fluorescent protein (GFP) so they can be differentiated from non-vital cells which exist within the myoma disc.
   (b) Non-adherent cells. Cancer cells can be also co-cultured with non-adherent cells such as peripheral blood mononuclear cells by adding these cells in the medium below the myoma disc. These cells can also be activated by adding different stimulants such as CD3 and CD28 antibodies, IL-2, ionomycin, phorbol 12-myristate 13-acetate, etc. to the medium. The number of the non-adherent cells can be decided depending on the aim of the study and the type of the cells.
6. In some cases, the medium flows on top of the myoma discs. Before adding the cells, remove any culture medium on top of the myoma.
7. When changing the media, conditioned media can be collected and stored at −20 °C for various analyses, e.g., for collagen degradation products during cancer cell invasion by radioimmunoassay kit.
8. Do not squeeze too big pieces of tissue into too small cassettes since this will result in poor penetration of fixative and possibly disturb the top cell layer.
9. Treat the images as research results. Save the original picture in TIFF form; JPEG is not recommended. Making simple adjustments is allowed (adjusting brightness, contrast and gamma—distribution). The settings must be identical when comparing images. Filters that improve image quality weaken the quality of the data. Intensities can be measured, if images have been modified as an entity and they have been calibrated for a known standard. You may lose some data while enlarging the image. Changes in the size of the image (number of pixels in *X* and *Y* axis) may cause folding artifacts.

Acknowledgments

This work was supported by Sigrid Juselius Foundation, the Finnish Cancer Foundation, the University of Helsinki Central Hospital, and the Health Science Council of the Academy of Finland (Centre of Excellence 2012–2017 Grant 251314). We thank Dr. Sini Nurmenniemi and Dr. Tatu Pirkola for developing the myoma model and the protocol of invasion quantification, respectively. We thank Mr. Donald Smart for the editorial assistance.

References

1. Benton G, Arnaoutova I, George J et al (2014) Matrigel: from discovery and ECM mimicry to assays and models for cancer research. Adv Drug Deliv Rev 79-80:3–18
2. Salo T, Sutinen M, al HAE e (2015) A novel human leiomyoma tissue derived matrix for cell culture studies. BMC Cancer 15:981
3. Teppo S, Sundquist E, Vered M et al (2013) The hypoxic tumor microenvironment regulates invasion of aggressive oral carcinoma cells. Exp Cell Res 319(4):376–389
4. Nurmenniemi S, Sinikumpu T, Alahuhta I et al (2009) A novel organotypic model mimics the tumor microenvironment. Am J Pathol 175(3):1281–1291
5. Sundquist E, Renko O, Salo S et al (2016) Neoplastic extracellular matrix environment promotes cancer invasion in vitro. Exp Cell Res 344(2):229–240
6. Alahuhta I, Aikio M, Väyrynen O et al (2015) Endostatin induces proliferation of oral carcinoma cells but its effect on invasion is modified by the tumor microenvironment. Exp Cell Res 336:130–140
7. Schindelin J, Arganda-Carreras I, Frise E et al (2012) Fiji: an open-source platform for biological-image analysis. Nat Methods 9(7):676–682

Chapter 20

Ear Sponge Assay: A Method to Investigate Angiogenesis and Lymphangiogenesis in Mice

Maureen Van de Velde, Melissa García-Caballero, Tania Durré, Frédéric Kridelka, and Agnès Noël

Abstract

Angiogenesis and lymphangiogenesis have become important research areas in the biomedical field. The outgrowth of new blood (angiogenesis) and lymphatic (lymphangiogenesis) vessels from preexisting ones is involved in many pathologies including cancer. In-depth investigations of molecular determinants such as proteases in these complex processes require reliable in vivo models. Here we present the ear sponge assay as an easy, rapid, quantitative and reproducible model of angiogenesis and lymphangiogenesis. In this system, a gelatin sponge soaked with tumor cells, cell-conditioned medium, or a compound to be tested is implanted, for 2–4 weeks, between the two mouse ear skin layers. The two vascular networks are next examined through histological procedures.

Key words Angiogenesis, Lymphangiogenesis, Ear sponge assay, Proteases, In vivo model

1 Introduction

Angiogenesis and lymphangiogenesis are critical processes that enable tumor progression and the formation of metastases, which remains the primary cause of cancer patient death [1–4]. The formation of new blood and lymphatic vessels closely correlate with metastasis and clinical outcome in various types of cancer [5–7]. Most researches are devoted to angiogenesis, and the lymphatic system remains often a somewhat forgotten part of the tumor vasculature. Although anti-angiogenic therapeutic drugs are currently used in clinic, no anti-lymphangiogenic compound is yet used. Nevertheless, encouraging data have been reported for the combination of anti-angiogenic and anti-lymphangiogenic treatments [8]. These complex biological processes are regulated by a large panel of molecules including at least growth factors, their cell

Maureen Van de Velde and Melissa García-Caballero contributed equally to this work.

Santiago Cal and Alvaro J. Obaya (eds.), *Proteases and Cancer: Methods and Protocols*, Methods in Molecular Biology, vol. 1731, https://doi.org/10.1007/978-1-4939-7595-2_20,

surface receptors, integrins, proteases, and their inhibitors. Although initially viewed as simple regulators of matrix degradation, matrix proteases (matrix metalloproteinases [MMPs], a disintegrin and metalloproteinases [ADAM], and a disintegrin and metalloproteinases with thrombospondin motifs [ADAM-TS]) are now considered as key players with a growing list of substrates [9, 10] and functions sometimes dual [11]. Reliable in vivo models are required to decipher the specific role played by all these molecular determinants during angiogenesis and lymphangiogenesis. For in vivo assessment of angiogenesis, the Matrigel plug assay was developed more than 20 years ago [12] and is still in wide use today because it is easy to set up [13]. Lymphangiogenesis is investigated by different in vivo assays: tumor transplantation, corneal assays [14, 15], spheroid-based human microvessel formation [16] and finally, genetic models of lymphatic vessel development [17, 18]. However, the main drawback of those in vivo models is the difficult quantification and/or the high intra-experimental variability. The ear sponge assay is an adaptation of Matrigel assays that has proved to be useful for studying these processes [13, 19]. The sponge assay takes advantage of the presence of dense blood and lymphatic vasculatures in the adult mice ear, allowing the concomitant analysis of both vascular networks. In this model, after mice anesthetization, a small incision is made on the external and basal part of the mice ears, and a gelatin sponge, soaked with either (lymph)angiogenic factors, inhibitors, tumor cells, or their conditioned medium, is implanted between the two ear skin layers. Two to four weeks later, sponges can be processed by different analyses including at least (1) histological examination of the neo-formed vascular networks, (2) flow cytometry to characterize infiltrated cells, or (3) evaluation of reporter gene activity through fluorescent or bioluminescent systems [20, 21] (Fig. 1). It is worth mentioning that the ear sponge model offers the possibility to perform a computerized quantification on 2D and 3D sponge images after specific stainings. This model is an ideal, rapid and reproducible approach for testing the in vivo potency of proteases or other molecules on tumor progression and metastatic events. Notably, this mouse-based assay can be applied to transgenic mice.

2 Materials

All soluble reagents are stored at 4 °C. Prepare all solutions using sterile buffers and under sterile conditions.

2.1 Sponge Preparation

1. A sterile compressed gelatin sponge (GELFOAM, Pfizer).
2. Puncher to cut cylindrical pieces (5 mm).
3. Interstitial collagen solution (this solution has to be prepared on ice): 7.5 volumes of interstitial type I collagen solution, 1

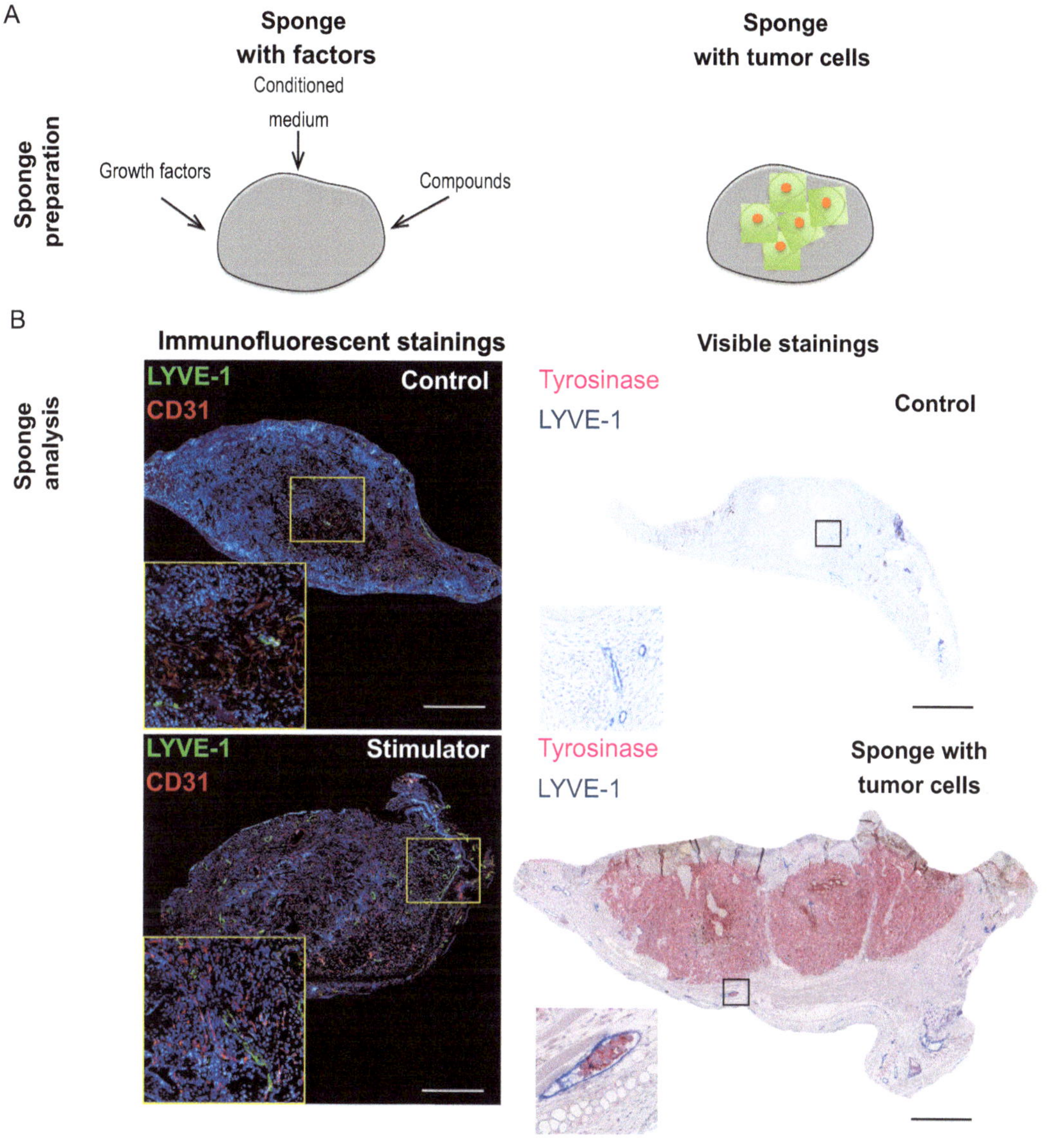

Fig. 1 Ear sponge assay applications and analysis. (**a**) Gelatin sponges are embedded with soluble compounds (growth factor as stimulator, drug, or cell-conditioned medium) (left part) or soaked with tumor cells (right part, in green). (**b**) Immunofluorescent (left) and visible (right) stainings of sponges resected 3 weeks post-implantation. Left: blood and lymphatic vessels are identified through CD31 and Lyve-1 stainings in sponges soaked with PBS (control) or with a growth factor used as a stimulator, respectively (left part). Angiogenesis and lymphangiogenesis. Cell nuclei appear in blue (DAPI). A zoom of the yellow square is represented. Scale bar = 1 mm. Right: illustrative visible staining of sponges soaked with tumor cells. The lymphatic vasculature is visualized by LYVE-1 staining (blue), and tumor cells appear in pink (tyrosinase is used as a marker of tumor cells). A zoom of the black square is presented. Scale bar = 1 mm

volume of 10× Hanks' balanced salt solution, 1.5 volume of 186 mM $NaHCO_3$. Adjust to pH 7.4 with a 1 M NaOH solution (*see* **Note 1**).

2.2 Mouse and Ear Preparation

1. Ketamine hydrochloride (100 mg/kg body weight).
2. Xylazine (10 mg/kg body weight).
3. Warming plate.
4. Microdissection instruments.

2.3 Cell Media and Cell Lines

1. Mouse melanoma B16F10 cells or similar according to the purpose of the study (*see* **Note 2**).
2. Dulbecco's Modified Eagle Medium (DMEM) or adapted medium according to the cell line used and the purpose of the study.
3. Medium conditioned by cells, growth factors, inhibitors, or any compound to be tested.
4. Trypsin.
5. Phosphate buffered saline (PBS).
6. Adapted medium according cell line used.
7. Glasstic slide with grids to count cells.
8. Amicon Ultra centrifugal filter of 3 kDa NMWL.

2.4 Sponge Implantation

It is necessary to perform chirurgical procedure under sterile conditions and use sterile materials.

1. Suture.
2. Warming plate.

2.5 Immunohistochemistry for Sample Processing

1. Polyclonal goat anti-mouse LYVE-1 (R&D Systems, AF2125).
2. Monoclonal rat anti-mouse CD31 (BD PharMingen, 557,355).
3. Rabbit anti-goat/Alexa Fluor 488.
4. Polyclonal goat anti-rat/Alexa Fluor 546.
5. Vectashield/DAPI mounting medium.
6. Medium for frozen section: Optimal Cutting Temperature (OCT).
7. Phosphate buffered saline (PBS).
8. Phosphate buffered saline (PBS)-1.5% milk.
9. Citrate buffer.
10. Protein block serum-free buffer.
11. Dako diluent solution (Dako, S2022).
12. Ferangi Blue chromogen kit (Biocare Medical FB8135).
13. Target buffer (Dako, S1699).

14. EnVision anti-rabbit/horseradish peroxidase (Dako K4003).
15. EnVision + System-HRP (DAB, Dako: K3468).
16. Entellan (Merck Millipore) or similar mounting medium.
17. Acetone.
18. Methanol.
19. Formalin.
20. Ethanol.
21. Isopropanol.
22. Xylene.
23. Paraffin.
24. H_2O_2.
25. Hematoxylin/eosin.

3 Methods

3.1 Sponge Preparation

Before any manipulations, sterilize all microdissection instruments and clean the work surface.

1. Cut gelatin sponges in small cylindrical pieces (around 3 mm^3) with a biopsia punch (*see* **Note 3**).
2. Place sponges in a 96-well plate, one sponge per well.
3. Prepare serum-free medium or phosphate buffered saline (PBS) for non-treated sponges and growth factor solutions, drug solutions, cell suspension, or cell-conditioned medium for treated sponges according to the experimental design.

3.1.1 For Drug and Growth Factor Solutions, the Procedure Is as Follows

1. Defrost drugs and/or growth factors on ice.
2. Dilute the compound to be tested in serum-free medium or PBS to obtain the requested concentration(s).
3. Mix the final solution by pipetting and keep it on ice.

3.1.2 For Cell Suspension Preparation, the Procedure Is as Follows

1. Culture cells in complete medium until reaching 80% of confluency.
2. Pre-warm at room temperature PBS, trypsin-EDTA (0.05% (wt/vol)) and the culture medium.
3. Remove the medium from the dish containing cultured cells.
4. Gently rinse 5 mL of pre-warmed PBS and aspirate PBS afterward.
5. Add 1.5 mL of trypsin-EDTA, shake the dish to cover the whole dish surface with the trypsin solution, and incubate the plate at 37 °C during 2–4 min.

6. Collect detached cells in medium supplemented with serum.
7. Centrifuge cell suspension at 260 × *g*, at room temperature for 10 min.
8. Remove supernatant and add 10 mL of serum-free medium.
9. Count cells and adjust their concentration.

3.1.3 For Cell-Conditioned Medium Preparation, the Procedure Is as Follows

1. Culture cells in complete medium until reaching 50% of confluency.
2. Pre-warm PBS and serum-free medium at room temperature before use.
3. Remove the culture medium, wash the cell culture with 5 mL of PBS, and aspirate PBS.
4. Incubate cells with 5 mL of serum-free medium for 10 min at 37 °C.
5. Remove the medium and repeat this step one more time.
6. Add 10 mL of fresh serum-free medium and culture cells for 48 h at 37 °C.
7. Collect the cell-conditioned medium, and concentrate it with an Amicon Ultra centrifugal filter placed in a 15 mL centrifuge tube and centrifuge at 2200 × *g*, 4 °C for 1.5 h.
8. Collect the concentrated medium from the filter and place it in a new tube.
9. Use the conditioned medium immediately or freeze it until use at −20 °C.
10. With a micropipette, add 20 μl of the solution to be tested as a drop on top of the sponge to allow a progressive diffusion of the solution into the sponge. Manipulate gently the plate in order to maintain the drop on the sponge (*see* **Note 4**).
11. Incubate the plate containing sponges at 37 °C for 30 min. During this incubation period, it is crucial to turn upside down each sponge in the same well, at least once (*see* **Note 5**).
12. Take each sponge with a forceps, embed it rapidly in a cold interstitial type I collagen solution, and place it immediately in a new well.
13. Incubate sponges at 37 °C for 30 min to allow collagen polymerization. Wait until complete collagen polymerization to ensure that the tested compound/cells remain(s) inside the sponge (*see* **Note 6**).

3.2 Mouse and Ear Preparation

Female mice of 6–8 weeks old are used (*see* **Note 7**).

1. Anesthetize mice with ketamine hydrochloride (100 mg/kg body weight) and xylazine (10 mg/kg body weight) by intraperitoneal injection with appropriate doses.

2. Wait for 4–6 min until the mouse is fully anesthetized.
3. Annotate clearly the cages and experimental groups (*see* **Note 8**).
4. A control group with sponges soaked with serum-free medium or PBS is applicable.
5. Sterilize the ear skin surfaces with a gauze soaked with 70% ethanol (vol/vol).

3.3 Sponge Implantation

1. Place the body of the mouse straight on a sterile support.
2. Make a little horizontal incision with a scissor in the basal, external, and central parts of the ear.
3. Detach smoothly both ear skin layers with a thin forceps, and make a hole of 5 mm^2. The ear skin layers are extremely thin, being possible to perforate them if this step is carried out too quickly. In case of perforation, exclude this ear (*see* **Note 9**).
4. Introduce the sponge into the ear hole with the help of a specific forceps trying to drive it at the end of the aperture. During the sponge implantation, the operator should push gently the sponge to avoid liquid loss.
5. Make two suture points in the incision part to join together the two ear edges.
6. Repeat the same procedure with the other mouse ear (identical treatment has to be applied to both ear of the same mouse).
7. After mouse operation, leave the animal on the warming plate (34 °C), and allow the mouse to recover from anesthesia.
8. Replace the mice to their appropriate annotated cages.

3.4 Sample Processing

1. After mice sacrifice, in accordance with the guideline of the local animal ethical committee, sponges can be harvested by cutting the surrounding skin. To visualize angiogenesis and lymphangiogenesis, sponges are collected 2–4 weeks post-implantation (*see* **Note 10**).
2. Sponges can be used for immunofluorescence and/or visible stainings according to the protocols detailed below (*see* **Note 11**).

3.4.1 For Immunofluorescent Stainings

1. Sponges are embedded in OCT and frozen in liquid nitrogen. The blocks are kept at −80 °C until use.
2. After cryosectioning in 10 μm sections, slides are kept at room temperature for 15 min.
3. Tissues are fixed first in acetone for 2 min at −20 °C and then in 80% methanol (vol/vol) for 5 min at 4 °C.
4. After washes in PBS (three times × 5 min), slides are incubated in PBS-1.5% milk for 30 min of blocking.
5. After the blocking step, slides are incubated with the primary antibodies. Antibodies raised against mouse LYVE-1 (diluted

1/100 in PBS; for lymphatic vessel detection) and/or mouse CD31 (diluted 1/400 in PBS; for blood vessel detection) are incubated for 2 h at room temperature.

6. Then, samples are washed in PBS (three times × 5 min) before the application of appropriate secondary antibodies conjugated to Alexa Fluor 488 (green) and/or Alexa Fluor 546 (red) (diluted 1/200 in PBS), for 30 and 45 min, respectively.
7. For double immunofluorescence-labeling studies, sections are first incubated with the two primary antibodies and then with Alexa Fluor 488 followed by the Alexa Fluor 546-conjugated secondary antibodies.
8. After three washes with PBS (each of 5 min), cell nuclei are counterstained with Vectashield/DAPI mounting medium.

3.4.2 For Visible Stainings

1. Sponges are fixed in 4% formalin overnight, followed by 70% ethanol (vol/vol), 96% ethanol (vol/vol), isopropanol, and xylene (two times × 1 h each step), and embedded into paraffin.
   (a) *For lymphatic vasculature detection*:
   - Sections of 5 μm are autoclaved for 11 min at 126 °C in citrate buffer.
   - Slides are washed with distilled water (two times × 5 min) and then, incubated with a protein block serum-free buffer, during 10 min.
   - Following the blocking step, slides are incubated with LYVE-1 antibody for 2 h (dilution 1/100 in Dako diluent solution) at room temperature.
   - Sections are then washed and revealed with the Ferangi Blue chromogen kit.

   (b) *For blood vasculature detection*:
   - Sections are autoclaved for 11 min at 126 °C in target buffer.
   - Slides are washed with distilled water (two times × 5 min) and incubated for 20 min at room temperature in H_2O_2 3% (diluted in distilled water) to block endogen peroxidase.
   - After two washes with distilled water (two times × 5 min), sections are incubated with the protein block serum-free buffer, during 10 min.
   - Following the blocking step, slides are incubated with CD31 antibody for 1 h (dilution 1/200 in Dako diluent solution) at room temperature.
   - Sections are then washed and revealed with the EnVision anti-rabbit/horseradish peroxidase and DAB.

2. Finally, in both cases, the samples are counterstained with hematoxylin/eosin, washed in water, dehydrated in graded alcohols, and mounted with Entellan mounting medium.

4 Notes

1. The use of color 10× HBSS is a color indicator to adjust the pH to 7.4. The addition of NaOH in collagen solution containing 10× HBSS induces a modification of HBSS color from yellow to purple. At this point, the pH of the collagen solution is adapted.
2. The ear sponge assay used with tumor cell expressing a reporter gene allows easily to follow tumor growth by the physical accessibility of the ear. For example, the bioluminescence of tumor cells luciferase positive is easily followed by luciferin intraperitoneal injection on mice.
3. The puncher has to be applied while turning on the sterile compressed gelatin sponge, not pushing. This ensures the structure of the sponge.
4. The addition of the drop at the top of the sponge is a crucial step of the ear sponge assay to allow a progressive diffusion of the solution into the sponge. It allows the precise amount of cells, conditioned medium, or compound used in the experimental procedure.
5. The sponge must be turned upside down to ensure the homogeneity of the cell suspension or compounds diffusion.
6. The collagen coating is a crucial element of the ear sponge assay. It allows to push gently the sponge between the two ear skin layers without a loss of the liquid embedded inside.
7. The ear sponge assay is applicable with female mice of 6–8 weeks old. We indeed observed higher result variability with males.
8. The implantation of sponge inside mice ear excludes the use of clip ear to identify animals. It is necessary to use well-annotated cages to follow experimental conditions.
9. It is important to check macroscopically the ear integrity to discard any mouse with lesions or damage in the ear tissue. Any perforations of ears impact to exclude the ear of the experiment. An alteration of the ear integrity could generate the loss of the implanted sponge.
10. Another disadvantage could be the sponge degradation after 4 weeks in the mouse ear. Although the (lymph)angiogenic tests to evaluate the effect of inhibitors/stimulators and to analyze the tumor cell proliferation/dissemination do not

need to keep sponges for more than 3–4 weeks, possible adaptations of this model for studies requiring more than 4 weeks cannot be performed.

11. Notable limitations of this assay include the involvement of inflammatory cells limiting the application to pathological conditions and not to the developmental context.

References

1. Reddy BY, Lim PK, Silverio K et al (2012) The microenvironmental effect in the progression, metastasis, and dormancy of breast cancer: a model system within bone marrow. Int J Breast Cancer 2012:721659. https://doi.org/10.1155/2012/721659
2. Hanahan D, Weinberg RA (2011) Hallmarks of cancer: the next generation. Cell 144(5): 646–674. https://doi.org/10.1016/j.cell.2011.02.013
3. Massague J, Obenauf AC (2016) Metastatic colonization by circulating tumour cells. Nature 529(7586):298–306. https://doi.org/10.1038/nature17038
4. Paupert J, Van de Velde M, Kridelka F et al (2014) Tumor angiogenesis and lymphangiogenesis: microenvironmental soil for tumor progression and metastatic dissemination. In: Feige JJ, Pagès G, Soncin F (eds) Molecular mechanisms of angiogenesis. Springer, Paris, pp 283–306. https://doi.org/10.1007/978-2-8178-0466-8
5. Balsat C, Blacher S, Signolle N et al (2011) Whole slide quantification of stromal lymphatic vessel distribution and peritumoral lymphatic vessel density in early invasive cervical cancer: a method description. ISRN Obstet Gynecol 2011:354861. https://doi.org/10.5402/2011/354861
6. Achen MG, McColl BK, Stacker SA (2005) Focus on lymphangiogenesis in tumor metastasis. Cancer Cell 7(2):121–127. https://doi.org/10.1016/j.ccr.2005.01.017
7. Shayan R, Karnezis T, Murali R et al (2012) Lymphatic vessel density in primary melanomas predicts sentinel lymph node status and risk of metastasis. Histopathology 61(4):702–710. https://doi.org/10.1111/j.1365-2559.2012.04310.x
8. Tampellini M, Sonetto C, Scagliotti GV (2016) Novel anti-angiogenic therapeutic strategies in colorectal cancer. Expert Opin Investig Drugs 25(5):507–520. https://doi.org/10.1517/13543784.2016.1161754
9. Overall CM, Lopez-Otin C (2002) Strategies for MMP inhibition in cancer: innovations for the post-trial era. Nat Rev Cancer 2(9): 657–672. https://doi.org/10.1038/nrc884
10. Page-McCaw A, Ewald AJ, Werb Z (2007) Matrix metalloproteinases and the regulation of tissue remodelling. Nat Rev Mol Cell Biol 8(3):221–233. https://doi.org/10.1038/nrm2125
11. Lopez-Otin C, Matrisian LM (2007) Emerging roles of proteases in tumour suppression. Nat Rev Cancer 7(10):800–808. https://doi.org/10.1038/nrc2228
12. Passaniti A (1992) Extracellular matrix-cell interactions: matrigel and complex cellular pattern formation. Lab Investig 67(6):804. author reply 804–808
13. Benton G, Arnaoutova I, George J et al (2014) Matrigel: from discovery and ECM mimicry to assays and models for cancer research. Adv Drug Deliv Rev 79-80:3–18. https://doi.org/10.1016/j.addr.2014.06.005
14. Cao R, Lim S, Ji H et al (2011) Mouse corneal lymphangiogenesis model. Nat Protoc 6(6):817–826. https://doi.org/10.1038/nprot.2011.359
15. Detry B, Blacher S, Erpicum C et al (2013) Sunitinib inhibits inflammatory corneal lymphangiogenesis. Invest Ophthalmol Vis Sci 54(5):3082–3093. https://doi.org/10.1167/iovs.12-10856
16. Laib AM, Bartol A, Alajati A et al (2009) Spheroid-based human endothelial cell microvessel formation in vivo. Nat Protoc 4(8):1202–1215. https://doi.org/10.1038/nprot.2009.96
17. Karpanen T, Schulte-Merker S (2011) Zebrafish provides a novel model for lymphatic vascular research. Methods Cell Biol 105:223–238. https://doi.org/10.1016/b978-0-12-381320-6.00009-6
18. Ny A, Vandevelde W, Hohensinner P et al (2013) A transgenic Xenopus laevis reporter model to study lymphangiogenesis. Biol Open 2(9):882–890. https://doi.org/10.1242/bio.20134739

19. Kibbey MC, Grant DS, Kleinman HK (1992) Role of the SIKVAV site of laminin in promotion of angiogenesis and tumor growth: an in vivo matrigel model. J Natl Cancer Inst 84(21):1633–1638
20. Garcia-Caballero M, Van de Velde M, Blacher S et al (2017) Modeling pre-metastatic lymphvascular niche in the mouse ear sponge assay. Sci Rep 7:41494. https://doi.org/10.1038/srep41494
21. Suarez-Carmona M, Bourcy M, Lesage J et al (2015) Soluble factors regulated by epithelial-mesenchymal transition mediate tumour angiogenesis and myeloid cell recruitment. J Pathol 236(4):491–504. https://doi.org/10.1002/path.4546

Chapter 21

Cancer Susceptibility Models in Protease-Deficient Mice

Alicia R. Folgueras, Sandra Freitas-Rodríguez, Yaiza Español, and Gloria Velasco

Abstract

For decades, proteases have been associated with cancer progression due to the ability of some members of this large group of enzymes to degrade tumor cell surroundings, thereby facilitating cancer invasion and dissemination. However, the generation of mouse models deficient in proteases has revealed the existence of a great variety of functions among proteolytic enzymes in cancer biology, including important tumor-suppressive roles. Therefore, in this chapter, we describe methods to chemically induce different types of cancer (lung adenocarcinoma, hepatocellular carcinoma, oral and esophageal carcinoma, colorectal carcinoma, skin cancer, and fibrosarcoma) in genetically modified mouse models to efficiently evaluate the specific pro- or antitumoral function of proteases in cancer.

Key words Protease, Cancer, Mouse models, Urethane, DEN, 4NQO, Azoxymethane, DMBA, MCA

1 Introduction

The annotation of human and mouse genomes at the beginning of this century allowed the first global view of the degradome, defined as the complete set of proteases that are produced at a specific moment by a cell, tissue, or organism [1, 2]. Since then, our understanding of the proteolytic systems has expanded enormously, mainly due to the valuable information provided by genetically engineered mouse models deficient in proteases. The generation of protease-deficient mice has demonstrated that these enzymes, initially considered as merely degradative agents, exert very complex and specific biological functions, as a consequence of the great diversity of bioactive substrates they can target through activating and inactivating proteolytic cleavages [3, 4]. Thus, proteases have emerged as key regulators of cellular behavior, being involved in cell proliferation, adhesion, differentiation, migration, and death, thereby influencing most biological processes. Accordingly, a

Santiago Cal and Alvaro J. Obaya (eds.), *Proteases and Cancer: Methods and Protocols*, Methods in Molecular Biology, vol. 1731, https://doi.org/10.1007/978-1-4939-7595-2_21,

deregulation of the proteolytic activity unleashes a variety of pathological conditions, including cancer [5–8].

Although uncontrolled proteolytic activity has long been associated with cancer progression, the improvement of our understanding of protease function has unveiled new roles for these enzymes in tumor development. Thus, the generation of genetically modified mouse models of gain or loss of protease function has provided definitive evidence of protease involvement in the earliest steps of malignant transformation, in addition to the classically attributed roles in invasion and metastatic dissemination [9–12]. Moreover, these animal models have been determinant to demonstrate for the first time the unexpected in vivo tumor-suppressive functions of certain extracellular proteases [13, 14].

In this chapter, we describe several protocols used in our laboratory to evaluate the specific pro- or antitumoral function of proteolytic enzymes in cancer development [15–19]. Thus, the methods described herein are suitable to chemically induce carcinogenic processes in mice that mimic most of the molecular and pathological features found in human cancers. We detail the following protocols to induce six different types of cancer in genetically modified mouse models:

1. The urethane model for induction of lung adenomas and adenocarcinomas (only in the most susceptible mouse strains). The intraperitoneal administration of this carcinogen causes activating mutations in the oncogene KRAS [20], which is frequently altered in non-small cell lung cancer [21].
2. The DEN (diethylnitrosamine) model for induction of hepatocarcinomas (HCC), which highly resembles the gene expression pattern of human HCCs with poor survival [22].
3. The 4NQO (4-Nitroquinoline-*N*-oxide) model, which recapitulates the pathogenic features of human oral and esophageal squamous cell carcinomas [23, 24].
4. The AOM (azoxymethane)/DSS (dextran sodium sulfate) model for induction of colitis-associated colorectal cancer. This method combines the administration of a single dose of the carcinogenic agent azoxymethane, which causes mutations that stabilize β-catenin [25], with several cycles of DSS treatment, which sustains a chronic inflammatory environment that promotes tumor progression [26, 27].
5. The DMBA (9,10-dimethyl-1,2-benzanthracene)/TPA (phorbol 12-myristate 13-acetate) model for induction of precancerous skin lesions (papillomas) and squamous cell carcinomas (SCC), which harbor the most frequent mutations in the RAS family found in human SCCs [28]. This two-step protocol combines the topical application of the carcinogen DMBA

with TPA, which enhances epidermal inflammation and proliferation.

6. The MCA (3-methylcholanthrene) model for induction of fibrosarcomas.

2 Materials

The reagents used in these protocols are classified as carcinogens, meaning that all solutions should be prepared following adequate handling and waste disposal regulations. Additional plans for mice cage labeling and bedding disposal may be required.

2.1 Lung Carcinogenesis Model

1. 100 mg/mL ethyl carbamate (also named urethane) solution in sterile saline (0.9% sodium chloride).
2. 1-mL syringe, 25-G needle, 5/8 in.

2.2 Liver Carcinogenesis Model

1. 2.5 mg/mL *N*-nitrosodiethylamine (also named diethylnitrosamine, DEN) solution in sterile saline (0.9% sodium chloride).
2. 1-mL syringe, 25-G needle, 5/8 in.

2.3 Oral and Esophageal Carcinogenesis Model

1. 5 mg/mL 4-nitroquinoline-*N*-oxide (4NQO) stock solution in propylene glycol.
2. Ultrasonic bath or probe-type sonicator.
3. Drinking water.

2.4 Colorectal Carcinogenesis Model

1. 1.25 mg/mL azoxymethane (AOM) solution in sterile saline (0.9% sodium chloride).
2. 1.5% dextran sulfate sodium salt (DSS) solution in drinking water.
3. 1-mL syringe, 25-G needle, 5/8 in.

2.5 Skin Carcinogenesis Model

1. 0.125 mg/mL 7,12-dimethylbenz[a]anthracene (also named 9,10-dimethyl-1,2-benzanthracene, DMBA) solution in acetone.
2. 0.02 mg/mL phorbol 12-myristate 13-acetate (also named 12-*O*-tetradecanoylphorbol-13-acetate, TPA) stock solution in acetone.
3. Trimmer.
4. 200 μL pipette.
5. Filter tips.
6. Inhalatory anesthetics (isoflurane).
7. Caliper.

2.6 Fibrosarcoma Carcinogenesis Model

1. 1 mg/mL 3-methylcholanthrene (MCA) solution in corn oil.
2. Ultrasonic bath or probe-type sonicator.
3. Inhalatory anesthetics (isoflurane).
4. 1-mL syringe, 25-G needle, 5/8 in.
5. Trimmer.
6. Caliper.

2.7 Necropsy and Sample Collection

1. Forceps and scissors.
2. Caliper.
3. Ruler.
4. Phosphate-buffered saline (PBS).
5. Petri dish.
6. Liquid nitrogen or dry ice.
7. 10% formalin solution, neutral buffered, or 4% w/v paraformaldehyde dissolved in PBS, pH 7.4.
8. OCT (optimal cutting temperature compound) and cryomolds.
9. Whatman paper (only for skin sample collection).

3 Methods

3.1 Lung Carcinogenesis Model

1. Dissolve urethane in sterile saline solution (0.9% sodium chloride) to a concentration of 100 mg/mL.
2. Inject 1 mg urethane/g body weight (b.w.) intraperitoneally into 8-week-old mice (*see* **Note 1**). For example, inject 100 μL of 100 mg/mL urethane solution (10 mg of urethane) into a 10-g mouse.
3. After 48 h, repeat **step 2** (*see* **Note 2**).
4. With the current protocol, tumors develop between 4 and 8 months after urethane injection in wild-type mice of sensitive strains (A/J > FVB/N > 129 > hybrid 129/C57). As the time for tumor development may also vary when working with genetically modified mouse models, it is highly recommended to monitor tumor progression by noninvasive imaging approaches (micro-CT scan, MRI) in order to determine the best time point to euthanize the mice.
5. When appropriate, weigh the experimental mouse, collect blood under anesthesia by cardiac puncture, and euthanize it to remove the lung.
6. Put the lung into a petri dish containing cold PBS to rinse the tissue.
7. Weigh the lung.

8. Take photographs of the lung using a ruler as scale reference.
9. Count the number of visible tumors and measure their size with a caliper.
10. Separate one or two specific lobes, and put them into formalin fixative overnight at 4 °C for paraffin embedding. Make sure that same lobes are consistently processed in the same way for histological analysis (*see* **Note 3**). Another lobe can be collected for cryo-embedding by placing the sample into a cryomold filled with OCT and freezing it onto a piece of dry ice.
11. Make separate aliquots of tumor-containing and tumor-free samples by dissecting the tissue from the remaining lobes using forceps and scissors. Snap freeze the aliquots in liquid nitrogen, and store them at −80 °C for further RNA and protein analysis.

3.2 Liver Carcinogenesis Model

1. Dissolve DEN in sterile saline solution (0.9% sodium chloride) to a concentration of 2.5 mg/mL.
2. Inject 25 mg DEN/kg b.w. intraperitoneally into 14-day-old mice. For example, inject 100 μL of 2.5 mg/mL DEN solution (0.25 mg of DEN) into a 10-g mouse (*see* **Note 4**).
3. Monitor liver tumor development by noninvasive imaging approaches (micro-CT scan, MRI, ultrasound). Tumors will develop between 6 and 10 months after DEN injection in wild-type mice.
4. When appropriate, euthanize the mice, and collect blood and liver samples following the procedures above-described in Subheading 3.1, **steps 5–11**.

3.3 Oral and Esophageal Carcinogenesis Model

1. Dissolve 4NQO in propylene glycol to a concentration of 5 mg/mL (*see* **Note 5**). 4NQO stock solution is then further diluted to a concentration of 100 μg/mL in drinking water.
2. Provide 7–8-week-old mice with weekly prepared drinking water containing 100 μg/mL 4NQO ad libitum for 20 weeks (*see* **Note 6**).
3. Monitor mouse weight regularly. If severe weight loss or any sign of discomfort is detected, mice should be euthanized.
4. Keep the mice untreated for 2 additional weeks, and euthanize them after blood collection.
5. Dissect the tongues and esophagi of mice.
6. Take photographs of the tongue and esophagus using a ruler as scale reference.
7. Count the number of visible tumors and measure their size with a caliper.

8. Separate one or two specific tumor-containing areas of the tongue and esophagus for cryo-embedding, as above-described in Subheading 3.1, **step 10**, and snap freezing (*see* Subheading 3.1, **step 11**).
9. Put the remaining tongue and esophagus into formalin fixative overnight at 4 °C for histological processing. Prior to paraffin embedding, cut each tissue in 4–5 mm transverse sections, and place the pieces oriented transversally into the same tissue cassette. After paraffin embedding, cut serial sections (spaced 100 μm) with a microtome for pathological evaluation. This protocol generates both precancerous and cancerous lesions, ranging from mild epithelial hyperplasia to invasive SCC, which can be further classified using established histopathological criteria.

3.4 Colorectal Carcinogenesis Model

1. Dissolve AOM in sterile saline solution (0.9% sodium chloride) to a concentration of 1.25 mg/mL.
2. Inject 12.5 mg AOM/kg b.w. intraperitoneally into 8-week-old mice. For example, inject 100 μL of 1.25 mg/mL azoxymethane solution (0.125 mg of AOM) into a 10-g mouse.
3. Let the mice recover for 5 days after AOM injection.
4. Provide mice with drinking water containing 1.5% DSS ad libitum for 5 consecutive days (*see* **Note 7**).
5. Provide mice with drinking water without DSS for 14 days.
6. Repeat **steps 4** and **5** two more times.
7. After a total of 3 cycles alternating 1.5% DSS exposure with water without DSS (Fig. 1), euthanize the mice after blood collection.
8. Dissect and unwrap the whole intestine, from stomach to anus. Remove the colon by cutting the intestine after the cecum. Remember the orientation of the colon (cecum end and rectal end).
9. Flush out the fecal content of the colon by using a syringe with PBS.
10. Measure the length of the colon.
11. Take one or two colon samples for snap freezing and cryo-embedding. Make sure that same intestinal areas are consistently processed in the same way.
12. Put the remaining colon into formalin fixative overnight at 4 °C, and follow the procedure above-described in Subheading 3.3, **step 9** for histological processing.

3.5 Skin Carcinogenesis Model

1. Shave the back of 7- to 8-week-old mice (*see* **Note 8**).
2. Let the mice rest 2 days after shaving.

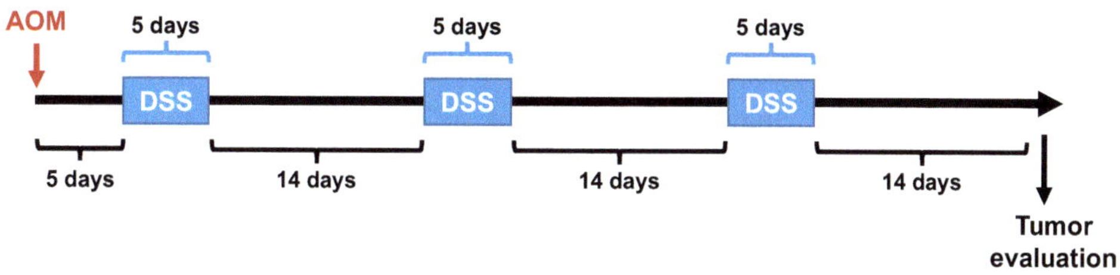

Fig. 1 Time course of the AOM/DSS carcinogenesis model for induction of colitis-associated colorectal cancer in mice

3. Dissolve DMBA in acetone to a concentration of 0.125 mg/mL. A 100× stock solution (12.5 mg/mL) may be stored at −20 °C. DMBA working solution should be made fresh on the day of the experiment and protected from light.
4. Anesthetize the recipient mouse with isoflurane.
5. Apply 200 μL of 0.125 mg/mL DMBA solution (25 μg of DMBA) onto the shaved back skin of the mice with a pipette (use filter tips), and wait a few min to allow acetone solution to evaporate. For the next 2 weeks, mice and bedding should be carefully handled following biohazard regulations.
6. Let the mice rest for 1 week.
7. Dissolve TPA in acetone to a concentration of 0.02 mg/mL. A 100× stock solution (2 mg/mL) may be stored at −20 °C for a month. TPA working solution should be made fresh on the day of the experiment.
8. Anesthetize the mice, apply 200 μL of 0.02 mg/mL TPA solution (4 μg of TPA) onto the dorsal skin of the mice with a pipette (use filter tips), and wait a few min to allow acetone solution to evaporate.
9. Repeat step 8 twice weekly for 24 weeks (*see* **Note 9**).
10. Approximately 6 weeks after first TPA administration, monitor tumor formation. Record the number of visible papillomas and measure their size with a caliper once weekly.
11. Monitor the conversion of papillomas to SCCs, which acquire a more flattened appearance.
12. Euthanize the mice 1 week after the last TPA application upon blood collection. If any wounds are detected in the course of the experiment, mice should be euthanized and removed from the experimental cohort since wounding may affect tumor progression.
13. Take photographs of the back skin.
14. Dissect tumor-containing and tumor-free skin areas, and take samples for paraffin embedding, cryo-embedding, and snap freezing (*see* **Note 10**).

3.6 Fibrosarcoma Carcinogenesis Model

1. Dissolve MCA in corn oil to a concentration of 1 mg/mL (*see* **Note 5**). MCA solution should be protected from light.
2. Shave one dorsal flank of 7- to 8-week-old male mice. Female mice are highly resistant to MCA-induced fibrosarcomas [15].
3. Anesthetize the recipient mouse with isoflurane.
4. Inject 100 μL of MCA solution (100 μg of MCA) subcutaneously into the flank of the mouse (load the syringe without the needle since corn oil is quite thick).
5. Record tumor initiation. Tumors will become palpable 10–12 weeks after MCA treatment in wild-type mice. Nevertheless, genetically modified mouse models may be more susceptible to tumor development, and tumors may arise earlier.
6. Monitor tumor growth with a caliper once weekly.
7. When appropriate (on the basis of tumor size according to ethical regulations), euthanize the mice, and collect blood and tumor samples for paraffin embedding, cryo-embedding, and snap freezing.

4 Notes

1. Urethane is an anesthetic. Provide mice with a heat source during recovery upon urethane administration.
2. The development of urethane-induced lung tumors depends on the susceptibility of the mouse strain used in the experiment. Thus, some strains such as inbred C57BL/6 are highly resistant to tumor development and require an alternative carcinogenesis protocol consisting in ten weekly urethane doses (1 mg/g b.w.) to reach a nearly 100% lung tumor incidence in wild-type mice [29].
3. Paraffin-embedded samples should be cut into serial sections (spaced 100 μm) with a microtome for pathological evaluation. In addition to tumor grade, tumor size may also be estimated on the basis of the number of cells present in the serial section showing the largest tumoral area.
4. In addition to variations in susceptibility to liver tumor development among mouse strains, being C3H the most susceptible and C57BL/6 the most resistant strain [30, 31], male mice develop more hepatic tumors than females [32].
5. To aid the carcinogen going into solution, use an ultrasonic bath or a probe-type sonicator.
6. Alternative methods consisting in 16 weeks of 4NQO administration and 12 weeks of observation after carcinogen treatment also reach 100% incidence in C57BL/6 mice [23].

7. This protocol provides reproducible results in C57BL/6 mice. Nevertheless, depending on the susceptibility of the mouse strain to DSS, concentration and length of DSS treatment should be adjusted (from 1% to 2.5% and 4–7 days, respectively) [33, 34].
8. Although standard protocols apply DMBA during the resting phase of the hair cycle (8-week-old mice), it has been described that proliferating cells are more susceptible to tumor initiation. Therefore, an alternative protocol based on the administration of DMBA onto anagen skin (4-week-old mice with a hair cycle in the proliferative phase) may be considered when working with mouse strains that are low sensitive to skin carcinogenesis [35].
9. The duration of the tumor promotion stage with TPA may be extended to increase the percentage of papillomas that progress to SCCs. Also, this percentage will vary depending on the susceptibility of the mouse strain [36, 37]. Alternatively, a high frequency of SCCs is achieved with a single-step protocol based on the weekly administration of 10 μg of DMBA for up to 25 weeks in the absence of TPA [38, 39].
10. Those skin biopsies that will undergo paraffin embedding or cryo-embedding should be cut into a rectangle following the anterior-posterior axis of the mouse. Additionally, it is important to place those skin samples onto a Whatman paper (dermal side down) in order to prevent the skin from curling. Finally, at the time of embedding, the rectangular piece of skin should stand in a 90° angle to the bottom of the cassette or cryo-mold and follow the long side axis in order to guarantee the right hair follicle orientation when sectioning.

Acknowledgments

We thank Dr. C. López-Otín for helpful comments and advice. Our work is supported by grants from Ministerio de Economía y Competitividad, Instituto de Salud Carlos III, CIBERONC, Plan Feder, and Progeria Research Foundation. S.F.-R. is recipient of an FPU Fellowship.

References

1. López-Otín C, Overall CM (2002) Protease degradomics: a new challenge for proteomics. Nat Rev Mol Cell Biol 3(7):509–519. https://doi.org/10.1038/nrm858
2. Puente XS, Sánchez LM, Overall CM et al (2003) Human and mouse proteases: a comparative genomic approach. Nat Rev Genet 4(7): 544–558. https://doi.org/10.1038/nrg1111
3. Mason SD, Joyce JA (2011) Proteolytic networks in cancer. Trends Cell Biol 21(4): 228–237. https://doi.org/10.1016/j.tcb.2010.12.002
4. Kruger A (2009) Functional genetic mouse models: promising tools for investigation of the proteolytic internet. Biol Chem 390(2):91–97. https://doi.org/10.1515/BC.2009.015

5. Quirós PM, Langer T, López-Otín C (2015) New roles for mitochondrial proteases in health, ageing and disease. Nat Rev Mol Cell Biol 16(6):345–359. https://doi.org/10.1038/nrm3984
6. Cal S, Lopez-Otin C (2015) ADAMTS proteases and cancer. Matrix Biol 44-46:77–85. https://doi.org/10.1016/j.matbio.2015.01.013
7. Fraile JM, Quesada V, Rodríguez D et al (2012) Deubiquitinases in cancer: new functions and therapeutic options. Oncogene 31(19):2373–2388. https://doi.org/10.1038/onc.2011.443
8. Freitas-Rodríguez S, Folgueras AR, López-Otín C (2017) The role of matrix metalloproteinases in aging: tissue remodeling and beyond. Biochim Biophys Acta 1864(11 Pt A):2015–2025
9. Folgueras AR, Pendás AM, Sánchez LM et al (2004) Matrix metalloproteinases in cancer: from new functions to improved inhibition strategies. Int J Dev Biol 48(5-6):411–424. https://doi.org/10.1387/ijdb.041811af
10. Affara NI, Andreu P, Coussens LM (2009) Delineating protease functions during cancer development. Methods Mol Biol 539:1–32. https://doi.org/10.1007/978-1-60327-003-8_1
11. Kessenbrock K, Plaks V, Werb Z (2010) Matrix metalloproteinases: regulators of the tumor microenvironment. Cell 141(1):52–67. https://doi.org/10.1016/j.cell.2010.03.015
12. Sevenich L, Joyce JA (2014) Pericellular proteolysis in cancer. Genes Dev 28(21):2331–2347. https://doi.org/10.1101/gad.250647.114
13. López-Otín C, Matrisian LM (2007) Emerging roles of proteases in tumour suppression. Nat Rev Cancer 7(10):800–808. https://doi.org/10.1038/nrc2228
14. Fanjul-Fernández M, Folgueras AR, Cabrera S et al (2010) Matrix metalloproteinases: evolution, gene regulation and functional analysis in mouse models. Biochim Biophys Acta 1803(1):3–19. https://doi.org/10.1016/j.bbamcr.2009.07.004
15. Balbín M, Fueyo A, Tester AM et al (2003) Loss of collagenase-2 confers increased skin tumor susceptibility to male mice. Nat Genet 35(3):252–257. https://doi.org/10.1038/ng1249
16. Fanjul-Fernández M, Folgueras AR, Fueyo A et al (2013) Matrix metalloproteinase Mmp-1a is dispensable for normal growth and fertility in mice and promotes lung cancer progression by modulating inflammatory responses. J Biol Chem 288(20):14647–14656. https://doi.org/10.1074/jbc.M112.439893
17. de la Rosa J, Freije JM, Cabanillas R et al (2013) Prelamin A causes progeria through cell-extrinsic mechanisms and prevents cancer invasion. Nat Commun 4:2268. https://doi.org/10.1038/ncomms3268
18. Fraile JM, Campos-Iglesias D, Rodríguez F et al (2016) The deubiquitinase USP54 is overexpressed in colorectal cancer stem cells and promotes intestinal tumorigenesis. Oncotarget 7(46):74427–74434. 10.18632/oncotarget.12769
19. Quirós PM, Español Y, Acín-Pérez R et al (2014) ATP-dependent Lon protease controls tumor bioenergetics by reprogramming mitochondrial activity. Cell Rep 8(2):542–556. https://doi.org/10.1016/j.celrep.2014.06.018
20. Westcott PM, Halliwill KD, To MD et al (2015) The mutational landscapes of genetic and chemical models of Kras-driven lung cancer. Nature 517(7535):489–492. https://doi.org/10.1038/nature13898
21. Naidoo J, Drilon A (2016) KRAS-mutant lung cancers in the era of targeted therapy. Adv Exp Med Biol 893:155–178. https://doi.org/10.1007/978-3-319-24223-1_8
22. Lee JS, Chu IS, Mikaelyan A et al (2004) Application of comparative functional genomics to identify best-fit mouse models to study human cancer. Nat Genet 36(12):1306–1311. https://doi.org/10.1038/ng1481
23. Tang XH, Knudsen B, Bemis D et al (2004) Oral cavity and esophageal carcinogenesis modeled in carcinogen-treated mice. Clin Cancer Res 10(1 Pt 1):301–313
24. Foy JP, Tortereau A, Caulin C et al (2016) The dynamics of gene expression changes in a mouse model of oral tumorigenesis may help refine prevention and treatment strategies in patients with oral cancer. Oncotarget 7(24):35932–35945. 10.18632/oncotarget.8321
25. Greten FR, Eckmann L, Greten TF et al (2004) IKKbeta links inflammation and tumorigenesis in a mouse model of colitis-associated cancer. Cell 118(3):285–296. https://doi.org/10.1016/j.cell.2004.07.013
26. Suzuki R, Kohno H, Sugie S et al (2004) Sequential observations on the occurrence of preneoplastic and neoplastic lesions in mouse colon treated with azoxymethane and dextran sodium sulfate. Cancer Sci 95(9):721–727
27. Tanaka T, Kohno H, Suzuki R et al (2003) A novel inflammation-related mouse colon carcinogenesis model induced by azoxymethane

and dextran sodium sulfate. Cancer Sci 94(11):965–973

28. Nassar D, Latil M, Boeckx B et al (2015) Genomic landscape of carcinogen-induced and genetically induced mouse skin squamous cell carcinoma. Nat Med 21(8):946–954. https://doi.org/10.1038/nm.3878
29. Miller YE, Dwyer-Nield LD, Keith RL et al (2003) Induction of a high incidence of lung tumors in C57BL/6 mice with multiple ethyl carbamate injections. Cancer Lett 198(2):139–144
30. Lee GH, Nomura K, Kanda H et al (1991) Strain specific sensitivity to diethylnitrosamine-induced carcinogenesis is maintained in hepatocytes of C3H/HeN in equilibrium with C57BL/6N chimeric mice. Cancer Res 51(12):3257–3260
31. Maronpot RR (2009) Biological basis of differential susceptibility to hepatocarcinogenesis among mouse strains. J Toxicol Pathol 22(1):11–33. https://doi.org/10.1293/tox.22.11
32. Poole TM, Drinkwater NR (1996) Strain dependent effects of sex hormones on hepatocarcinogenesis in mice. Carcinogenesis 17(2):191–196
33. Suzuki R, Kohno H, Sugie S et al (2006) Strain differences in the susceptibility to azoxymethane and dextran sodium sulfate-induced colon carcinogenesis in mice. Carcinogenesis 27(1):162–169. https://doi.org/10.1093/carcin/bgi205
34. Neufert C, Becker C, Neurath MF (2007) An inducible mouse model of colon carcinogenesis for the analysis of sporadic and inflammation-driven tumor progression. Nat Protoc 2(8):1998–2004. https://doi.org/10.1038/nprot.2007.279
35. Miller SJ, Wei ZG, Wilson C et al (1993) Mouse skin is particularly susceptible to tumor initiation during early anagen of the hair cycle: possible involvement of hair follicle stem cells. J Invest Dermatol 101(4):591–594
36. Abel EL, Angel JM, Kiguchi K et al (2009) Multi-stage chemical carcinogenesis in mouse skin: fundamentals and applications. Nat Protoc 4(9):1350–1362. https://doi.org/10.1038/nprot.2009.120
37. Sundberg JP, Sundberg BA, Beamer WG (1997) Comparison of chemical carcinogen skin tumor induction efficacy in inbred, mutant, and hybrid strains of mice: morphologic variations of induced tumors and absence of a papillomavirus cocarcinogen. Mol Carcinog 20(1): 19–32
38. Schober M, Fuchs E (2011) Tumor-initiating stem cells of squamous cell carcinomas and their control by TGF-beta and integrin/focal adhesion kinase (FAK) signaling. Proc Natl Acad Sci U S A 108(26):10544–10549. https://doi.org/10.1073/pnas.1107807108
39. Hennings H, Glick AB, Lowry DT et al (1993) FVB/N mice: an inbred strain sensitive to the chemical induction of squamous cell carcinomas in the skin. Carcinogenesis 14(11):2353 2358

Chapter 22

Imaging Proteolytic Activities in Mouse Models of Cancer

Anupama Pal and Alnawaz Rehemtulla

Abstract

Proteases are "protein-cleaving" enzymes, which, in addition to their non-specific degrading function, also catalyze the highly specific and regulated process of proteolytic processing, thus regulating multiple biological functions. Alterations in proteolytic activity occur during pathological conditions such as cancer. One of the major deregulated classes of proteases in cancer is caspases, the proteolytic initiators and mediators of the apoptotic machinery. The ability to image apoptosis noninvasively in living cells and animal models of cancer can not only provide new insight into the biological basis of the disease but can also be used as a quantitative tool to screen and evaluate novel therapeutic strategies. Optical molecular imaging such as bioluminescence-based genetically engineered biosensors has been developed in our laboratory and exploited to study protease activity in animal models with a high signal to noise. Using the circularly permuted form of firefly luciferase, we have developed a reporter for Caspase 3/7, referred to as Caspase 3/7 GloSensor. Here, we discuss the use of the Caspase 3/7 GloSensor for imaging apoptotic activity in mouse xenografts and genetically engineered mouse models of cancer and present the potential of this powerful platform technology to image the proteolytic activity of numerous other proteases.

Key words Caspase 3/7, GloSensor, Firefly luciferase, Proteases, Mouse models, Cancer

1 Introduction

Proteases are enzymes that cleave the peptide bond between two amino acids and were originally identified as destructive enzymes essential for protein catabolism [1]. Subsequently, in addition to their non-specific degradative function, a role for proteases in catalyzing a substrate-specific proteolytic cleavage resulting in the production of new protein products has become appreciated [2]. There is hardly a signaling process in a living cell that is not associated with protease activity in one way or another. Besides regulating the localization and activity of proteins, proteases create new bioactive molecules as well as generate, transduce, and amplify cellular signals through modulation of protein-protein interactions [3]. Thus proteases regulate multiple biological processes including cell proliferation, differentiation and morphogenesis, DNA replication and transcription, tissue morphogenesis and remodeling,

Santiago Cal and Alvaro J. Obaya (eds.), *Proteases and Cancer: Methods and Protocols*, Methods in Molecular Biology, vol. 1731, https://doi.org/10.1007/978-1-4939-7595-2_22, © Springer Science+Business Media, LLC 2018

autophagy, apoptosis, etc. [4–11]. Considering the multitude of cellular functions performed by proteases, it is no surprise that alterations in proteolytic systems occur during several pathological conditions such as cancer, neurodegenerative disorders, inflammation, and cardiovascular diseases.

Apoptosis or programmed cell death is a genetically regulated process to self-destruct unwanted and damaged cells [12]. Apoptosis can be activated extrinsically through the activation of cell surface death receptors like TNF-α or intrinsically through mitochondria-mediated release of cytochrome c. Irrespective of extrinsically or intrinsically activated apoptosis, the two pathways converge on activation of terminal, effector caspases, culminating in cell death [12]. Caspases are a family of cysteine-aspartic proteases that drive the process of apoptosis by cleaving essential proteins and thus dismantling the unwanted or damaged cell [13]. Caspases 3 and 7 are effector caspases that are activated in response to initiator caspases, caspases 8 and 9, which are activated in response to an extrinsic or intrinsic signal, respectively [13, 14]. Caspase 3/7 activation is used as a surrogate marker for apoptosis [15, 16]. Activation of the proteolytic activity of Caspase 3/7 has been used to design assays to interrogate the initiation of apoptosis and its deregulation in cancer [17, 18].

Bioluminescence is the emission of light by a chemiluminescent reaction involving light-generating enzymes called luciferases, which are a large family of enzymes that catalyze the oxidation of a substrate, luciferin, into oxyluciferin, with the concomitant production of light [19, 20]. At the cellular level, this light can be captured and detected using an extremely sensitive cooled charge-coupled device (CCD) camera or a photomultiplier. With the current advancement of instrumentation, bioluminescence imaging can be used to carry out real-time functional imaging of biological processes like protein-protein interactions, kinase activities, cellular trafficking, disease progression and response to therapy, etc. [21]. This is achieved by using a reporter gene that is genetically engineered and encodes the light-generating enzyme luciferase in a form such that its catalytic activity is modulated in context of a protein modifying activity (e.g., protease or a kinase). In the presence of a substrate, luciferase-expressing cells emit a blue to yellow-green light with an emission spectra peaking at a wavelength between 490 and 620 nm. This noninvasive imaging modality is extremely sensitive over a broad dynamic range with an exceptionally large signal-to-noise ratio. Presently, more than 30 luciferase-luciferin systems are known, but the most frequently used luciferase for in vivo molecular imaging is the ATP-dependent firefly (*Photinus pyralis*) luciferase [19]. The main advantage of using firefly luciferase is the high signal-to-noise ratio as 30% of the light produced by firefly luciferase has an emission spectrum above 600 nm, a region with the least amount of signal attenuation due to absorbing and scattering properties of live mammalian tissue [19]. More recently, a smaller but very bright luciferase NanoLuc from deep sea shrimp (*Oplophorus gracilirostris*) has been successfully engineered [22]. NanoLuc uses a new substrate to produce light which is 100-fold brighter than that of firefly luciferase [23].

In addition to studies wherein the luciferase reporter technology is used to interrogate transcriptional activity of promoters, protein complementation assays are becoming a method of choice to detect the activity of an enzyme or protein in response to therapeutics. Conceptually, protein complementation technology involves reporter gene manipulation, wherein a monomeric reporter is split into two inactive components, which when brought together can reconstitute a functionally active molecule. Split-luciferase reporters where the luciferase has been divided into two halves (N-Luc and C-Luc) have been developed to study protein-protein interactions. These split-luciferase reporters are based on either the intermolecular or intramolecular complementation of the luciferase fragments to generate signal in response to cellular cues [24, 25]. In our laboratory we have utilized the split-luciferase technology to develop reporters for the activities of several kinases including AKT [26, 27], GSK3β [28], CK1α [28], and ATM [29] and more recently proteases like Caspase 3/7 [30].

Previously, we have reported the generation of a hybrid polypeptide that noninvasively reports on Caspase-3 activity in living cells and animals [31]. This reporter, called as ANLucBCLuc, comprised of a fusion of two small interacting peptides, peptide A and peptide B, with NLuc and CLuc fragments of luciferase on their N terminals, respectively, with an intervening Caspase-3 cleavage site (DEVD) between pepANLuc (ANLuc) and pepB-CLuc (BCLuc) [31]. In response to apoptosis, activated Caspase 3 cleaves the engineered reporter, enabling dissociation of ANLuc from BCLuc and thus facilitating the high-affinity interaction between peptide A and peptide B. This interaction restores luciferase enzymatic activity by NLuc and CLuc complementation resulting in the generation of light in the presence of substrate, luciferin [31]. The reporter was found to be very useful in vivo but had limitations in high-throughput screens in vitro due to its significant background signal. Continuing our efforts to develop an effective and highly sensitive imaging reporter for Caspase 3/7 activity, we utilized recent advances in biosensor research including circularly permuted forms of firefly luciferase and thermostable *Photinus pyralis* luciferases [32–34]. In collaboration with Promega Corporation, we screened a library of randomly mutated thermally stable luciferase constructs permuted at residue 358 and found a reporter with >50-fold induction of bioluminescence activity following stimulation. The reporter has been further engineered such that the magnitude of the luminescence increase is directly proportional to the amount of analyte or protease activity present and has been made commercially available as GloSensor™ luciferase [35]. This reporter has been used by several investigators to generate biosensors for the activity of various other proteases. Li et al. used the GloSensor technology to develop biosensors for the proteolytic activity of granzyme B/Caspase 8 and used it in combination with the Caspase 3/7 reporter to examine the distinct pattern of caspase activation cascade induced by granzyme B vs Fas [36]. Kilianski et al. utilized the GloSensor reporter to develop reporters for imaging the activity of papain-like protease and chymotrypsin-like protease [37]. These reporters were then used to identify potential inhibitors of Middle East respiratory syndrome coronavirus (MERS-CoV) [37]. These studies exemplify a wide applicability of this powerful technology to image the activity of many specific and regulated proteases.

In this chapter we discuss the generation of GloSensor Caspase 3/7, its validation in vitro in cell culture and in high-throughput screens and its application in imaging proteolytic activity in mouse models.

2 Materials

2.1 Vector Construction

1. pGloSensor plasmid pGlo-30F (Promega, WI).
2. Oligonucleotides corresponding to the amino sequence DEVD for Caspase 3/7, IETD for granzyme b/Caspase 8, etc.
3. Restriction enzymes BamHI and HindIII.
4. Expression vectors and packaging plasmids for generating lentiviral particles (optional).
5. High-fidelity polymerases (Pfu), dNTP, primers for cloning and sequencing, buffers, thermocycler, restriction endonuclease, DNA ligase, pipettes, filter tips, etc.
6. High-efficiency competent cells, antibiotic, bacterial growth media (LB, SOC), agar plates, plasmid DNA extraction kits, DNA gel purification and sequencing kits, etc.

2.2 Cell Culture

1. RPMI 1640.
2. Fetal bovine serum (FBS).
3. Trypsin-EDTA.
4. D54-MG and MDA-MB-231-1833 cells maintained in 10% FBS-RPMI 1640.
5. Antibiotic G418 for selection of stable clones.
6. FuGENE 6 for transfection.
7. Flat bottom 96-well culture plates.
8. 10 cm culture dishes.
9. Tissue culture supplies.

2.3 Cell Imaging

1. Translucent black- or white-walled 96-well clear bottom plates.
2. GloSensor c-AMP reagent at 40 mg/mL stock concentration in 1× PBS, stored in dark-colored vials at −80 °C.
3. Drugs for treating cells: TRAIL, CV3988, docetaxel, anti-Fas antibody, and pan-Caspase inhibitor Z-VAD-FMK.
4. DMSO for control.
5. Luminometer to image bioluminescence.
6. Liquid handling instrument, plate handling robot, and a cell culture incubator compatible with high-throughput instruments for high-throughput assays (optional).

2.4 Animal Imaging

1. Immunocompromised mice (athymic nude or NOD/SCID) for human tumor xenografts.
2. Calipers for tumor measurement. Calculate the tumor volume using the formula $V = (W(2) \times L)/2$, where V is tumor volume, W is tumor width, and L is tumor length.
3. pCLEX vector with CAG and floxed GFP/stop cassette.
4. FVB/N females.
5. Tissue-specific Cre-recombinase mouse (CMV-Cre or p48-Cre).
6. Primers for CMV-Cre.

   Forward oIMR1084 5′-GCGGTCTGGCAGTAAAAACTATC-3′.

   Reverse oIMR1085 5′-GTGAAACAGCATTGCTGTCACTT-3′.
7. Primers for p48Cre.

   Forward p48 GT-Cre 5′-CATGCTTCATCGTCGGTCC-3′.

   Reverse p48 GT-Cre 5′-GATCATCAGCTACACCAGAG-3′.
8. Primers for reporter mouse.

   Forward 358 F 5′-AGTTTCAACAGCCAAATGG-3′.

   Reverse 358 R 5′-CCGGAATAGCTGCATAACGAGAT-3′.
9. Cerulein for inducing pancreatitis.
10. Luciferin (VivoGlo Luciferin) at 4 mg/mL in sterile 1× PBS as stock concentration. The stock can be stored in dark tubes at −20 or −80 °C.
11. 1 mL insulin syringes for intraperitoneal (i.p.) luciferin injection in mice.
12. IVIS imaging system with temperature-controlled platform and isoflurane anesthesia injection and controller system.

3 Methods

3.1 Construction of Biosensor Expression Plasmid

1. The GloSensor Caspase 3/7 biosensor is encoded by the pGLS-30F construct and is also commercially available (GLS Caspase 3/7, Promega). The GLS.DEVD version is based in a thermal stable variant of *Photuris pennsylvanica* luciferase that has been evolved for enhanced detection of Caspase 3/7 activity.
2. To construct plasmids for Caspase 3/7 or any other desired proteolytic activity, anneal and ligate the oligonucleotides corresponding to the amino sequence of the protease of interest, e.g., DEVD for Caspase 3/7, IETD for granzyme B/Caspase 8, RLKGG for papain-like protease, or VRLQS for chymotrypsin-like protease into the BamHI/HindIII sites of pGLC-30F plasmid (*see* **Note 1**).

3.2 Generation of Stable Transfectants Expressing Caspase 3/7 Reporter

1. Transfect Caspase 3/7 reporter into desired cell lines like D54-MG and MDA-MB-231/1833 using FuGENE reagent following manufacturer's protocol (*see* **Note 2**).
2. Selection can be started after 48 h by placing the cells in selection media (400 μg/mL G418 in 10% FBS-RPMI 1640).
3. Single-cell clones can be selected by limited dilution method by plating the transfected cell population at a density of 0.3 cells/well using 96-well culture plates (*see* **Note 3**).
4. Once single-cell clones are selected, they can be tested for reporter expression by Western blotting with luciferase antibody and for bioluminescence. In response to apoptosis, Caspase 3/7 activation will lead to an increase in bioluminescence as compared to untreated control cells (Figs. 1 and 2). Clones with similar reporter expression and bioluminescence activity can be selected for further experiments.
5. Expand and freeze 3–4 best reporter expressing stable clones at low passage for future use.
6. Revive and maintain cells in 10 cm dishes in 10% FBS-RPMI 1640 with appropriate amount of G418 (*see* **Note 4**).

3.3 Cell-Based Bioluminescence Assay

1. It is important to carry out cell-based and in vivo bioluminescence assays using the reporter expressing stable cell lines.
2. Select the cell lines which represent appropriate cellular and biological context as desired.
3. Stable cell lines expressing Caspase 3/7 reporter are plated overnight in black-walled or white-walled, clear bottom 96-well plates for live cell assays at a density of 1–2 × 10^4 cells/well 24 h prior to treatment.

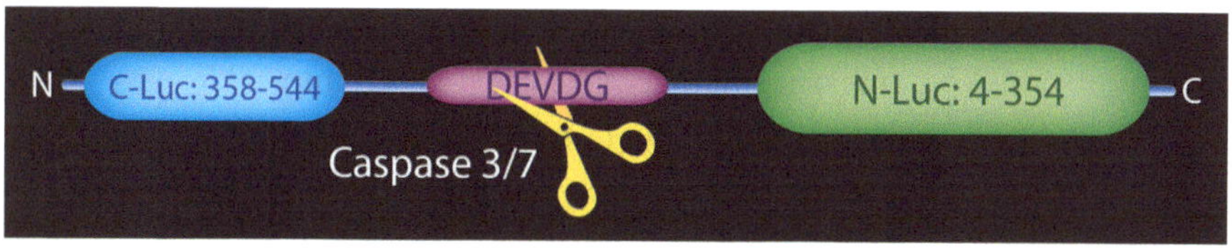

Fig. 1 Schematic representation of the GloSensor Caspase 3/7 reporter. The reporter comprises of an N-terminal domain coding for the C terminus (358–544) of luciferase and C-terminal domain coding for the N terminus (4–354) of firefly luciferase with an intervening Caspase 3/7 recognition sequence DEVD

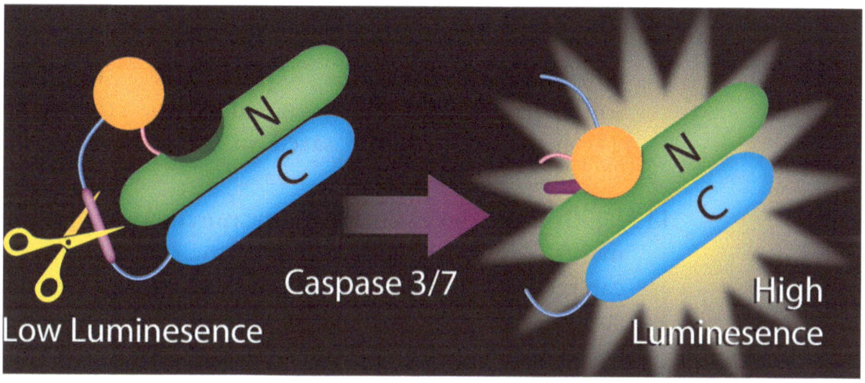

Fig. 2 Schematic diagram showing the mechanistic basis for the GloSensor Caspase 3/7 reporter. In response to apoptosis, activation of Caspase 3/7 leads to cleavage of the intervening peptide DEVD in the GloSensor Caspase 3/7 reporter. This caspase-mediated cleavage of the DEVD sequence results in the reconstitution of the enzymatic activity and a resultant increase in bioluminescence in the presence of luciferin substrate (shown in purple)

4. Treat the cells with the drug of interest like 100–200 ng/mL TRAIL, 12.5 μM CV3988, 50 μM docetaxel, or 25–100 ng/mL anti-Fas antibody in fresh media.
5. For studies evaluating the specificity of the reporter, protease inhibitors such as the pan-Caspase inhibitor Z-VAD-FMK can be utilized. Cells should be preincubated with 20 μM Z-VAD-FMK or DMSO (vehicle control) 1 h prior to treatment.
6. Add 100 μg/mL GloSensor cAMP reagent to the assay media, and perform live cell imaging at desired time points.
7. If cells are to be imaged at multiple time points, cells can be incubated with 100 mL of CO_2-independent media containing 300 μg/mL of GloSensor cAMP reagent for 2 h prior to the beginning of the treatment. Photon counts can be acquired over time pre- and posttreatment using the EnVision Luminometer (*see* **Notes 5–7**).
8. Image the black-walled 96-well plates on the live cell imaging system (such as Xenogen IVIS) immediately after adding the

substrate at medium binning for 30–60 s. For a time course measurement, image every 3–10 min.

9. The white-walled plates can be read on the live cell plate reader (such as EnVision) right after addition of the substrate. Typically each well of the plate is read for 0.01–1.0 s. For a time course activity measurement, the images can be acquired with a delay of 15–60 min between each read. If using high throughput system, for each read the robot takes the plate out from the incubator, loads it on the reader where the plate is read, and transfers it back to the incubator until the next time point.
10. Quantify bioluminescence acquired on the IVIS imaging system by region-of-interest (ROI) analysis using Living Image software. The bioluminescence data from the live cell plate reader is automatically saved in quantitative form in tab-delimited file format.
11. Validate the bioluminescence measurements in parallel experiments by immunoblot analysis of the cleavage products. This can include cleavage of the reporter or cleavage of cellular substrates of the protease (e.g., PARP).

3.4 In Vivo Imaging of Caspase 3 Activity

1. For flank xenografts, expand low-passage D54-MG cells expressing Caspase 3/7. Trypsinize and resuspend in RPMI 1640 media at 40 × 10^6 cells/mL. Inject 50 μL of this suspension subcutaneously into each flank (2 × 10^6 cells) of NOD/SCID mice. Monitor tumor size by caliper measurements, and start the treatment once the tumor size reaches around 100 mm^3.
2. For breast cancer bone metastasis model, implant MDA-MB-231/1833 cells stably expressing the Caspase 3/7 GloSensor into the tibia of SCID mice. Follow tumor growth by MRI, and start the treatment when tumor reaches size 5–15 mm^3.
3. For in vivo bioluminescence imaging, anesthetize the mice using 2% isoflurane/air mixture, and inject with a single i.p. dose of 150 mg/kg VivoGlo Luciferin (*see* **Note 8**).
4. Acquire baseline bioluminescence measurements 6 h before starting the treatment.
5. Transfer mice to the bioluminescence instrument while maintaining under anesthesia. A maximum of five mice can be imaged at once isolated by a plastic separator. Acquire bioluminescence images using a 15–30 s acquisition time at medium sensitivity to begin with. Adjust the settings depending on the signal. To account for the variation in signal intensity between tumors and in order to be able to acquire bioluminescence at its peak signal, it is helpful to do sequential acquisition of 10–20 reads with a 1–2 min delay between the reads (*see* **Note 9**).

6. Remove mice from the imaging instrument, and monitor for complete recovery from anesthesia.
7. Treat the mice with appropriate inhibitors or activators, and again monitor bioluminescence over time (*see* **Note 10**).
8. Acquire images posttreatment at required time points. It is important to give a 4–6 h gap between consecutive imaging so that the bioluminescence signal from the previous substrate injection has dissipated.
9. Quantify imaging data by ROI analysis of bioluminescence produced by the tumor using units of photon flux (*see* **Notes 11–14**).
10. Fold induction of bioluminescence activation can be calculated by normalizing posttreatment values to pretreatment values of each individual animal.

3.5 Generation of Caspase Bioluminescence Transgenic Reporter Mouse

1. Caspase 3/7 reporter can be conditionally activated in a tissue-specific manner in mice to visualize apoptosis in real time but noninvasively.
2. A transgenic construct for Caspase 3/7 reporter can be generated by cloning the Caspase 3/7 reporter in pCLEX vector with CAG and floxed GFP/stop cassette. Constitutively active CAG promoter drives the expression of green fluorescent protein EGFP to determine the expression of transgene in various tissues. The EGFP coding sequence is flanked by loxP sites and a polyA signal with a strong termination sequence preventing the transcription of the downstream-located bioluminescent reporter construct (Fig. 3).
3. The transgenic Caspase 3/7 reporter mice can be generated by pronuclear microinjection of the transgene containing the apoptosis reporter into fertilized eggs obtained from FVB/N females.
4. Intercross the transgene reporter mice with a tissue-specific Cre-recombinase mouse (CMV-Cre or p48-Cre). Upon Cre-mediated recombination driven by CMV or p48 Cre expression, the EGFP lox-stop-lox cassette will be excised thus allowing for transcription of the reporter in Cre-expressing cells (Fig. 3).
5. Genotyping can be done using the primers specified above (in Subheading 2.4) for CMV-Cre, p48Cre, and apoptosis reporter mice.
6. To evaluate reporter activity, treat the mice with an agent that initiates the activation of apoptosis. In mice wherein the reporter is expressed within the pancreas (due to pancreatic expression of the Cre-recombinase in the P48-Cre animals), two series of 6 hourly intraperitoneal injections of cerulein can induce pancreatitis (75 μg/kg, total 12 injections in 48 h) [30].

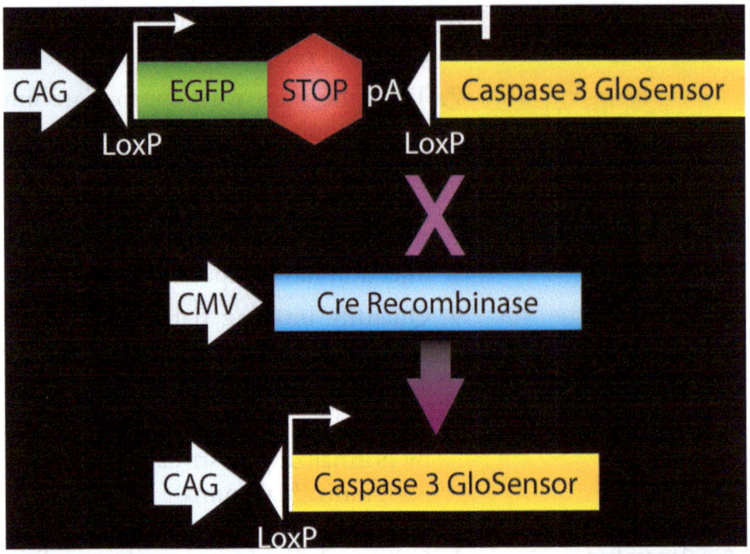

Fig. 3 Development of transgenic mice conditional for the Caspase 3/7 GloSensor reporter. A genetically engineered transgenic mouse was generated using an expression cassette wherein the GloSensor Caspase 3/7 reporter was preceded by a floxable GFP/stop cassette in pCLEX vector driven by CAG promoter. Reporter expression is achieved in a Cre-dependent manner which can simultaneously be detected by the loss of EGFP expression

7. Perform bioluminescence imaging prior to treatment and 30 h posttreatment using the methodology described as above for imaging the xenografts [30] (*see* **Note 15**).

4 Notes

1. Substrate sequence for the construction of the reporter for any protease should be determined considering the specificity of the substrate and based on published literature.
2. The selection of a specific cell line for creating a reporter-expressing stable line should be based on the specific biological question being interrogated and the intrinsic activity and detectability of the proteases and the substrates in the cell line. The cell lines should be selected based on literature search and experimentally.
3. Clonal selection can be done by limited dilution method in 96-well plates. Alternately for picking up the clones, complete growth media with antibiotic is aspirated from the tissue culture dishes containing single-cell clones. Transfer sterilized filter paper discs pre-wetted in trypsin to the clones using sterilized forceps in a laminar flow hood. After 4–5 min, using

sterilized forceps transfer the discs from the tissue culture plate to 24-well plate containing complete growth media with half the concentration of antibiotic used for clonal selection. Generally 12–24 single-cell clones are picked. Forceps can be sterilized by ethanol or by heating. Wait for the ethanol to evaporate before using the forceps to pick up the clones.

4. The G418 concentration for stable clone selection should be empirically decided. For maintaining the stable cell lines, it is preferable to use half the concentration of G418 than that is used for selection.
5. Perform all the bioluminescence acquisitions at 37 °C as the N-Luc and C-Luc fragments used in the construction of the complementation-based reporters have been optimized in mammalian cells at the physiological temperature (37 °C).
6. The reporter is based on the complementation of the light-generating enzyme luciferase, and it works only in live cells under physiological conditions. Methods wherein cell lysates are used to measure the bioluminescence signal may be incompatible with this reporter system and may not be able to yield a desired signal to background (under different treatment conditions).
7. The EnVision system is built with ultrasensitive luminescence detection technology. Even 0.01–0.1 s measurements for each well are usually sufficient. Also, the bioluminescence signal from GloSensor cAMP reagent is stable for a prolonged period of time and facilitates measurement of the protease activity for long-term studies.
8. We have found that 400 μg luciferin/mouse gives the best signal-to-background bioluminescence readings for split firefly luciferase-based reporters. However amount of luciferin can be increased to 150 mg/kg body weight (i.e., 3.5–4 mg/mouse with 20–25 g average mouse weight) in case of smaller tumors or tumors generated from cell lines expressing very low levels of reporter.
9. Generally 4–5 mice can be used in an experimental group for bioluminescence data acquisition on the IVIS imaging system. A stage level, i.e., the distance of the CCD camera from the subject, is selected and kept consistent for the entire experiment. Changing the stage level would lead to variations in photon counts, making it hard to analyze the data.
10. It is important to test 2–3 different concentrations of the drug in the mouse tumor xenograft model to find the optimal concentration which gives highest-fold change over vehicle control without being toxic to animals.
11. For analyzing the bioluminescence data, it is advisable to create similar ROIs for each tumor. The same ROI can be copied

and pasted for each tumor for counting total photon flux for all the time points. However, the positioning of the ROI can be adjusted so that it covers the tumor without overlapping with the ROI of any adjacent tumor.

12. The photon flux should be acquired without any saturated pixels. Data from saturated pixels cannot be accurately analyzed.
13. Since luciferin bioavailability and peak intra-tumoral concentration vary from mouse to mouse, we consider only the maximum photon flux emitted from each tumor for analysis. Since each tumor may show the maximum emittance at different time points, it is helpful to perform sequential reads with a delay between each read.
14. As a limitation of sensitivity of the imaging system, a minimal background signal is always observed in nude and SCID mice. If using a mouse strain with hair, the optical scatter can be minimized by shaving off the hair which will reduce the background.
15. Any data obtained using bioluminescence images acquired in a mouse xenograft model should be independently validated by biochemical methods such as Western blotting or immunohistochemistry (IHC). For validation of the bioluminescence data for Caspase 3/7, tumor tissue should be analyzed using antibodies specific for activated Caspase 3 or PARP antibodies.

Acknowledgments

We would like to acknowledge our lab members Amy Delaney and Liu Yajing for critical review of the manuscript and Steven Kronenberg for helping with the figures. This work was supported by the National Institutes of Health grants R01CA193690, P01CA085878, and U01CA216449.

References

1. Levene PA (1905) The cleavage products of proteases. J Biol Chem 1(1):45–58
2. Lopez-Otin C, Bond JS (2008) Proteases: multifunctional enzymes in life and disease. J Biol Chem 283(45):30433–30437. https://doi.org/10.1074/jbc.R800035200
3. Ehrmann M, Clausen T (2004) Proteolysis as a regulatory mechanism. Annu Rev Genet 38:709–724. https://doi.org/10.1146/annurev.genet.38.072902.093416
4. Sternlicht MD, Werb Z (2001) How matrix metalloproteinases regulate cell behavior. Annu Rev Cell Dev Biol 17:463–516. https://doi.org/10.1146/annurev.cellbio.17.1.463
5. Ciechanover A (2005) Proteolysis: from the lysosome to ubiquitin and the proteasome. Nat Rev Mol Cell Biol 6(1):79–87. https://doi.org/10.1038/nrm1552
6. Lopez-Otin C, Overall CM (2002) Protease degradomics: a new challenge for proteomics. Nat Rev Mol Cell Biol 3(7):509–519. https://doi.org/10.1038/nrm858
7. Marino G, Uria JA, Puente XS et al (2003) Human autophagins, a family of cysteine proteinases potentially implicated in cell degradation by autophagy. J Biol Chem 278(6):3671–3678. https://doi.org/10.1074/jbc.M208247200

8. Page-McCaw A, Ewald AJ, Werb Z (2007) Matrix metalloproteinases and the regulation of tissue remodelling. Nat Rev Mol Cell Biol 8(3):221–233. https://doi.org/10.1038/nrm2125
9. Sauer RT, Bolon DN, Burton BM et al (2004) Sculpting the proteome with AAA(+) proteases and disassembly machines. Cell 119(1):9–18. https://doi.org/10.1016/j.cell.2004.09.020
10. Siegel RM (2006) Caspases at the crossroads of immune-cell life and death. Nat Rev Immunol 6(4):308–317. https://doi.org/10.1038/nri1809
11. Hollenberg MD (2005) Physiology and pathophysiology of proteinase-activated receptors (PARs): proteinases as hormone-like signal messengers: PARs and more. J Pharmacol Sci 97(1):8–13
12. Koff JL, Ramachandiran S, Bernal-Mizrachi L (2015) A time to kill: targeting apoptosis in cancer. Int J Mol Sci 16(2):2942–2955. https://doi.org/10.3390/ijms16022942
13. Shalini S, Dorstyn L, Dawar S et al (2015) Old, new and emerging functions of caspases. Cell Death Differ 22(4):526–539. https://doi.org/10.1038/cdd.2014.216
14. Duclos C, Lavoie C, Denault JB (2017) Caspases rule the intracellular trafficking cartel. FEBS J 284(10):1394–1420. https://doi.org/10.1111/febs.14071
15. Vermeulen K, Van Bockstaele DR, Berneman ZN (2005) Apoptosis: mechanisms and relevance in cancer. Ann Hematol 84(10):627–639. https://doi.org/10.1007/s00277-005-1065-x
16. Zhivotovsky B (2003) Caspases: the enzymes of death. Essays Biochem 39:25
17. Julien O, Wells JA (2017) Caspases and their substrates. Cell Death Differ. https://doi.org/10.1038/cdd.2017.44
18. Edgington LE, Berger AB, Blum G et al (2009) Noninvasive optical imaging of apoptosis by caspase-targeted activity-based probes. Nat Med 15(8):967–973. doi:http://www.nature.com/nm/journal/v15/n8/suppinfo/nm.1938_S1.html
19. Sato A, Klaunberg B, Tolwani R (2004) In vivo bioluminescence imaging. Comp Med 54(6):631–634
20. Choy G, Choyke P, Libutti SK (2003) Current advances in molecular imaging: noninvasive in vivo bioluminescent and fluorescent optical imaging in cancer research. Mol Imaging 2(4):303–312
21. Close DM, Xu T, Sayler GS et al (2011) In vivo bioluminescent imaging (BLI): noninvasive visualization and interrogation of biological processes in living animals. Sensors (Basel) 11(1):180–206. https://doi.org/10.3390/s110100180
22. Stacer AC, Nyati S, Moudgil P et al (2013) NanoLuc reporter for dual luciferase imaging in living animals. Mol Imaging 12(7):1–13
23. England CG, Ehlerding EB, Cai W (2016) NanoLuc: a small luciferase is brightening up the field of bioluminescence. Bioconjug Chem 27(5):1175 1187. https://doi.org/10.1021/acs.bioconjchem.6b00112
24. Godinat A, Budin G, Molares AR et al (2014) A biocompatible "split luciferin" reaction and its application for non-invasive bioluminescent imaging of protease activity in living animals. Curr Protoc Chem Biol 6(3):169–189. https://doi.org/10.1002/9780470559277.ch140047
25. Luker KE, Smith MC, Luker GD et al (2004) Kinetics of regulated protein-protein interactions revealed with firefly luciferase complementation imaging in cells and living animals. Proc Natl Acad Sci U S A 101(33):12288–12293. https://doi.org/10.1073/pnas.0404041101
26. Zhang L, Lee KC, Bhojani MS et al (2007) Molecular imaging of Akt kinase activity. Nat Med 13(9):1114–1119
27. Wang H, Galbán S, Wu R et al (2013) Molecular imaging reveals a role for AKT in resistance to cisplatin for ovarian endometrioid adenocarcinoma. Clin Cancer Res 19(1):158
28. Nyati S, Ranga R, Ross BD et al (2010) Molecular imaging of glycogen synthase kinase-3beta and casein kinase-1alpha kinases. Anal Biochem 405(2):246–254. https://doi.org/10.1016/j.ab.2010.06.020
29. Williams TM, Nyati S, Ross BD et al (2013) Molecular imaging of the ATM kinase activity. Int J Radiat Oncol Biol Phys 86(5):969–977. https://doi.org/10.1016/j.ijrobp.2013.04.028
30. Galbán S, Jeon YH, Bowman BM et al (2013) Imaging proteolytic activity in live cells and animal models. PLoS One 8(6):e66248. https://doi.org/10.1371/journal.pone.0066248
31. Khanna D, Hamilton CA, Bhojani MS et al (2010) A transgenic mouse for imaging caspase-dependent apoptosis within the skin. J Invest Dermatol 130(7):1797–1806. https://doi.org/10.1038/jid.2010.55
32. Fan F, Binkowski BF, Butler BL et al (2008) Novel genetically encoded biosensors using firefly luciferase. ACS Chem Biol 3(6):346–351. https://doi.org/10.1021/cb8000414
33. Cheraghi R, Hosseinkhani S, Davoodi J et al (2013) Structural and functional effects of circular permutation on firefly luciferase: In vitro

assay of caspase 3/7. Int J Biol Macromol 58:336–342. https://doi.org/10.1016/j.ijbiomac.2013.04.015

34. Wigdal SS, Anderson JL, Vidugiris GJ et al (2008) A novel bioluminescent protease assay using engineered firefly luciferase. Curr Chem Genomics 2:16–28. https://doi.org/10.2174/1875397300802010016

35. Binkowski J, Butler J (2014) A real-time assay of caspase-3/7 activity in cell culture and animal models. Promega Corporation, Madison, WI

36. Li J, Figueira SK, Vrazo ACA et al (2014) Real time detection of cytotoxic lymphocyte function reveals distinct patterns of caspase activation mediated by Fas versus granzyme B. J Immunol 193(2):519–528. https://doi.org/10.4049/jimmunol.1301668

37. Kilianski A, Mielech AM, Deng X et al (2013) Assessing activity and inhibition of middle east respiratory syndrome coronavirus papain-like and 3C-like proteases using luciferase-based biosensors. J Virol 87(21):11955–11962. https://doi.org/10.1128/JVI.02105-13

Chapter 23

Protease Silencing to Explore the Molecular Mechanisms of Cancer and Aging

Julia M. Fraile, Diana Campos-Iglesias, and José M.P. Freije

Abstract

Proteases play key roles in the execution and regulation of most if not all biological functions, and alterations in their activity, expression, or location are associated with multiple pathological conditions, including cancer and aging. In this regard, the use of RNA interference-based approaches to specifically target the expression of individual proteases constitutes an invaluable tool to identify enzymes involved in central aspects of these processes and to explore their potential as targets of therapeutic interventions. Here we describe simple protocols to optimize and monitor the specific silencing of cancer- and aging-related proteases.

Key words Degradome, Proteases, shRNA, siRNA, Lentiviral vectors, ZMPSTE24, Nuclear lamina, Deubiquitinases, USP39, qRT-PCR, Immunofluorescence

1 Introduction

Cancer and aging constitute two biological problems of paramount biomedical importance. Both processes seem to be inevitable consequences of the eventual malfunction of the genetic, epigenetic, and metabolic circuitries of multicellular organisms and involve a complex and diverse set of molecular and cellular alterations that can provide opportunities of intervention to prevent or control cancer and to alleviate or delay the manifestations of old age [1, 2]. Like most biological processes, cancer and aging involve multiple changes in the cellular proteome, resulting from transcriptional or translational reprogramming as well as from the action of the cellular machinery involved in posttranslational modification of proteins [3]. In this regard, protease-mediated hydrolysis of the peptide bond is one of the most common posttranslational modifications undergone by cellular proteins, with consequences ranging from their activation or subcellular relocation to their final destruction and recycling. Mammalian degradomes, the repertoire of proteases encoded in their genomes, comprise more than 500

Santiago Cal and Alvaro J. Obaya (eds.), *Proteases and Cancer: Methods and Protocols*, Methods in Molecular Biology, vol. 1731, https://doi.org/10.1007/978-1-4939-7595-2_23,

different proteolytic enzymes, many of which play causal roles in aging and in an overwhelming variety of human diseases, including cancer and more than 120 hereditary diseases [4–6].

The elucidation of the importance of particular proteases in different processes usually involves the experimental manipulation of their levels in cellular or animal models. RNA interference (RNAi) allows to specifically downregulate the expression of genes of interest with double-stranded RNA molecules, which guide the cellular RNA-induced silencing complex (RISC) to cleave the corresponding mRNAs or inhibit their translation [7, 8]. RNAi can be achieved with two different approaches: by administering synthetic double-stranded small interfering RNA (siRNA) or by using plasmid constructs encoding short hairpin RNAs (shRNA), under the control of RNA polymerase II or III promoters [9]. In the latter case, inserting the shRNA sequences into an endogenous miRNA backbone leads to the production of RNAs that are recognized as natural substrates of the RNAi pathway, with optimal efficacy and reduced toxicity [10]. The power and specificity of RNAi and the development of efficient delivery systems based on lentiviral vectors [11] have enabled the implementation of genome-wide RNAi screens for the functional annotation of mammalian genomes [12] and the identification of specific vulnerabilities of cancer cells [13–15]. Here we describe detailed protocols to optimize the knockdown of genes encoding proteases involved in aging, *ZMPSTE24*, also known as *FACE-1* [16, 17], and cancer, *USP39* [15], using siRNA- and shRNA-based approaches, respectively. We also describe the procedures for monitoring silencing efficiency, based on the quantitation of the protease transcript by qRT-PCR or the detection of substrate accumulation at the cell level by immunofluorescence.

2 Materials

2.1 Reagents and Solutions

1. Cells: Human cancer cell lines, such as HCT116, T47D, and Hs578T, purchased from the American Type Culture Collection (ATCC).
2. Lentiviral packaging cells, such as human embryo kidney cell line HEK 293T, obtained from the ATCC.
3. Dulbecco's modified Eagle's medium (DMEM). Store at 4 °C.
4. Growth medium: DMEM, 10% fetal bovine serum (FBS), 100 U/mL penicillin, and 100 μg/mL streptomycin. Store at 4 °C.
5. Selection medium: growth medium and 1 μg/mL of puromycin.
6. Opti-MEM reduced-serum medium.

7. 1× Dulbecco's phosphate-buffered saline (DPBS) without Ca^{2+} and Mg^{2+}. Store at room temperature (RT).
8. VSVG-based package system (kindly provided by Dr. J. M. Silva, Columbia University, New York, USA).
9. *USP39*-specific shRNA and empty (pLKO.1) vectors obtained from Open Biosystems, Thermo Scientific.
10. *ZMPSTE24*-specific stealth RNAi™ siRNA (Invitrogen, HSS115697) and silencer negative control siRNA (Ambion, AM4611).
11. Lipofectamine and PLUS reagent (Invitrogen).
12. Lipofectamine™ RNAiMAX (Invitrogen).
13. Polybrene.
14. Fixation solution: 4% paraformaldehyde solution (PFA) (v/v) prepared in DPBS. Store at RT.
15. Permeabilization solution: 0.5% Triton X-100 (v/v) prepared in DPBS. Store at RT.
16. Blocking solution: 15% goat serum solution (v/v) prepared in DPBS.
17. Primary antibody solution: 1% goat polyclonal anti-prelamin A antibody (C-20, sc-6214, Santa Cruz Biotechnology) in blocking solution.
18. Secondary antibody solution: 0.2% Alexa Fluor-594 donkey anti-goat IgG (Invitrogen) in blocking solution.
19. TBS-T buffer: 20 mM Tris–HCl pH 7.4, 150 mM NaCl, 0.05% Tween 20.
20. DAPI-mounting media: 1 μg/mL DAPI (4,6′ diamidino-2-phenylindole dihydrochloride) in mounting media. Store at 4 °C.
21. TRIzol reagent (Life Technologies).
22. Chloroform.
23. 2-Propanol.
24. ThermoScript RT-PCR System (Life Technologies), including 10 mM dNTP mix, random hexamers (50 ng/μL), 0.1 M dithiothreitol (DTT), RNaseOUT (40 units/μL), ThermoScript™ RT (15 units/μL), and 5× cDNA synthesis buffer.
25. RT-Master reaction mix: 1 μL diethyl pyrocarbonate-treated (DEPC) water, 1 μL DTT, 1 μL RNaseOUT, 1 μL ThermoScript™ RT, and 4 μL of 5× cDNA synthesis buffer per sample. Remember to vortex 5× cDNA synthesis buffer before use.
26. Power SYBR Green PCR Master Mix (Life Technologies).

27. *USP39*-specific primers: 5′-GCTCTGCACTCAGCTCT-GGGG-3′ and 5′-TGCTGGCAGATCAGGATGGGGA-3′.
28. β-actin-specific primers: 5′-CACAGAGCCTCGCCTTTGCC-GAT-3′ and 5′-CGAGCGCGGCGATATCATCATCC-3′.
29. Ethanol.
30. RNase-free water.
31. Distilled water.

2.2 Equipment

1. Cell culture incubator (37 °C and 5% CO_2).
2. Tissue culture 6- and 12-well plates (polystyrene flat bottom).
3. Eppendorf tubes: 1.5 and 2 mL.
4. 0.45 μm sterile filters.
5. Microscope slide glass.
6. Cover glasses (18 mm × 18 mm).
7. Hemocytometer.
8. Tweezers.
9. Absorbent paper.
10. Nail varnish.
11. Confocal or fluorescent microscope.
12. NanoDrop ND-1000 spectrophotometer.
13. Thermal cycler.
14. Applied Biosystems 7300HT Real-Time PCR System or similar.

3 Methods

3.1 Validation of FACE-1 Silencing Through Immunofluorescence

3.1.1 Cell Growth and Transfection

1. Place sterilized 18 mm × 18 mm cover glasses in the corresponding wells of a 12-well plate.
2. Seed T47D and Hs578 cells with growth medium without antibiotic to be 50–60% confluent at transfection.
3. Next day, dilute 2.5–7.5 μL Lipofectamine RNAiMAX reagent in 250 μL of Opti-MEM reduced-serum medium (*see* **Note 1**).
4. Dilute 3–150 pmol *ZMPSTE24*-specific stealth RNAi™ siRNA or silencer negative control siRNA in 250 μL of Opti-MEM reduced-serum medium.
5. After 5 min, add diluted siRNA to diluted Lipofectamine RNAiMAX reagent (1:1 ratio).
6. Incubate for 15 min at RT.
7. Add 500 μL of siRNA-lipid complex to cells.
8. Remove transfection medium and add fresh growth medium 6 h after transfection.

3.1.2 Prelamin A Immunofluorescence

1. After 72 h, remove growth medium, wash cells twice with DPBS, and fix them with fixation solution for 10 min at RT.
2. Wash twice with DPBS and incubate with permeabilization solution for 5 min at RT.
3. Discard the permeabilization solution, wash twice with DPBS, and incubate with blocking solution for 1 h at 37 °C.
4. Aspirate blocking solution and incubate cells with primary antibody solution for 1 h at RT.
5. Wash cells twice with TBS-T.
6. Incubate cells with secondary antibody solution for 1 h in the dark.
7. Aspirate the secondary antibody solution and wash twice with TBS-T.

3.1.3 DAPI Staining, Mounting of Fluorescence Preparations, and Microscope Analysis

1. Add 10 μL of DAPI-mounting media on the slide glass.
2. Hold carefully the cover glasses with tweezers, wash with distilled water, and place it on the correspondent slide with DAPI-mounting media.
3. Eliminate the excess of DAPI-mounting media by pressing gently but firmly the cover glass against the slide over a piece of absorbent paper. Then, seal the edges with varnish or similar, and keep the slides in the dark at 4 °C until observation (*see* **Note 2**).
4. Analyze the preparation using a confocal or fluorescent microscope to verify prelamin A accumulation as a consequence of *ZMPSTE24* downregulation (Fig. 1). Slides can be stored in a dark place at 4 °C for up to 1 year.

3.2 USP39-Specific shRNA Efficiency by qRT-PCR

3.2.1 Lentiviral Production

1. Seed HEK 293T cells to be 90% confluent at transfection in 6-well plates.
2. Next day, dilute 4 μL of Lipofectamine reagent in 100 μL of DMEM (without FBS) per condition (*see* **Note 3**).
3. Dilute 1 μg of *USP39*-specific shRNA or pLKO.1 and 1 μg of VSVG-based package system in 100 μL of DMEM (without FBS). Then, add 6 μL of PLUS reagent and incubate for 15 min at RT (*see* **Note 4**).
4. Add diluted DNA to diluted Lipofectamine reagent (1:1 ratio) and incubate for 15 min at RT.
5. Add DNA-lipid complex to cells and incubate for 3 h at 37 °C and 5% CO_2.
6. Remove transfection medium and add fresh growth medium.
7. After 24 h and 48 h, collect the viral supernatant and filter it through a 0.45 μm sterile filter.

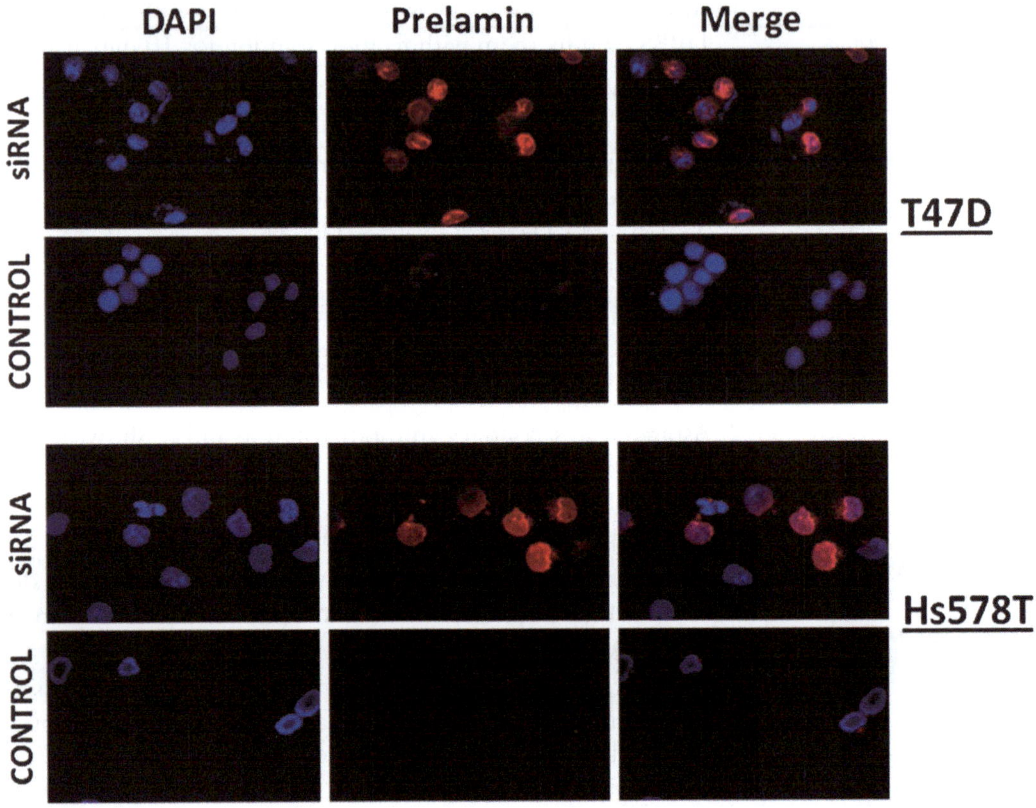

Fig. 1 Prelamin A immunofluorescence demonstrates *ZMPSTE24* downregulation in human breast cancer cells. *ZMPSTE24* siRNA efficiency is evaluated at the cell level by analyzing the accumulation of its substrate prelamin A through immunofluorescence (red color). Nuclei are visualized with DAPI staining (blue color). Prelamin A is specifically accumulated in T47D and Hs578T cells transfected with *ZMPSTE24*-specific siRNA, compared to the same cells transfected with a negative control

3.2.2 Cell Infection and Antibiotic Selection

1. Seed human cancer cells, such as HCT116, in 6-well plates at 20–30% confluence 24 h before infection (2 mL per well).
2. Next day, add 1 mL of viral supernatant to each well supplemented with 5 mg/mL of polybrene, and incubate for 24 h at 37 °C and 5% CO_2.
3. Remove viral supernatant, add 2 mL of growth medium and 1 mL of viral supernatant to each well supplemented with 5 mg/mL of polybrene, and incubate for 24 h at 37 °C and 5% CO_2.
4. Remove viral supernatant and leave the cells recovering for 24 h in growth medium (*see* **Note 5**).
5. Add selection medium and incubate for 24 h at 37 °C and 5% CO_2.
6. Repeat the step with fresh selection medium.

3.2.3 RNA Preparation

1. After puromycin selection, remove growth medium, wash the cells twice with DPBS, and add 1 mL of TRIzol reagent to lyse the cells. Put the solution in an Eppendorf tube (2 mL). Incubate for 5 min at RT.
2. Add 200 μL of chloroform and mix. Incubate for 3 min at RT.
3. Centrifuge samples for 15 min at 12,000 × *g* at 4 °C. The mixture separates into a lower red phenol-chloroform, an interphase and an upper aqueous phase.
4. Collect the aqueous phase containing the RNA in a new Eppendorf tube (1.5 mL).
5. Add 500 μL of 2-propanol and mix carefully. Store at −80 °C overnight.
6. Centrifuge samples for 10 min at 12,000 × *g* at 4 °C.
7. Total RNA is precipitated in a pellet at the bottom of the tube. Discard the supernatant and wash with ethanol 70%.
8. Centrifuge samples for 5 min at 7500 × *g* at 4 °C.
9. Discard the supernatant and air-dry the RNA pellet for 5 min.
10. Resuspend the pellet in 20–50 μL of RNase-free water, and incubate for 10 min at 55 °C. Store at −80 °C.

3.2.4 Real-Time Quantitative PCR (qRT-PCR) Analysis

1. Quantify RNA samples and evaluate their purity (260/280 nm ratio) with a NanoDrop ND-1000 spectrophotometer. Then, mix 10 pg to 5 μg of RNA with 1 μL of random hexamers and 2 μL of dNTP mix (final volume = 12 μL) (*see* **Note 6**).
2. Denaturalize RNA and primers by incubating for 5 min at 65 °C. Then, place the samples on ice.
3. Add 8 μL of RT-Master reaction mix into each reaction tube on ice.
4. Transfer the samples to a thermal cycler and incubate for 10 min at 25 °C, followed by 50 min at 50 °C, and a final step of 5 min at 85 °C. Samples can be stored at −20 °C.
5. Dilute cDNA 1:10 and add 4 μL of each cDNA to PCR tubes by triplicate. Add 5 μL of Power SYBR Green PCR Master Mix and 0.5 μL of each *USP39*-specific primer at 10 μM (final volume = 10 μL).
6. Add 4 μL of the same cDNA by triplicate, and mix them with 5 μL of Power SYBR Green PCR Master Mix and 0.5 μL of each β-actin-specific primers (final volume = 10 μL).
7. Transfer the samples to an Applied Biosystems 7300HT Real-Time PCR System or similar.
8. Analyze *USP39* gene expression normalized to the β-actin gene, and represent relative expression using RQ value: $RQ = 2^{-(\Delta Ct\ shRNA - \Delta Ct\ pLKO.1)}$, where ΔCt = Ct sample – Ct β-actin (Fig. 2).

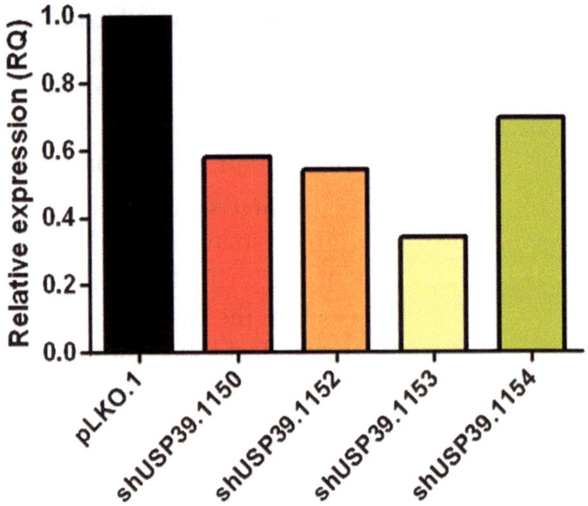

Fig. 2 shRNA-mediated *USP39* silencing is confirmed through qRT-PCR. *USP39* gene expression of *USP39* wild-type and *USP39*-silenced HCT116 cells is analyzed by qRT-PCR in order to evaluate the efficiency of each shRNA. In this case, shUSP39.1152 and shUSP39.1153 are the best shRNAs from the set

4 Notes

1. Cells can be transfected in different tissue culture formats, and consequently, the amounts of Lipofectamine™ RNAiMAX, RNAi duplex, and medium used must vary in proportion to the relative surface area.
2. This protocol can be performed in other types of adherent cells, although some aspects, such as the number of seeded cells, could be variable depending on each cell line.
3. As explained before with Lipofectamine™ RNAiMAX, the amounts of reagents must be modified depending on tissue culture formats.
4. It is extremely important to add PLUS reagent after DNA is resuspended to avoid precipitation.
5. Puromycin action requires cells to be proliferating. Therefore, if cells are confluent at this point, trypsinize and seed them on a larger surface.
6. Note that different types of primers can be used in this protocol: Random Hexamers (total RNA), oligo(dT) primers (poly(A)$^{+}$–selected RNA), or a gene-specific primer. Each condition requires different parameters at the thermal cycler.

Acknowledgments

We thank C. López-Otín and G. Velasco for their support and assistance. This work was supported by grants from Ministerio de Economía y Competitividad, Instituto de Salud Carlos III (CIBERONC), Principado de Asturias, and EDP Foundation. Instituto Universitario de Oncología is supported by Fundación Bancaria Caja de Ahorros de Asturias.

References

1. Hanahan D, Weinberg RA (2011) Hallmarks of cancer: the next generation. Cell 144(5):646–674. https://doi.org/10.1016/j.cell.2011.02.013
2. Lopez-Otin C, Blasco MA, Partridge L et al (2013) The hallmarks of aging. Cell 153(6): 1194–1217. https://doi.org/10.1016/j.cell.2013.05.039
3. Sendoel A, Dunn JG, Rodriguez EH et al (2017) Translation from unconventional 5′ start sites drives tumour initiation. Nature 541(7638):494–499. https://doi.org/10.1038/nature21036
4. Perez-Silva JG, Espanol Y, Velasco G et al (2016) The degradome database: expanding roles of mammalian proteases in life and disease. Nucleic Acids Res 44(D1):D351–D355. https://doi.org/10.1093/nar/gkv1201
5. Freije JM, Fraile JM, Lopez-Otin C (2011) Protease addiction and synthetic lethality in cancer. Front Oncol 1:25. https://doi.org/10.3389/fonc.2011.00025
6. Freitas-Rodriguez S, Folgueras AR, Lopez-Otin C (2017) The role of matrix metalloproteinases in aging: tissue remodeling and beyond. Biochim Biophys Acta. https://doi.org/10.1016/j.bbamcr.2017.05.007
7. Fire A, Xu S, Montgomery MK et al (1998) Potent and specific genetic interference by double-stranded RNA in Caenorhabditis elegans. Nature 391(6669):806–811. https://doi.org/10.1038/35888
8. Hannon GJ (2002) RNA interference. Nature 418(6894):244–251. https://doi.org/10.1038/418244a
9. Rao DD, Vorhies JS, Senzer N et al (2009) siRNA vs. shRNA: similarities and differences. Adv Drug Deliv Rev 61(9):746–759. https://doi.org/10.1016/j.addr.2009.04.004
10. Boudreau RL, Martins I, Davidson BL (2009) Artificial microRNAs as siRNA shuttles: improved safety as compared to shRNAs in vitro and in vivo. Mol Ther 17(1):169–175. https://doi.org/10.1038/mt.2008.231
11. Manjunath N, Wu H, Subramanya S et al (2009) Lentiviral delivery of short hairpin RNAs. Adv Drug Deliv Rev 61(9):732–745. https://doi.org/10.1016/j.addr.2009.03.004
12. Moffat J, Grueneberg DA, Yang X et al (2006) A lentiviral RNAi library for human and mouse genes applied to an arrayed viral high-content screen. Cell 124(6):1283–1298. https://doi.org/10.1016/j.cell.2006.01.040
13. Luo J, Emanuele MJ, Li D et al (2009) A genome-wide RNAi screen identifies multiple synthetic lethal interactions with the Ras oncogene. Cell 137(5):835–848. https://doi.org/10.1016/j.cell.2009.05.006
14. Hsu TY, Simon LM, Neill NJ et al (2015) The spliceosome is a therapeutic vulnerability in MYC-driven cancer. Nature 525(7569):384–388. https://doi.org/10.1038/nature14985
15. Fraile JM, Manchado E, Lujambio A et al (2017) USP39 deubiquitinase is essential for KRAS oncogene-driven cancer. J Biol Chem 292(10):4164–4175. https://doi.org/10.1074/jbc.M116.762757
16. Freije JM, Blay P, Pendas AM et al (1999) Identification and chromosomal location of two human genes encoding enzymes potentially involved in proteolytic maturation of farnesylated proteins. Genomics 58(3):270–280. https://doi.org/10.1006/geno.1999.5834
17. Varela I, Cadinanos J, Pendas AM et al (2005) Accelerated ageing in mice deficient in Zmpste24 protease is linked to p53 signalling activation. Nature 437(7058):564–568. https://doi.org/10.1038/nature04019

Chapter 24

Analysis of Somatic DNA Methylation Alterations of Genes Encoding Cell Surface Metallopeptidases in Colorectal Cancer

Sergio Alonso, Beatriz González, Andreu Alibés, and Manuel Perucho

Abstract

The genome of cancer cells accumulates numerous genetic and epigenetic somatic alterations ultimately conferring capabilities for unrestrained growth, invasion of local tissues, migration, and colonization of distant organs. Many of these new capabilities require the disruption of the cell-to-cell interactions between the cancer cell and its microenvironment. These interactions are mediated, among other factors, by the activity of extracellular enzymes that reshape not only the extracellular compartment of the cancer cells but also that of the neighboring non-cancerous stroma cells. Cell surface metallopeptidases play a crucial role in this process, by cleaving and modifying fundamental components of the extracellular compartment. The transcriptional profile of cell surface metallopeptidases becomes deregulated in several human cancers by genetic and epigenetic alterations, contributing to the tumor phenotype. In this article, we describe two common strategies to analyze somatic epigenetic alterations of cell surface metallopeptidases, i.e., high-resolution single locus analysis and high-throughput multi-loci analysis, presenting several illustrative analyses performed on our CRC collection. These analyses demonstrate that cell surface metallopeptidases, particularly those belonging to the ADAMTS gene family, frequently undergo somatic DNA hypermethylation in CRC suggesting the existence of an underlying mechanism or a strong selection process favoring the transcriptional silencing of these genes.

Key words Extracellular metallopeptidases, Colorectal cancer, Epigenetic alterations, Genetic alterations

1 Introduction

Metallopeptidases (MPs) are enzymes that catalyze the cleavage of peptide bonds in a single-step reaction, without the formation of covalent bonds, mediated by a catalytic metal site in their active center. The majority of the human metallopeptidases require zinc or, less frequently, cobalt atoms in their catalytic domain. Most of the MPs exert their functions at the cell membrane or the extracellular matrix (ECM) compartment, playing a key role in the

Santiago Cal and Alvaro J. Obaya (eds.), *Proteases and Cancer: Methods and Protocols*, Methods in Molecular Biology, vol. 1731, https://doi.org/10.1007/978-1-4939-7595-2_24, © Springer Science+Business Media, LLC 2018

interactions between cells and their microenviroment [1, 2]. These tightly regulated interactions become disrupted in cancer cells, conferring them the ability to reshape their microenvironment and facilitating invasion of local organs, migration to distant organs, and adaptation to grow in those new niches. Remodeling of the ECM is thus an essential process in tumor progression that directly contributes to primary and secondary tumor development [3]. Improving our understanding of the different mechanisms that participate in the deregulation of the ECM may open interesting avenues for cancer patient stratification, prognosis, and treatment.

The human genome encodes more than 600 known or putative peptidases [4]. Of these, 186 encode proteins classified as MPs, subclassified into 26 subfamilies. A number of these MPs have been found to undergo somatic alterations that affect their expression or functionality in human cancer, frequently involving DNA hypermethylation of their promoter sequences [5–9].

As a rule of thumb, hypermethylated gene promoters associate to a closed chromatin state and transcriptional silencing, while unmethylated promoters are accessible to the transcriptional machinery and their expression is modulated by transcriptional factors. Given the direct effect that loss of ECM homeostasis exerts in the interaction between cancer cells and their microenvironment, the analysis of DNA methylation alterations affecting cell surface metallopeptidases, mainly comprising matrix metallopeptidases (MMPs), is important for a comprehensive characterization of the molecular profile that ultimately dictates essential malignant capabilities of the cancer cell.

In the last decades, a wide range of technical approaches to detect and quantify DNA methylation changes have been devised, producing very detailed profiles of epigenetic alterations in cancer [10–12]. Most of the current methods rely on the conversion of DNA with sodium bisulfite. This treatment deaminates non-methylated cytosine, transforming it into uracil [13, 14]. On the other hand, 5-methylcytosine is more resistant to deamination and remains mostly unaltered [15–17]. The uracil residues can be subsequently detected by PCR amplification and sequencing [18, 19]. A wide variety of bisulfite-based protocols have been designed [12, 20], capable to interrogate from just one single CpG site or short sequences with several in *cis* CpG sites by PCR [18, 19, 21–23], up to hundreds of thousands of CpG sites using microarray platforms [24–26], and even genome-wide single-nucleotide resolution CpG methylation profiles by using next-generation sequencing platforms [27–29].

In this article, we describe two of the most common techniques to analyze DNA methylation changes. The first one, bisulfite sequencing, was first introduced in the early 1990s [18, 19]. This technique interrogates a single *locus*, typically a sequence shorter than 250 bp containing several CpG sites in *cis*. Despite its limited throughput, bisulfite sequencing provides a good resolution *vs* cost balance, thus being suitable for the analysis of a limited number of genes in a large number of samples. Bisulfite sequencing is a very informative strategy providing single-nucleotide resolution of the methylation pattern in individual DNA segments. Essentially, the locus of interest is amplified by PCR after bisulfite conversion. The PCR amplification product is subsequently cloned into a plasmid vector and sequenced. The methylation of the CpG sites can be inferred from the PCR-amplified sequence. If they remain unaltered, it is considered that they were originally methylated and therefore protected from the bisulfite transformation. The unmethylated cytosine will be transformed to uracil and will appear as thymine in the amplification products [18, 19]. Since methylation outside of CpG sites is extremely uncommon (although not completely absent) in somatic human cells, it can be assumed that all the cytosines outside CpG sites should have been transformed to thymines, providing an internal control of the conversion efficiency of the bisulfite treatment. Other routinely used PCR-based methods, such as methylation-sensitive PCR (MSP) [22] and combined bisulfite and restriction analysis (COBRA) [23], will be also briefly discussed.

The second technique is the Illumina HM450K BeadChip [25], arguably the most prevalent commercial genome-wide methylation analysis platform, used in several large studies of the International Cancer Genome Consortium (ICGC) [30]. In contrast with bisulfite sequencing, microarray platforms provide a much larger coverage of the genome albeit with lower resolution per *locus*, making them ideal for exploratory analyses. The HM450K array interrogates more than 450,000 individual CpG sites in the human genome. The latest release of the Illumina Methylation BeadChip, i.e., the MethylationEPIC array, has increased that resolution up to over 850,000 CpG sites [26]. The higher throughput, however, is accompanied by a significantly higher cost that can become a limiting factor to analyze a large number of samples.

2 Materials

1. DNA extraction kit: Qiagen DNAeasy Blood and Tissue Kit or similar.
2. DNA bisulfite treatment kit: Zymo Research EZ DNA Methylation™ Kit or similar.
3. PCR Amplification Kit: Qiagen Taq PCR Master Mix Kit (250 U) or similar.

4. Thermocycler, preferentially equipped with a gradient-enabled thermoblock.
5. Restriction enzymes: BstUI, TaqI, MaeII/HpyCH4IV, and Bsh1236I.
6. DNA restoration kit: Illumina Infinium HD FFPE DNA Restore Kit (24 samples) or similar.
7. DNA quality control kit: Illumina FFPE QC Kit or similar.
8. Methylation array: Illumina HumanMethylation450 DNA Analysis BeadChip Kit (24 samples) or similar.
9. Tris-EDTA (TE) 0.1× Buffer: 1 mM Tris–HCl, 0.1 mM EDTA, pH 8.0.
10. Computational requirements: personal computer with Windows, MacOS, or Linux operating system. RnBeads (multiplatform, freeware, available at http://rnbeads.mpi-inf.mpg.de/). RStudio (multiplatform, freeware, available at https://www.rstudio.com/).

3 Methods

3.1 DNA Extraction

1. DNA quality is extremely important for the subsequent procedures. We regularly employ DNA extraction kits from Qiagen following the protocol provided with the kit, but many different methods and commercial kits are available. Describing all suitable protocols would exceed the scope of this article, but regardless of the method employed, we strongly encourage to quantify the concentration and quality of the purified DNA by spectrophotometry before proceeding with the bisulfite treatment.

3.2 DNA Restoration of FFPE Samples

1. For formalin-fixed paraffin-embedded (FFPE) samples, specific procedures should be performed prior to bisulfite treatment, particularly if the DNA is going to be employed for microarray analysis. Specific protocols for DNA restoration can be found at Illumina's website [31].

3.3 Bisulfite Treatment of DNA

Both methods presented in this article are based on the bisulfite transformation of DNA. Several protocols are available. In our laboratory, we regularly employ the EZ Bisulfite Conversion Kit (D5001, Zymo Research), with excellent results for genomic DNA obtained from in vitro cultured cell lines and freshly frozen tissues. The complete protocol is available at Zymo Research website [32]. We transcribe it in here to include several modifications and notes, some already suggested by the manufacturer and some that we have found to improve the DNA recovery yield.

3.3.1 Preparation of CT Conversion Reagent

The CT Conversion Reagent supplied within the Zymo Research EZ Methylation kit is a solid mixture and must be prepared prior to first use. Prepare as follows:

1. Add 750 μL water and 210 μL of M-Dilution Buffer to a tube of CT Conversion Reagent.
2. Mix at room temperature with frequent vortexing or shaking for 10 min.

It is normal to see trace amounts of undissolved reagent in the CT Conversion Reagent. Each tube of CT Conversion Reagent is designed for ten separate DNA treatments.

The CT Conversion Reagent is light sensitive, so minimize its exposure to light. For best results, the CT Conversion Reagent should be used immediately following preparation. If not used immediately, the CT Conversion Reagent solution can be stored overnight at room temperature, 1 week at 4 °C or up to 1 month at −20 °C. Stored CT Conversion Reagent solution must be warmed to 37 °C and then mixed by vortexing prior to use.

3.3.2 Preparation of M-Wash Buffer

1. Add 24 mL of 100% ethanol to the 6 mL M-Wash Buffer concentrate or 96 mL of 100% ethanol to the 24 mL M-Wash Buffer concentrate before use.

3.3.3 Bisulfite Transformation

1. Add 5 μL of M-Dilution Buffer to the DNA sample (500 pg to 2 μg), and adjust the total volume to 50 μL with water. Mix the sample by flicking or pipetting up and down.
2. Incubate the sample at 37 °C for 15 min.
3. After the above incubation, add 100 μL of the prepared CT Conversion Reagent to each sample and mix.
4. Incubate the sample in the dark at 50 °C for 12–16 h (*see* **Note 1**).
5. Incubate the sample at 0–4 °C (e.g., on ice) for 10 min.
6. Add 400 μL of M-Binding Buffer to a Zymo-Spin™ IC Column, and place the column into a provided collection tube.
7. Load the sample (from **step 5**) into the Zymo-Spin™ IC Column containing the M-Binding Buffer. Close the cap and mix it by inverting the column several times.
8. Centrifuge at full speed (>10,000 × *g*) for 30 s. Discard the flow-through.
9. Add 100 μL of M-Wash Buffer to the column. Centrifuge at full speed for 30 s.
10. Add 200 μL of M-Desulphonation Buffer to the column, and let it stand at room temperature (20–30 °C) for 15–20 min. After the incubation, centrifuge at full speed for 30 s.

11. Add 200 μL of M-Wash Buffer to the column. Centrifuge at full speed for 30 s. Add another 200 μL of M-Wash Buffer, and centrifuge for an additional 30 s.
12. Place the column into a 1.5 mL microcentrifuge tube. Add 10–20 μL of M-Elution Buffer (pre-warmed at 60 °C) directly to the column matrix. Incubate for 5 min and centrifuge for 30 s at full speed to elute the DNA.
13. For maximum DNA recovery, repeat **step 12** on a second 1.5 mL microcentrifuge tube. This second elution will have substantially lower DNA concentration than the first elution but still high enough for most PCR-based analytical methods.
14. The treated DNA is ready for immediate analysis or can be stored at or below −20 °C for later use. For long-term storage, store at or below −70 °C.

3.4 Bisulfite Sequencing and Related Techniques

There are many bisulfite-based methods commonly used to analyze the methylation of a single locus. In here, we describe bisulfite sequencing, which interrogates the methylation status of a short sequence at single-nucleotide resolution [18, 19]. Essentially, the method employs a pair of PCR primers that amplify the *locus* of interest irrespective of its methylation status. The PCR amplicons are then cloned into plasmid vectors, transformed into *E. coli* cells, isolated, and individually sequenced. In contrast with other very common single-locus analysis methods based on PCR-amplification of bisulfite-transformed DNA, such as methylation-sensitive PCR (MSP) [22], combined restriction and methylation analysis (COBRA) [23], MethyLight [33], or pyrosequencing [34], bisulfite sequencing provides a single-nucleotide analysis of every CpG site within the amplified region while maintaining at the same time the intramolecular methylation information. This method is also semiquantitative, providing an estimation of the proportion of methylated *vs* unmethylated molecules, albeit one must be aware of biases that might occur during PCR amplification and/or cloning efficiency that can affect the accuracy of the quantification. In comparison with the aforementioned single-locus methods, however, bisulfite sequencing is considerably more laborious and expensive, because in order to obtain a reliable view of the methylation status of the studied locus, a minimum of ten sequences per sample, often even more, are generally required.

In any case, bisulfite sequencing is a sensible first approach to investigate the pattern of the methylation changes in a particular *locus* in a reduced number of samples that can be later complemented with other less laborious, faster, and more economical techniques to extend the study to a larger number of samples. In this regard, the same PCR amplicons obtained for bisulfite sequencing can be readily employed for combined restriction and methylation analysis (COBRA), if the internal sequence includes CpG-containing restriction sites susceptible to the bisulfite conversion (see below).

3.5 Bisulfite Sequencing: Primer Design

Bisulfite-sequencing PCR primers must anneal onto sequences devoid of CpG sites and surrounding the CpG sites to be interrogated [35].

The first step of primer design is the in silico transformation of the original sequence mimicking the effect of the bisulfite conversion. This process can be done using free web tools, e.g. http://www.zymoresearch.com/tools/bisulfite-primer-seeker, or any word processor by simply substituting all CG dinucleotides in the original sequence by NG and then substituting the remaining C by T. One particular consideration is that the in silico transformation must be performed separately on the two strands of the *locus* of interest, because after bisulfite conversion they are no longer complementary, and very often primer design is easier to achieve in one of the strands than in the other.

Primer design might be particularly challenging due to the extreme DNA sequence composition after bisulfite modification and the constraints on the primers and their location on the template. In addition, PCR amplification of bisulfite-treated DNA very often generates unspecific products due to the sequence complexity reduction of the bisulfite-treated genome, which allows the primers to anneal at unexpected locations.

Our group has routinely and successfully relied on the free web tool Primer3 [36, 37] to design all of our primers, but there is specific software to facilitate the design of primers for bisulfite-sequencing and methylation-specific PCR, such as MethPrimer [38]. Essentially we aim for a primer length larger than 22 mer, with a GC content over 40%, and targeting a sequence of 100–250 bp. Amplification of longer sequences is possible but not recommended, because the bisulfite treatment degrades the DNA hampering the amplification of very large DNA molecules.

To achieve methylation-independent amplification, bisulfite-sequencing primers must avoid CpG sites within their annealing sequences, especially at their 3′ end. If completely unavoidable, some CpG sites at the 5′ end of bisulfite sequencing might be tolerated (coded as YG or CR in the primer sequence, depending on the target strand, being Y and R the IUPAC codes for pyrimidine or purine, respectively). The internal part of the amplified sequence should contain the CpG sites to be interrogated (we suggest to include as many as possible). If the product is going to be later analyzed by enzymatic restriction by COBRA, it must contain the restriction sites to be interrogated, most typically BstUI (CGCG), TaqI (TCGA), or MaeII (ACGT). Restriction enzymes with longer target sequences can also be employed, taking into account that any unmethylated cytosine will be transformed to thymine after bisulfite treatment and PCR amplification.

To overcome the typical challenges of bisulfite-sequencing PCRs, we routinely design two forward (F1 and F2) and two reversal (R1 and R2) primers for every region to be analyzed. This set of primers allows testing four different combinations, i.e., F1-R1, F2-R2, F1-R2, and F2-R1, as well as nested or semi-nested strategies for the PCR amplification (see below).

Primers and conditions for DNA bisulfite sequencing are valid for several types of downstream analysis (see below). In contrast, the also popular methylation-sensitive PCR (MSP) and its quantitative-derived variants employ primers purposely targeting CpG sites. It is imperative that the 3′ end of the MSP primers anneals directly on the interrogated CpGs. Therefore, for MSP two different set of primers must be designed: one to amplify the methylated molecules and the other to amplify the unmethylated molecules, and the methylation status is determined by the PCR amplification itself rather than by the analysis of the amplified product composition.

3.6 PCR Amplification Strategy

PCR setup might be notably difficult and must be empirically determined for each analyzed *locus* [39]. As an initial attempt, we regularly test the abovementioned four primer combinations at different annealing temperatures within the ±5 °C range of their predicted annealing temperature, using a gradient-enabled thermocycler. We routinely perform all PCR reactions with Qiagen HotStart Kit, in 25 μL of 1× buffer, 0.5× Q-Solution, 0.125 mM dNTPs, 0.4 μM of each primer, 100 ng of bisulfite-treated genomic DNA (*see* **Note 2**), and 1 unit of polymerase. Other thermostable polymerases, primer, or dNTP concentrations might be used [39]. The amplification of a unique and specific PCR product must be verified by agarose gel electrophoresis.

If complete specificity is not achieved by any of the four primer combinations in the tested annealing temperature range, we generally attempt a touchdown program in which the annealing temperature starts at 70 °C and progressively decreases to 55 °C in the first ten cycles, to continue at 55 °C for the rest of the amplification cycles (again 25–35, depending on the target sequence), with the abovementioned template, buffer, dNTPs, and primer concentrations. If complete specificity is still not achieved by the touchdown program, we resort to nested or semi-nested PCR strategy, in which the bisulfite-treated DNA is first subjected to PCR with the most external primers pair for a limited number of cycles (ideally less than 15), and one tenth of this reaction is used as template for a second PCR. This strategy, however, increases the total number of amplification cycles and might introduce undesirable bias toward the methylated or unmethylated molecules.

3.7 Bisulfite-PCR Product Analysis: Cloning, Direct Sequencing, Enzymatic Restriction, and Melting Temperature Profiling

3.7.1 Cloning

Once the PCR conditions are set and the amplification of a unique and specific product is verified, several options are available for the analysis. The traditional option, which we suggest as a first choice since it provides the most comprehensive information, is to clone the PCR product into a plasmid vector, transform it into *E. coli* cells, select a number (between 10 and 20) of colonies harboring recombinant plasmids, and sequence the cloned inserts (Fig. 1a–c). We regularly employed pCDNA3.2 TOPO-TA cloning kit (Qiagen) or the StrataClone PCR cloning kit (Agilent Technologies), following manufacturer's instructions. Albeit the same primers employed for the bisulfite PCR might be used for the sequencing of the insert, it is advisable to use external primers annealing onto the vector, such as the M13, T7, or T3 primers (depending on the vector), for longer and better quality sequencing results.

3.7.2 PCR Direct Sequencing

Alternatively, the PCR product can be purified and directly sequenced using one of the amplification primers (Fig. 1d). This option, albeit faster and more economical than sequencing of individual clones, has some disadvantages. First, while still providing single-nucleotide resolution information, the within-molecule information is disregarded, i.e., direct sequencing cannot discern whether the methylation is heterogeneous within every molecule or there is a mixture of methylated and unmethylated molecules. In addition, the conversion of unmethylated cytosine into thymine often results in long stretches of mononucleotides, prone to undergo random deletions and insertions during the PCR amplification due to the slippage of the Taq polymerase. These deletions and insertions generally result in poor-quality sequencing results downstream the mononucleotide tracts. To overcome the presence of mononucleotide tracts, the PCR product might be sequenced from both ends, although this not always solves the issue if two (or more) mononucleotide tracts are present surrounding the CpGs of interest. Moreover, the amplification primers might not be very efficient for sequencing, increasing the probability of poor-quality results. Finally, although the height of the Sanger sequencing electropherogram profile peaks is often used to estimate the proportion of methylated vs unmethylated molecules, it has to be noted that Sanger sequencing is not truly quantitative and therefore it does not accurately reflect this proportion.

A more quantitative approach for the direct sequencing strategy, which at the same time overcomes the problem caused by the mononucleotide tracts, is employing pyrosequencing to estimate the proportion of methylated vs unmethylated cytosines at every CpG site within the amplified sequence [40]. Pyrosequencing, however, requires specialized equipment, is slightly more expensive, and generates shorter sequences than Sanger sequencing.

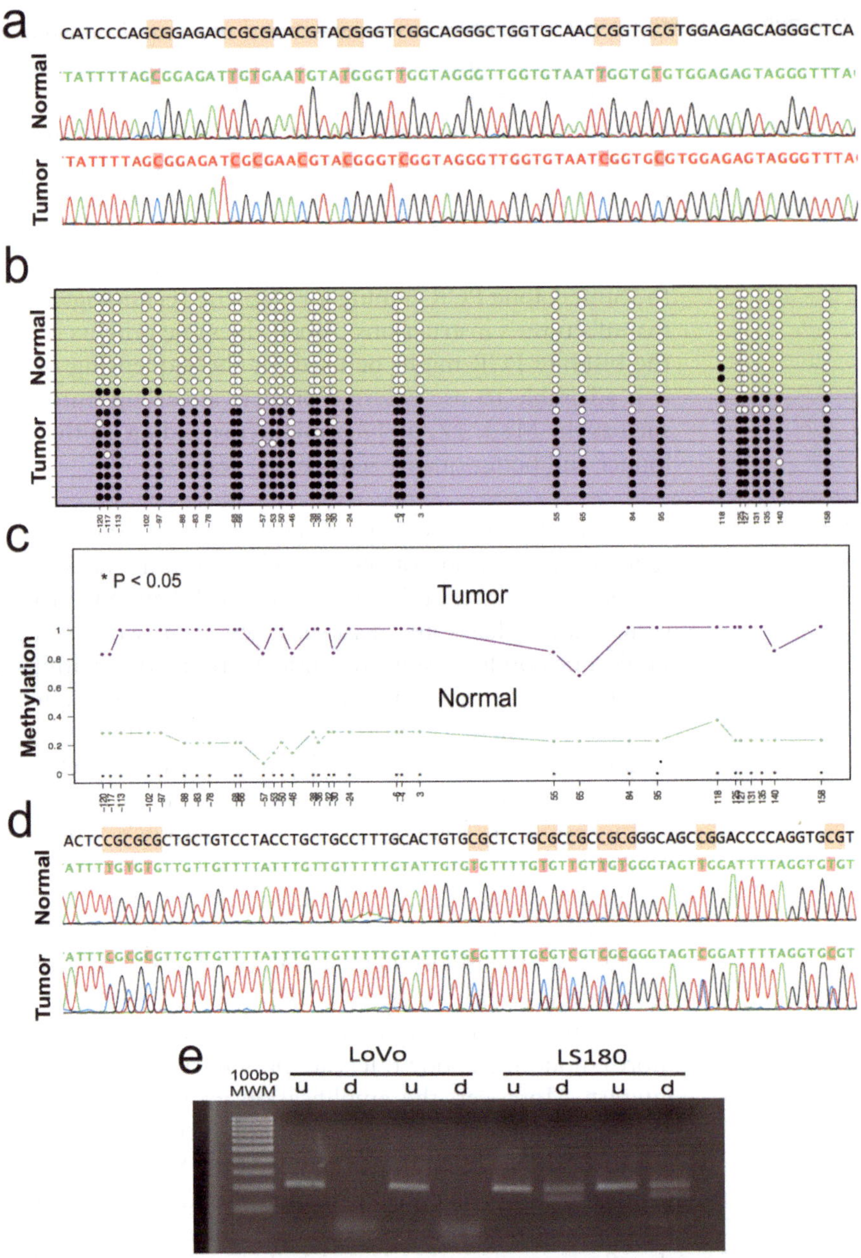

Fig. 1 Bisulfite-sequencing analysis of *ADAMTS14* and *ADAMTS19* genes. (**a**) In black font a 71-bp sequence within the *ADAMTS19* promoter containing eight CpG sites (shaded in orange). Below, the sequences and electropherogram profiles obtained after bisulfite sequencing of an unmethylated molecule from a normal sample (green) and a methylated molecule from a tumor sample (red). Note that all cytosines outside CpG sites have been converted to thymine in the transformed sequences. (**b**) Graphical representation of the methylation status of a 280 bp sequence containing 28 CpG sites within the *ADAMTS19* promoter in ten clones from a normal sample (green-shaded area) and ten clones from a tumor sample (purple-shaded area). White circles represent unmethylated CpG sites. Black circles represent methylated CpG sites. (**c**) Average methylation levels per CpG site in the same sequence presented in panel **b**. The clones derived from the tumor sample exhibited much higher levels of methylation than those derived from the normal sample, in all the interrogated CpG sites ($P < 0.05$, Mann–Whitney test).

Hence, direct PCR sequencing is a valid option for rapid scanning of samples that are not expected to exhibit excessively heterogeneous methylation and do not have long mononucleotide tracts that might complicate the reading of the sequence.

3.7.3 Combined Bisulfite and Restriction Analysis (COBRA)

A very fast and economical alternative is treating the bisulfite PCR product with restriction enzymes [23]. Restriction sites containing CG dinucleotides will be transformed by the bisulfite treatment if they were originally unmethylated, but not if methylated. Thus, the incubation with an appropriate restriction enzyme will generate different restriction fragments depending on the original methylation status of the molecule. These restriction fragments are subsequently resolved by agarose gel electrophoresis (Fig. 1e). Generally, the selected enzymes will cut the originally methylated sites that retained the CG dinucleotide within their recognition sequence, but not the originally unmethylated sites, which after bisulfite conversion contain TG instead of CG. This strategy, however, does not provide single-nucleotide information because it is restricted to the interrogated restrictions sites.

3.7.4 Melting Temperature Analysis

Lastly, if a real-time thermocycler is available, methylation status can be inferred by the different melting temperature exhibited by the PCR products from originally methylated molecules, with higher proportion of GC base pairs, vs those from originally unmethylated molecules, where the GC base pairs have been substituted by AT [41]. This approach does not provide single-nucleotide resolution but rather estimates the global content of methylated cytosines within the studied sequence. The amplification product of originally methylated molecules would contain a larger proportion of GC pairs and would typically exhibit higher melting temperature. Although this is a fast and very capable approach to distinguish between methylated vs unmethylated samples if they are homogeneous, in our experience the analysis of heterogeneous samples, such as those from tumor biopsies where there is frequent and unavoidable contaminantion with non-tumoral cells, might generate complex melting curves that make their interpretation more challenging. This is due to the inherent differences in the

Fig. 1 (continued) (**d**) Bisulfite PCR direct sequencing of a 80 bp sequence within the *ADAMTS14* promoter containing ten CpG sites (shaded in orange). The PCR product derived from the normal sample showed no traces of methylation in any of the interrogated CpG sites, while the product derived from the tumor sample exhibited a mix of methylated and unmethylated molecules (a mix of T and C peaks in the electropherogram). As in panel a, note that all cytosines outside CpG sites have been converted to thymine in the transformed sequences. (**e**) COBRA results of a 214 bp PCR product from the *ADAMTS14* promoter region derived from two CRC cell lines: LoVo, highly methylated, and LS180, with low levels of methylation. The original PCR products (lanes u) became completely digested by BstUI (lanes d) in LoVo but only partially digested in LS180

melting profiles in the mixture of amplification products derived from both methylated and unmethylated molecules, as well as the generation of heteroduplex molecules in the last cycles of the PCR that exhibit yet a different melting profile [42].

3.7.5 Bisulfite Sequencing Data Representation

For bisulfite sequencing data representation, we suggest using the Methylation Plotter web server (http://maplab.imppc.org/methylation_plotter/), a platform-independent tool to visualize continuous methylation data generating lollipop or grid graphics [43]. This user-friendly web tool provides very comprehensive and detailed visual information required by most of wet lab researchers analyzing the methylation of single (or a limited number) of *loci* (Fig. 2).

3.7.6 Typical Results

As examples of the typical results, we present the analyses of two ADAMTS genes, i.e., *ADAMTS14* and *ADAMTS19* (Fig. 1). The amplification of *ADAMTS14* was achieved with a simple PCR program that consisted of 15 min at 95 °C to activate the polymerase; 35 cycles of 30 s at 95 °C, 30 s at 55 °C, and 30 s at 72 °C; and a

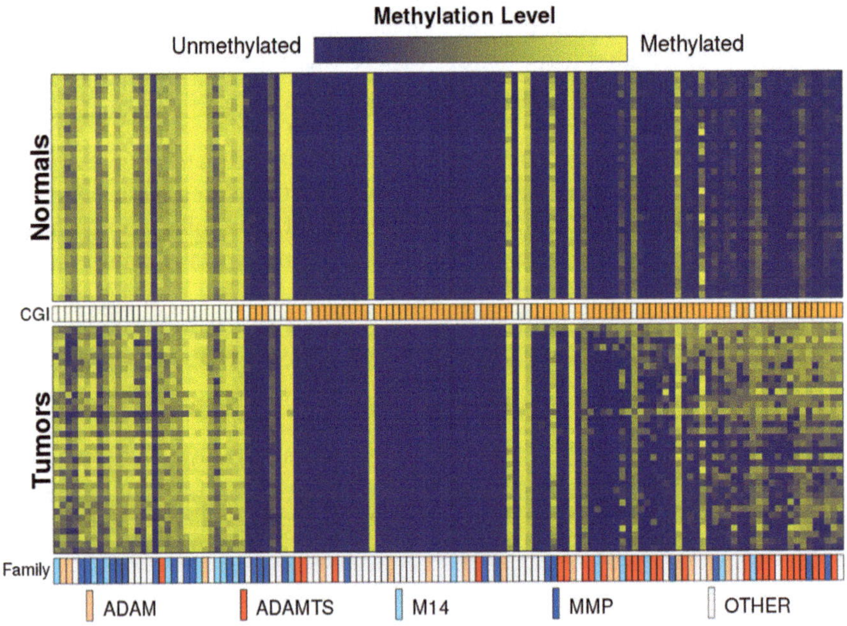

Fig. 2 Methylation profile of extracellular metallopeptidase-encoding genes in normal and tumor samples from 35 CRC patients. Methylation is shown from blue to yellow gradient. Normal samples on top, tumor samples below. In the *x*-axis genes and in the *y*-axis samples, both ordered according to their somatic methylation change (difference between tumor and normal). The CGI row between the two upper heatmaps indicates genes with (in orange) or without (in yellow) promoter-associated CGI. The bottom row indicates the gene family according to the color scheme shown in the legend. Note the overrepresentation of ADAMTS genes (red) among the frequently hypermethylated genes

final extension of 10 min at 72 °C, using primers 5′-GTTTTTAGTTT GGGATTTGG-3′ and 5′-AACAACCTTAAACCACCCTAAC-3′. The PCR conditions for amplification of *ADAMTS14* promoter region were very robust, so much in fact that this PCR is regularly employed in our laboratory as a control test to verify the efficiency of bisulfite transformation on newly treated samples.

ADAMTS19 required a two-step nested amplification strategy. The first PCR program consisted of 1 cycle at 95 °C for 15 min to activate the enzyme, followed by 20 cycles of denaturation at 95 °C for 30 s, annealing at 55 °C for 30 s, and extension at 72 °C for 60 s, ending at 72 °C for 5 min to complete extension, using the primers 5′-TTGGTTGTGGGTTTGTTTTG-3′ and 5′-CCCC TTAACCTACACCTCAAAC-3′. The product of the first amplification was diluted 1:20 (v/v) in TE 0.1×. One microliter of the dilution was used as template for a second reaction with the same conditions than the previous one but using primers 5′-GGTAGA TAAAGGGTTTGGGTAAAT-3′ and 5′-CCCACTAAACCCTAC TCTCCAC-3′ and 25 cycles.

Both *ADAMTS14* and *ADAMTS19* were first analyzed by bisulfite sequencing in a limited number of samples, and when the methylation pattern of the samples was clearly determined to be bimodal, i.e., a mix of molecules harboring almost every CpG site methylated and molecules almost completely unmethylated, we continued the analyses by the much faster and cheaper COBRA strategy, using BstUI (NEB, cuts at 60 °C) or its isoschizomer Bsh1236I (ThermoFisher, cuts at 37 °C), in a larger number of samples (Fig. 1).

3.7.7 Genome-Wide Methylation Analysis

There are several commercial options to analyze the methylation of hundreds of thousands of CpG sites in the human genome. As abovementioned, Illumina methylation chips are arguably the most common microarray platform nowadays, offering a reasonable balance between cost and throughput. These arrays are based on the Illumina's proprietary Infinium technology. A very detailed information about these arrays is available on the Illumina website [44]. Sample processing in these arrays requires very specific equipment, software, and technical knowledge, generally restricted to support units and commercial service providers, well above the typical capabilities of a basic research laboratory. We recommend these steps to be performed by a facility with the required equipment and ample experience. Thus, this article will not discuss the sample preparation, scanning, and initial data processing for the analysis of Illumina HM450K arrays.

3.7.8 Computational Analysis

In our laboratory, Illumina HM450K array secondary processing is performed using the freeware software RnBeads [45]. This software performs essential normalization and filtering steps and generates very comprehensive reports including some basic analyses, such as sample group comparison, chromosome-by-chromosome analysis, clustering, and gene-centered analysis. Subsequent, ad hoc computational analyses can be performed using free software: R, Rstudio, and Bioconductor [46, 47]. Substantial knowledge in bioinformatics is required to implement the typical HM450K methylation post-analysis. In here we succinctly describe the procedures that we have performed to analyze somatic methylation changes of extracellular metallopeptidases in 35 CRC patients. A complete set of R-scripts to replicate the analysis is available upon request.

3.7.9 Selection of Extracellular Metallopeptidase-Encoding Genes

A list of 649 peptidase-encoding human genes is available from the MEROPS database [4]. Of these, 187 encode proteins classified as metallopeptidases, subclassified into 26 families. Querying the ENSEMBL [48] using the BiomaRt R package [49] for the gene ontology term "metallopeptidase activity" (GO:0008237) retrieves 169 unique genes. The list of these 169 genes contains 19 genes not present in the MEROPS database. To be as inclusive as possible, these 19 genes were considered in our analyses, yielding a total of 206 metallopeptidase-encoding genes. This list was further refined by selecting the 128 genes that had any of the following gene ontology annotations regarding their cellular compartment location: extracellular matrix (GO:0031012), extracellular region (GO:0005576), plasma membrane (G:0005886), cell adhesion (GO:0007155), or cell junction (GO:0030054) (Table 1).

We classified the genes into five groups: ADAMTS, comprising the *ADAMTS*, *ADAMTSL*, and *PAPLN* genes (panther family PTHR13723); ADAM, comprising the *ADAM* and *ADAMDEC* genes (panther family PTHR11905); M14, comprising primarily carboxypeptidase-encoding genes (panther families PTHR11532, PTHR11705, and PTHR12756); MMP, comprising the MMP genes (panther family PTHR10201); and OTHER, comprising the rest of extracellular metallopeptidases not included in any of the previous families.

3.7.10 Selection of HM450K Probes Interrogating Genes Encoding Extracellular Metallopeptidases

A numerical matrix with the methylation values of all the HM450K probes for 35 colorectal cancers and their matching normal mucosas was obtained from the HTML report generated by RnBeads [45].

For every one of the 128 extracellular metallopeptidase-encoding genes, we calculated the average methylation of HM450K probes within the ±1.5 kb sequence surrounding the transcriptional start site (TSS) of their canonical transcripts. If a CGI overlapped that region, i.e., a TSS-associated CGI, the average methylation of probes within that CGI was used to represent the average methylation of the gene promoter. For genes with two TSS-associated CGIs (*ADAM11*, *ADAMTS1*, *ADAMTS3*, *ADAMTS10*, *MMP15*, *and*

Table 1
List of human genes encoding extracellular matrix metallopeptidases

Gene	Ensembl geneID	Entrez geneID	Ensembl transcriptID	Trans-cript biotype	External transcript name	Transcript appris	Transcript tsl	Transcript start	Transcript end	Chromo-some	Strand	Panther family	Family
LNPEP	ENSG00000113441	4012	ENST00000231368	Protein_coding	LNPEP-001	Principal1	tsl1	96935464	97037515	chr5	1	PTHR11533	OTHER
MMP28	ENSG00000271447	79148	ENST00000605424	Protein_coding	MMP28-005	Principal1	tsl1	35766340	35795582	chr17	−1	PTHR10201	MMP
BMP1	ENSG00000168487	649	ENST00000306385	Protein_coding	BMP1-001	Principal1	tsl1	22164736	22212326	chr8	1	PTHR10127	OTHER
MMP25	ENSG00000008516	64386	ENST00000336577	Protein_coding	MMP25-001	Principal1	tsl1	3046681	3060726	chr16	1	PTHR10201	MMP
NLN	ENSG00000123213	57486	ENST00000380985	Protein_coding	NLN-001	Principal1	tsl1	65722196	65829283	chr5	1	PTHR11804	OTHER
MMP19	ENSG00000123342	4327	ENST00000322569	Protein_coding	MMP19-001	Principal1	tsl1	55836426	55842922	chr12	−1	PTHR10201	MMP
MMP11	ENSG00000099953	4320	ENST00000215743	Protein_coding	MMP11-001	Principal1	tsl1	23772819	23784316	chr22	1	PTHR10201	MMP
CLCA2	ENSG00000137975	9635	ENST00000370565	Protein_coding	CLCA2-001	Principal1	tsl1	86424086	86456558	chr1	1	PTHR10579	OTHER
CLCA4	ENSG00000016602	22802	ENST00000370563	Protein_coding	CLCA4-001	Principal1	tsl1	86547078	86580754	chr1	1	PTHR10579	OTHER
AEBP1	ENSG00000106624	165	ENST00000223357	Protein_coding	AEBP1-001	Principal1	tsl1	44104361	44114560	chr7	1	PTHR11532	M14
ADAMTS18	ENSG00000140873	170692	ENST00000282849	Protein_coding	ADAMTS18-001	Principal1	tsl1	77282128	77435114	chr16	−1	PTHR13723	ADAMTS
ADAMTS17	ENSG00000140470	170691	ENST00000268070	Protein_coding	ADAMTS17-001	Principal1	tsl1	99971589	100342005	chr15	−1	PTHR13723	ADAMTS
ADAM23	ENSG00000114948	8745	ENST00000264377	Protein_coding	ADAM23-001	Principal2	tsl1	206443539	206621130	chr2	1	PTHR11905	ADAM
ADAMTS1	ENSG00000154734	9510	ENST00000284984	Protein_coding	ADAMTS1-001	Principal1	tsl1	26835747	26845409	chr21	−1	PTHR13723	ADAMTS
ADAMTS5	ENSG00000154736	11096	ENST00000284987	Protein_coding	ADAMTS5-001	Principal1	tsl1	26917912	26966513	chr21	−1	PTHR13723	ADAMTS
PSMD14	ENSG00000115233	10213	ENST00000409682	Protein_coding	PSMD14-001	Principal1	tsl1	161308038	161411717	chr2	1	PTHR10410	OTHER
ADAMTS4	ENSG00000158859	9507	ENST00000367996	Protein_coding	ADAMTS4-001	Principal1	tsl1	161184308	161199056	chr1	−1	PTHR13723	ADAMTS
QPCT	ENSG00000115828	25797	ENST00000338415	Protein_coding	QPCT-001	Principal1	tsl1	37344574	37373322	chr2	1	PTHR12283	OTHER
CPA3	ENSG00000163751	1359	ENST00000296046	Protein_coding	CPA3-001	Principal1	tsl1	148865256	148897196	chr3	1	PTHR11705	M14
MMP2	ENSG00000087245	4313	ENST00000219070	Protein_coding	MMP2-001	Principal1	tsl1	55478971	55506691	chr16	1	PTHR10201	MMP
MEP1B	ENSG00000141434	4225	ENST00000269202	Protein_coding	MEP1B-001	Principal1	tsl1	32190024	32220404	chr18	1	PTHR10127	OTHER
ADAMTS12	ENSG00000151388	81792	ENST00000504830	Protein_coding	ADAMTS12-002	Principal1	tsl1	33523535	33892192	chr5	−1	PTHR13723	ADAMTS

(continued)

Table 1
(continued)

Gene	Ensembl geneID	Entrez geneID	Ensembl transcriptID	Trans-cript biotype	External transcript name	Transcript appris	Transcript tsl	Transcript start	Transcript end	Chromo-some	Strand	Panther family	Family
CPXM1	ENSG00000088882	56265	ENST00000380605	Protein_coding	CPXM1-001	Principal1	tsl1	2794069	2800637	chr20	−1	PTHR11532	M14
ADAMTS7	ENSG00000136378	11173	ENST00000388820	Protein_coding	ADAMTS7-001	Principal1	tsl1	78759203	78811431	chr15	−1	PTHR13723	ADAMTS
ADAMTSL1	ENSG00000178031	92949	ENST00000380548	Protein_coding	ADAMTSL1-012	Principal1	tsl5	18473894	18910950	chr9	1	PTHR13723	ADAMTS
ERAP1	ENSG00000164307	51752	ENST00000443439	Protein_coding	ERAP1-002	Principal1	tsl1	96774484	96807909	chr5	−1	PTHR11533	OTHER
PAPLN	ENSG00000100767	89932	ENST00000340738	Protein_coding	PAPLN-001	Principal2	tsl5	73237497	73274640	chr14	1	PTHR13723	ADAMTS
MMP24	ENSG00000125966	10893	ENST00000246186	Protein_coding	MMP24-001	Principal1	tsl1	35226654	35277000	chr20	1	PTHR10201	MMP
CPZ	ENSG00000109625	8532	ENST00000315782	Protein_coding	CPZ-001	Principal3	tsl1	8592756	8619749	chr4	1	PTHR11532	M14
MMP9	ENSG00000100985	4318	ENST00000372330	Protein_coding	MMP9-001	Principal1	tsl1	46008908	46016561	chr20	1	PTHR10201	MMP
CPN1	ENSG00000120054	1369	ENST00000370418	Protein_coding	CPN1-001	Principal1	tsl1	100042193	100081877	chr10	−1	PTHR11532	M14
IDE	ENSG00000119912	3416	ENST00000265986	Protein_coding	IDE-001	Principal1	tsl1	92451684	92574076	chr10	−1	PTHR11851	OTHER
PA2G4	ENSG00000170515	5036	ENST00000303305	Protein_coding	PA2G4-001	Principal1	tsl1	56104319	56113861	chr12	1	PTHR10804	OTHER
LTA4H	ENSG00000111144	4048	ENST00000228740	Protein_coding	LTA4H-001	Principal1	tsl1	96000828	96035661	chr12	−1	PTHR11533	OTHER
PAPPA	ENSG00000182752	5069	ENST00000328252	Protein_coding	PAPPA-001	Principal1	tsl1	116153804	116402322	chr9	1	PTHR19325	OTHER
ADAMTS20	ENSG00000173157	80070	ENST00000389420	Protein_coding	ADAMTS20-001	Principal1	tsl1	43353866	43551921	chr12	−1	PTHR13723	ADAMTS
CPE	ENSG00000109472	1363	ENST00000402744	Protein_coding	CPE-001	Principal1	tsl1	165378942	165498320	chr4	1	PTHR11532	M14
CNDP1	ENSG00000150656	84735	ENST00000358821	Protein_coding	CNDP1-001	Principal2	tsl1	74534440	74585025	chr18	1	PTHR11014	OTHER
TLL1	ENSG00000038295	7092	ENST00000061240	Protein_coding	TLL1-001	Principal1	tsl1	165873258	166103895	chr4	1	PTHR10127	OTHER
ADAMTS16	ENSG00000145536	170690	ENST00000274181	Protein_coding	ADAMTS16-001	Principal1	tsl2	5140330	5320304	chr5	1	PTHR13723	ADAMTS
MMEL1	ENSG00000142606	79258	ENST00000378412	Protein_coding	MMEL1-001	Principal1	tsl2	2590643	2632990	chr1	−1	PTHR11733	OTHER
ADAM9	ENSG00000168615	8754	ENST00000487273	Protein_coding	ADAM9-001	Principal1	tsl1	38996986	39105001	chr8	1	PTHR11905	ADAM
ADAMTS9	ENSG00000163638	56999	ENST00000498707	Protein_coding	ADAMTS9-001	Principal1	tsl1	64515654	64688000	chr3	−1	PTHR13723	ADAMTS
MMP21	ENSG00000154485	118856	ENST00000368808	Protein_coding	MMP21-001	Principal1	tsl1	125766453	125775821	chr10	−1	PTHR10201	MMP

PSMD7	ENSG00000103035	5713	ENST00000219313	Protein_coding	PSMD7-001	Principal1	tsl1	74296775	74306288	chr16	1	PTHR10540	OTHER
MMP7	ENSG00000137673	4316	ENST00000260227	Protein_coding	MMP7-001	Principal1	tsl1	102520508	102530753	chr11	−1	PTHR10201	MMP
MMP20	ENSG00000137674	9313	ENST00000260228	Protein_coding	MMP20-001	Principal1	tsl1	102576835	102625332	chr11	−1	PTHR10201	MMP
MMP8	ENSG00000118113	4317	ENST00000236826	Protein_coding	MMP8-001	Principal1	tsl1	102711795	102724954	chr11	−1	PTHR10201	MMP
MMP3	ENSG00000149968	4314	ENST00000299855	Protein_coding	MMP3-001	Principal1	tsl1	102835801	102843803	chr11	−1	PTHR10201	MMP
MMP10	ENSG00000166670	4319	ENST00000279441	Protein_coding	MMP10-001	Principal1	tsl1	102770503	102780628	chr11	−1	PTHR10201	MMP
MMP1	ENSG00000196611	4312	ENST00000315274	Protein_coding	MMP1-001	Principal1	tsl1	102789920	102798160	chr11	−1	PTHR10201	MMP
MMP12	ENSG00000262406	4321	ENST00000571244	Protein_coding	MMP12-001	Principal1	tsl1	102862736	102875034	chr11	−1	PTHR10201	MMP
MMP13	ENSG00000137745	4322	ENST00000260302	Protein_coding	MMP13-001	Principal1	tsl1	102942995	102955734	chr11	−1	PTHR10201	MMP
ADAMTSL5	ENSG00000185761	339366	ENST00000330475	Protein_coding	ADAMTSL5-001	Principal1	tsl2	1505018	1513189	chr19	−1	PTHR13723	ADAMTS
ADAMTS14	ENSG00000138316	140766	ENST00000373208	Protein_coding	ADAMTS14-001	Principal4	tsl2	70672803	70762441	chr10	1	PTHR13723	ADAMTS
CPB2	ENSG00000080618	1361	ENST00000181383	Protein_coding	CPB2-001	Principal1	tsl1	46053186	46105026	chr13	−1	PTHR11705	M14
TLL2	ENSG00000095587	7093	ENST00000357947	Protein_coding	TLL2-001	Principal1	tsl1	96364606	96513911	chr10	−1	PTHR10127	OTHER
CPA2	ENSG00000158516	1358	ENST00000222481	Protein_coding	CPA2-001	Principal1	tsl1	130266827	130289798	chr7	1	PTHR11705	M14
CPA4	ENSG00000128510	51200	ENST00000222482	Protein_coding	CPA4-001	Principal1	tsl1	130293153	130324179	chr7	1	PTHR11705	M14
ADAMTS2	ENSG00000087116	9509	ENST00000251582	Protein_coding	ADAMTS2-001	Principal1	tsl1	179110851	179345430	chr5	−1	PTHR13723	ADAMTS
ADAM12	ENSG00000148848	8038	ENST00000368679	Protein_coding	ADAM12-001	Principal4	tsl1	126012381	126388455	chr10	−1	PTHR11905	ADAM
MMP17	ENSG00000198598	4326	ENST00000360564	Protein_coding	MMP17-001	Principal2	tsl1	131828393	131851771	chr12	1	PTHR10201	MMP
CPA1	ENSG00000091704	1357	ENST00000011292	Protein_coding	CPA1-001	Principal1	tsl1	130380371	130388088	chr7	1	PTHR11705	M14
ADAMTSL3	ENSG00000156218	57188	ENST00000286744	Protein_coding	ADAMTSL3-001	Principal3	tsl1	83654086	84039842	chr15	1	PTHR13723	ADAMTS
ADAMTS6	ENSG00000049192	11174	ENST00000381055	Protein_coding	ADAMTS6-007	Principal1	tsl1	65148736	65481920	chr5	−1	PTHR13723	ADAMTS
XPNPEP2	ENSG00000122121	7512	ENST00000371106	Protein_coding	XPNPEP2-001	Principal1	tsl1	129739022	129769538	chrX	1	PTHR10804	OTHER
RNPEP	ENSG00000176393	6051	ENST00000295640	Protein_coding	RNPEP-001	Principal1	tsl1	201982624	202006147	chr1	1	PTHR11533	OTHER
PAPPA2	ENSG00000116183	60676	ENST00000367662	Protein_coding	PAPPA2-001	Principal1	tsl1	176463171	176845605	chr1	1	PTHR19325	OTHER
ADAMTS13	ENSG00000160323	11093	ENST00000371929	Protein_coding	ADAMTS13-001	Principal4	tsl1	133422000	133459386	chr9	1	PTHR13723	ADAMTS
MMP16	ENSG00000156103	4325	ENST00000286614	Protein_coding	MMP16-001	Principal1	tsl1	88032009	88327488	chr8	−1	PTHR10201	MMP

(continued)

Table 1 (continued)

Gene	Ensembl geneID	Entrez geneID	Ensembl transcriptID	Trans-cript biotype	External transcript name	Transcript appris	Transcript tsl	Transcript start	Transcript end	Chromo-some	Strand	Panther family	Family
PM20D1	ENSG00000162877	148811	ENST00000367136	Protein_coding	PM20D1-001	Principal1	tsl1	205828022	205850117	chr1	−1	PTHR11014	OTHER
ACE	ENSG00000159640	1636	ENST00000290866	Protein_coding	ACE-001	Principal1	tsl1	63477071	63498380	chr17	1	PTHR10514	OTHER
CPQ	ENSG00000104324	10404	ENST00000220763	Protein_coding	CPQ-001	Principal1	tsl1	96645227	97143501	chr8	1	PTHR12053	OTHER
ADAM28	ENSG00000042980	10863	ENST00000265769	Protein_coding	ADAM28-001	Principal1	tsl1	24294040	24359018	chr8	1	PTHR11905	ADAM
ADAMDEC1	ENSG00000134028	27299	ENST00000256412	Protein_coding	ADAMDEC1-001	Principal3	tsl1	24384285	24406013	chr8	1	PTHR11905	ADAM
CPA6	ENSG00000165078	57094	ENST00000297770	Protein_coding	CPA6-001	Principal1	tsl1 (assigned to previous version 8)	67422072	67746385	chr8	−1	PTHR11705	M14
ADAMTS8	ENSG00000134917	11095	ENST00000257359	Protein_coding	ADAMTS8-001	Principal1	tsl1	130404925	130428993	chr11	−1	PTHR13723	ADAMTS
ADAMTS15	ENSG00000166106	170689	ENST00000299164	Protein_coding	ADAMTS15-001	Principal1	tsl1	130448974	130476641	chr11	1	PTHR13723	ADAMTS
ADAM17	ENSG00000151694	6868	ENST00000310823	Protein_coding	ADAM17-001	Principal1	tsl1	9488486	9555788	chr2	−1	PTHR11905	ADAM
ADAM15	ENSG00000143537	8751	ENST00000356955	Protein_coding	ADAM15-019	Principal4	tsl1	155051286	155062758	chr1	1	PTHR11905	ADAM
ENPEP	ENSG00000138792	2028	ENST00000265162	Protein_coding	ENPEP-001	Principal1	tsl1	110476073	110565285	chr4	1	PTHR11533	OTHER
ASTL	ENSG00000188886	431705	ENST00000342380	Protein_coding	ASTL-001	Principal1	tsl1	96123850	96138436	chr2	−1	PTHR10127	OTHER
ADAM10	ENSG00000137845	102	ENST00000260408	Protein_coding	ADAM10-001	Principal1	tsl1	58588807	58749978	chr15	−1	PTHR11905	ADAM
MYSM1	ENSG00000162601	114803	ENST00000472487	Protein_coding	MYSM1-001	Principal1	tsl2	58654739	58700092	chr1	−1	PTHR12802	OTHER
DPYSL2	ENSG00000092964	1808	ENST00000311151	Protein_coding	DPYSL2-001	Principal3	tsl1	26577843	26658178	chr8	1	PTHR11647	OTHER
CPO	ENSG00000144410	130749	ENST00000272852	Protein_coding	CPO-001	Principal1	tsl1	206939554	206969474	chr2	1	PTHR11705	M14
DPP3	ENSG00000254986	10072	ENST00000541961	Protein_coding	DPP3-005	Principal1	tsl5	66480431	66509657	chr11	1	PTHR23422	OTHER
ADAM22	ENSG00000008277	53616	ENST00000398209	Protein_coding	ADAM22-002	Principal4	tsl1	87934420	88202889	chr7	1	PTHR11905	ADAM
NAALAD2	ENSG00000077616	10003	ENST00000534061	Protein_coding	NAALAD2-001	Principal1	tsl1	90134529	90192894	chr11	1	PTHR10404	OTHER
ADAM11	ENSG00000073670	4185	ENST00000200557	Protein_coding	ADAM11-001	Principal1	tsl1	44759031	44781846	chr17	1	PTHR11905	ADAM
ADAM20	ENSG00000134007	8748	ENST00000256389	Protein_coding	ADAM20-001	Principal1	tsl1	70522358	70535015	chr14	−1	PTHR11905	ADAM

ADAM21	ENSG00000139985	8747	ENST00000603540	Protein_coding	ADAM21-001	Principal1	tsl3	70452157	70459899	chr14	1	PTHR11905	ADAM
ECE1	ENSG00000117298	1889	ENST00000264205	Protein_coding	ECE1-006	Principal4	tsl1	21219937	21290257	chr1	−1	PTHR11733	OTHER
ADAM8	ENSG00000151651	101	ENST00000445355	Protein_coding	ADAM8-001	Principal3	tsl1	133262403	133276868	chr10	−1	PTHR11905	ADAM
MMP15	ENSG00000102996	4324	ENST00000219271	Protein_coding	MMP15-001	Principal1	tsl1	58025566	58046901	chr16	1	PTHR10201	MMP
ANPEP	ENSG00000166825	290	ENST00000300060	Protein_coding	ANPEP-001	Principal1	tsl1	89784889	89814862	chr15	−1	PTHR11533	OTHER
TRABD2B	ENSG00000269113	388630	ENST00000606738	Protein_coding	TRABD2B-001	Principal1	tsl1	47760528	47996895	chr1	−1	PTHR31120	OTHER
MMP14	ENSG00000157227	4323	ENST00000311852	Protein_coding	MMP14-001	Principal1	tsl1	22836557	22847761	chr14	1	PTHR10201	MMP
ADAM2	ENSG00000104755	2515	ENST00000265708	Protein_coding	ADAM2-001	Principal3	tsl1	39743735	39838289	chr8	−1	PTHR11905	ADAM
ADAM30	ENSG00000134249	11085	ENST00000369400	Protein_coding	ADAM30-001	Principal1	tslNA	119893533	119896495	chr1	−1	PTHR11905	ADAM
KEL	ENSG00000197993	3792	ENST00000355265	Protein_coding	KEL-001	Principal1	tsl1	142941114	142962681	chr7	−1	PTHR11733	OTHER
CPD	ENSG00000108582	1362	ENST00000225719	Protein_coding	CPD-001	Principal1	tsl1	30378905	30469989	chr17	1	PTHR11532	M14
PHEX	ENSG00000102174	5251	ENST00000379374	Protein_coding	PHEX-001	Principal1	tsl1	22032441	22251310	chrX	1	PTHR11733	OTHER
ATP23	ENSG00000166896	91419	ENST00000300145	Protein_coding	ATP23-001	Principal1	tsl1	57941577	57957269	chr12	1	PTHR21711	OTHER
ADAM7	ENSG00000069206	8756	ENST00000175238	Protein_coding	ADAM7-001	Principal2	tsl1	24441026	24509565	chr8	1	PTHR11905	ADAM
NAALADL1	ENSG00000168060	10004	ENST00000358658	Protein_coding	NAALADL1-001	Principal1	tsl1	65044823	65058549	chr11	−1	PTHR10404	OTHER
METAP2	ENSG00000111142	10988	ENST00000323666	Protein_coding	METAP2-001	Principal3	tsl1	95473951	95515839	chr12	1	PTHR10804	OTHER
LMLN	ENSG00000185621	89782	ENST00000420910	Protein_coding	LMLN-004	Principal2	tsl1	197960222	198039011	chr3	1	PTHR10942	OTHER
COPS5	ENSG00000121022	10987	ENST00000357849	Protein_coding	COPS5-001	Principal1	tsl1	67043079	67062317	chr8	−1	PTHR10410	OTHER
MMP23B	ENSG00000189409	8510	ENST00000356026	Protein_coding	MMP23B-001	Principal1	tsl1	1632095	1634654	chr1	1	PTHR10201	MMP
MMP27	ENSG00000137675	64066	ENST00000260229	Protein_coding	MMP27-001	Principal1	tsl1	102691487	102705806	chr11	−1	PTHR10201	MMP
ADAMTS3	ENSG00000156140	9508	ENST00000286657	Protein_coding	ADAMTS3-001	Principal1	tsl1	72280969	72569386	chr4	−1	PTHR13723	ADAMTS
ADAMTSL2	ENSG00000197859	9719	ENST00000354484	Protein_coding	ADAMTSL2-001	Principal1	tsl1	133532164	133575519	chr9	1	PTHR13723	ADAMTS
TFRC	ENSG00000072274	7037	ENST00000360110	Protein_coding	TFRC-001	Principal3	tsl1	196049284	196082189	chr3	−1	PTHR10404	OTHER
CLCA1	ENSG00000016490	1179	ENST00000234701	Protein_coding	CLCA1-001	Principal1	tsl1	86468368	86500259	chr1	1	PTHR10579	OTHER
ACE2	ENSG00000130234	59272	ENST00000252519	Protein_coding	ACE2-001	Principal1	tsl1	15561033	15601014	chrX	−1	PTHR10514	OTHER
CPB1	ENSG00000153002	1360	ENST00000491148	Protein_coding	CPB1-001	Principal1	tsl5	148791102	148860187	chr3	1	PTHR11705	M14

(continued)

Table 1
(continued)

Gene	Ensembl geneID	Entrez geneID	Ensembl transcriptID	Trans-cript biotype	External transcript name	Transcript appris	Transcript tsl	Transcript start	Transcript end	Chromo-some	Strand	Panther family	Family
ADAMTS19	ENSG00000145808	171019	ENST00000274487	Protein_coding	ADAMTS19-001		tsl1	129460265	129738683	chr5	1	PTHR13723	ADAMTS
CPM	ENSG00000135678	1368	ENST00000551568	Protein_coding	CPM-001	Principal1	tsl1	68851175	68933199	chr12	−1	PTHR11532	M14
CPA5	ENSG00000158525	93979	ENST00000485477	Protein_coding	CPA5-001	Principal1	tsl1	130344847	130368730	chr7	1	PTHR11705	M14
MMP26	ENSG00000167346	56547	ENST00000380390	Protein_coding	MMP26-001	Principal1	tsl5	4767270	4992429	chr11	1	PTHR10201	MMP
DPEP1	ENSG00000015413	1800	ENST00000261615	Protein_coding	DPEP1-001	Principal1	tsl1	89630289	89638456	chr16	1	PTHR10443	OTHER
STAMBP	ENSG00000124356	10617	ENST00000394070	Protein_coding	STAMBP-001	Principal1	tsl1	73829020	73867172	chr2	1	PTHR12947	OTHER
MME	ENSG00000196549	4311	ENST00000460393	Protein_coding	MME-001	Principal1	tsl1	155079647	155183708	chr3	1	PTHR11733	OTHER
TFR2	ENSG00000106327	7036	ENST00000462107	Protein_coding	TFR2-001	Principal1	tsl5	100620420	100642721	chr7	−1	PTHR10404	OTHER
ADAMTS10	ENSG00000142303	81794	ENST00000597188	Protein_coding	ADAMTS10-001	Principal1	tsl5	8580727	8610700	chr19	−1	PTHR13723	ADAMTS
TRABD2A	ENSG00000186854	129293	ENST00000335459	Protein_coding	TRABD2A-001		tsl1	84821650	84881245	chr2	−1	PTHR31120	OTHER
FOLH1	ENSG00000086205	2346	ENST00000256999	Protein_coding	FOLH1-001	Principal1	tsl1	49146635	49208670	chr11	−1	PTHR10404	OTHER

MMP21), both CGIs were examined separately. To avoid confounding results due to gain or loss of imprinted genes, those encoded in the chromosome X (*ACE2*, *PHEX*, and *XPNPEP2*) were excluded. *ADAM20*, *ADAM21*, *CPB1*, and *DPEP1* were also excluded because no CGI or probes were located within the TSS ±1.5 kb region. For every *locus*, the methylation value of the selected probes was averaged after *M*-value transformation [50] to yield a single methylation value (*see* **Note 3**).

3.7.11 HM450K Methylation Data Representation

DNA methylation is generally represented in the form of a heatmap showing the β-values in a color scale (*see* **Note 3**). There are no formal guidelines regarding the color code to represent the level of methylation. However, the current consensus is to use a blue (unmethylated) to yellow (methylated) gradient (Fig. 2). In R, heatmaps can be generated very easily and efficiently using the command heatmap.2 from the package gplots [51], providing also the option of clustering and representation of dendrograms.

As an example, we show two heatmaps summarizing the methylation information of extracellular metallopeptidase-encoding genes in normal and tumor tissues from 35 CRC patients (Fig. 2). In agreement with the general model, genes without promoter-associated CGI tend to be methylated in normal tissues and loss methylation in tumors. In contrast, genes with promoter-associated CGI are generally unmethylated in normal tissues and, in some cases, become hypermethylated in tumors. Ordering the genes according to their somatic change value, i.e., the difference in methylation between tumors and normal tissues, reveals that ADAMTS genes tend to undergo somatic hypermethylation, while MMP genes tend to undergo somatic hypomethylation. Of note, hypermethylation of ADAMTS genes did not associate with the highly methylated cancers of the right colon (which in turn associate with microsatellite instability due to hypermethylation of *hMLH1*). Therefore the observed DNA hypermethylation cannot be a consequence of the so-called CpG island methylator phenotype previously proposed [52] that we challenged [53]. Whether the observed hypermethylation reflects an inconsequential higher tendency of ADAMTS genes to become epigenetically silenced or responds to a selection pressure preceding or accompanying tumor progression remains to be elucidated. However, there is a substantial body of evidence suggesting that these genes are not merely passive actors in the tumorigenesis and tumor progression processes but important contributors to the tumor development and final phenotype [7].

4 Notes

1. Transformation efficiency can be improved by incubating the sample(s) in a thermocycler during 16 cycles of 95 °C for 30 s and 50 °C for 60 min and then holding the temperature at 4 °C. This is strongly recommended when using Illumina Infinium® Methylation arrays.
2. The original Zymo Research protocol recommends using 1–4 μL of eluted DNA for each PCR and even up to 10 μL if necessary. In our hands, however, most of the PCRs impeccably worked with a much lower amount. Hence, we routinely dilute the bisulfite-treated DNA 1:10 or even 1:20 and employ 1.5–2 μL of the diluted sample as template for PCR amplification.
3. The results generated by Illumina Methylation arrays are generally represented as β-values, i.e., a continuous value representing the proportion of methylated molecules at the studied *locus*, ranging between 0 (complete demethylation) and 1 (complete methylation). β-values are very intuitive and therefore preferred for graphical representation of methylation. However, for statistical analysis it is advisable to transform it into M-values, which are more appropriate for parametric tests than β-values due to their reduced heteroscedasticity [50]. Transformation between β- and M-values is straightforward using the following equations:

$$M = \log_2\left(\frac{\beta}{1-\beta}\right)$$

$$\beta = \frac{2^M}{1+2^M}$$

Acknowledgments

This work was supported by the Spanish Ministry of Health Plan Nacional de $I + D + I$, FEDER, FIS PI09/02444, and Plan Estatal de $I + D + I$, ISCIII, FEDER, FIS PI12/00511, and ISCIII, FEDER, FIS PI15/01763.

References

1. Kessenbrock K, Plaks V, Werb Z (2010) Matrix metalloproteinases: regulators of the tumor microenvironment. Cell 141(1):52–67
2. Noël A, Gutierrez-Fernandez A, Sounni NE et al (2012) New and paradoxical roles of matrix metalloproteinases in the tumor microenvironment. Front Pharmacol 3:140
3. Noël A, Jost M, Maquoi E (2008) Matrix metalloproteinases at cancer tumor-host interface. Semin Cell Dev Biol 19(1):52–60
4. Rawlings ND, Barrett AJ, Finn R (2016) Twenty years of the MEROPS database of proteolytic enzymes, their substrates and inhibitors. Nucleic Acids Res 44(D1):D343–D350

5. Rocks N, Paulissen G, El Hour M et al (2008) Emerging roles of ADAM and ADAMTS metalloproteinases in cancer. Biochimie 90(2): 369–379
6. Turner SL, Blair-Zajdel ME, Bunning RA (2009) ADAMs and ADAMTSs in cancer. Br J Biomed Sci 66(2):117–128
7. Cal S, Lopez-Otin C (2015) ADAMTS proteases and cancer. Matrix Biol 44-46:77–85
8. Alonso S, Gonzalez B, Ruiz-Larroya T et al (2015) Epigenetic inactivation of the extracellular matrix metallopeptidase ADAMTS19 gene and the metastatic spread in colorectal cancer. Clin Epigenetics 7:124
9. Alonso S, Dai Y, Yamashita K et al (2015) Methylation of MGMT and ADAMTS14 in normal colon mucosa: biomarkers of a field defect for cancerization preferentially targeting elder African-Americans. Oncotarget 6(5): 3420–3431
10. Jorda M, Peinado MA (2010) Methods for DNA methylation analysis and applications in colon cancer. Mutat Res 693(1–2):84–93
11. Samuelsson JK, Alonso S, Yamamoto F et al (2010) DNA fingerprinting techniques for the analysis of genetic and epigenetic alterations in colorectal cancer. Mutat Res 693(1–2):61–76
12. Harrison A, Parle-McDermott A (2011) DNA methylation: a timeline of methods and applications. Front Genet 2:74
13. Shapiro R, Servis RE, Welcher M (1970) Reactions of uracil and cytosine derivatives with sodium bisulfite. A specific deamination method. J Am Chem Soc 92:422–424
14. Hayatsu H, Wataya Y, Kazushige K (1970) The addition of sodium bisulfite to uracil and to cytosine. J Am Chem Soc 92:724–726
15. Hayatsu H, Wataya Y, Kai K et al (1970) Reaction of sodium bisulfite with uracil, cytosine, and their derivatives. Biochemistry 9:2858–2865
16. Wang RY, Gehrke CW, Ehrlich M (1980) Comparison of bisulfite modification of 5-methyldeoxycytidine and deoxycytidine residues. Nucleic Acids Res 8(20):4777–4790
17. Hayatsu H (2008) Discovery of bisulfite-mediated cytosine conversion to uracil, the key reaction for DNA methylation analysis—a personal account. Proc Jpn Acad Ser B Phys Biol Sci 84(8):321–330
18. Frommer M, McDonald LE, Millar DS et al (1992) A genomic sequencing protocol that yields a positive display of 5-methylcytosine residues in individual DNA strands. Proc Natl Acad Sci U S A 89(5):1827–1831
19. Clark SJ, Harrison J, Paul CL et al (1994) High sensitivity mapping of methylated cytosines. Nucleic Acids Res 22(15):2990–2997
20. Lister R, Ecker JR (2009) Finding the fifth base: genome-wide sequencing of cytosine methylation. Genome Res 19(6):959–966
21. Gonzalgo ML, Jones PA (1997) Rapid quantitation of methylation differences at specific sites using methylation-sensitive single nucleotide primer extension (Ms-SNuPE). Nucleic Acids Res 25(12):2529–2531
22. Herman JG, Graff JR, Myohanen S et al (1996) Methylation-specific PCR: a novel PCR assay for methylation status of CpG islands. Proc Natl Acad Sci U S A 93(18):9821–9826
23. Xiong Z, Laird PW (1997) COBRA: a sensitive and quantitative DNA methylation assay. Nucleic Acids Res 25(12):2532–2534
24. Bibikova M, Le J, Barnes B et al (2009) Genome-wide DNA methylation profiling using Infinium(R) assay. Epigenomics 1(1):177–200
25. Bibikova M, Barnes B, Tsan C et al (2011) High density DNA methylation array with single CpG site resolution. Genomics 98(4):288–295
26. Pidsley R, Zotenko E, Peters TJ et al (2016) Critical evaluation of the Illumina MethylationEPIC BeadChip microarray for whole-genome DNA methylation profiling. Genome Biol 17(1):208
27. Lister R, Pelizzola M, Dowen RH et al (2009) Human DNA methylomes at base resolution show widespread epigenomic differences. Nature 462(7271):315–322
28. Reinders J, Paszkowski J (2010) Bisulfite methylation profiling of large genomes. Epigenomics 2(2):209–220
29. Walker DL, Bhagwate AV, Baheti S et al (2015) DNA methylation profiling: comparison of genome-wide sequencing methods and the infinium human methylation 450 bead chip. Epigenomics 7(8):1287–1302
30. International Cancer Genome Consortium, Hudson TJ, Anderson W et al (2010) International network of cancer genome projects. Nature 464(7291):993–998
31. Illumina (2017) Analyzing FFPE samples with Infinium® microarrays. https://www.illumina.com/content/dam/illumina-marketing/documents/products/technotes/technote-infinium-ffpe-sample-analysis.pdf
32. Zymo Research (2017) EZ DNA Methylation™ kit. http://www.zymoresearch.com/downloads/dl/file/id/56/d5001i.pdf
33. Eads CA, Danenberg KD, Kawakami K et al (2000) MethyLight: a high-throughput assay to measure DNA methylation. Nucleic Acids Res 28(8):E32
34. Tost J, Gut IG (2007) Analysis of gene-specific DNA methylation patterns by pyrosequencing technology. Methods Mol Biol 373:89–102

35. Wani K, Aldape KD (2016) PCR techniques in characterizing DNA methylation. Methods Mol Biol 1392:177–186
36. Untergasser A, Cutcutache I, Koressaar T et al (2012) Primer3—new capabilities and interfaces. Nucleic Acids Res 40(15):e115
37. Rozen S, Skaletsky H (2000) Primer3 on the WWW for general users and for biologist programmers. Methods Mol Biol 132:365–386
38. Li LC (2007) Designing PCR primer for DNA methylation mapping. Methods Mol Biol 402:371–384
39. Roux KH (2009) Optimization and troubleshooting in PCR. Cold Spring Harb Protoc 2009(15):pdb ip66
40. Colella S, Shen L, Baggerly KA et al (2003) Sensitive and quantitative universal pyrosequencing methylation analysis of CpG sites. BioTechniques 35(1):146–150
41. Wojdacz TK, Dobrovic A (2009) Melting curve assays for DNA methylation analysis. Methods Mol Biol 507:229–240
42. Guldberg P, Worm J, Gronbaek K (2002) Profiling DNA methylation by melting analysis. Methods 27(2):121–127
43. Mallona I, Diez-Villanueva A, Peinado MA (2014) Methylation plotter: a web tool for dynamic visualization of DNA methylation data. Source code. Biol Med 9:11
44. Illumina Infinium MethylationEPIC BeadChip
45. Assenov Y, Muller F, Lutsik P et al (2014) Comprehensive analysis of DNA methylation data with RnBeads. Nat Methods 11(11): 1138–1140
46. Gentleman RC, Carey VJ, Bates DM et al (2004) Bioconductor: open software development for computational biology and bioinformatics. Genome Biol 5(10):R80
47. Core Team R (2015) R: a language and environment for statistical computing. R Foundation for Statistical Computing, Vienna
48. Yates A, Akanni W, Amode MR et al (2016) Ensembl 2016. Nucleic Acids Res 44(D1):D710–D716
49. Durinck S, Moreau Y, Kasprzyk A et al (2005) BioMart and bioconductor: a powerful link between biological databases and microarray data analysis. Bioinformatics 21(16):3439–3440
50. Du P, Zhang X, Huang CC et al (2010) Comparison of beta-value and M-value methods for quantifying methylation levels by microarray analysis. BMC Bioinformatics 11:587
51. Warnes GR, Bolker B Bonebakker L et al 2016 gplots: various R programming tools for plotting data R package version 30.1.
52. Toyota M, Ahuja N, Ohe-Toyota M et al (1999) CpG island methylator phenotype in colorectal cancer. Proc Natl Acad Sci U S A 96(15):8681–8686
53. Yamashita K, Dai T, Dai Y et al (2003) Genetics supersedes epigenetics in colon cancer phenotype. Cancer Cell 4(2):121–131

Chapter 25

Targeting Deubiquitinases in Cancer

Joseph S. Bednash and Rama K. Mallampalli

Abstract

The ubiquitin-proteasome system (UPS) is a complex and robust metabolic pathway that contributes to the regulation of many key cellular processes including the cell cycle, cell division, and response to external stimuli. Ubiquitin ligases, which tag proteins with ubiquitin, are opposed by deubiquitinase enzymes (DUBs). The relative activity of these enzymes allows for a dynamic balance that determines the abundance and activity of cellular proteins. Targeting the UPS in cancer has proven successful, as evidenced by use of bortezomib, a proteasome inhibitor, in multiple myeloma. However, no pharmacologic inhibitor of the upstream enzymes has yet to reach clinical trials for the treatment of malignancy. Here we present an in vitro DUB assay for use in drug discovery and development that provides a biologically relevant platform for screening and developing lead or tool compounds targeting DUBs.

Key words Ubiquitin, Deubiquitinase, DUB, Cancer

1 Introduction

In 2003, the FDA approved bortezomib (marketed as Velcade by Millennium Pharmaceuticals) for the treatment of multiple myeloma (MM). A hematologic malignancy, MM is characterized by clonal proliferation of B cell-derived plasma cells that produce monoclonal antibodies. Clinically, patients with MM experience bone pain, increased susceptibility to infection, anemia, renal failure, and blood hyperviscosity. Prior to bortezomib, treatment options were few; MM was a devastating, aggressive, and fatal diagnosis. Treatment with bortezomib provided a new life-prolonging therapy in patients with refractory MM [1]. Induction therapy with bortezomib proved superior to conventional therapies in achieving remissions [2]. Through inhibition of the proteolytic activity of the 26S proteasome, bortezomib targets the ubiquitin-proteasome system (UPS) to change the balance of pro- and antiapoptotic proteins in cancer [3]. Further research has led to two more FDA-approved proteasome inhibitors (carfilzomib [4, 5] and ixazomib [6]) for use in MM. In a broader sense, these proteasome inhibitors provide proof of concept for further development of pharmaceuticals targeting the UPS in cancer and other diseases.

Santiago Cal and Alvaro J. Obaya (eds.), *Proteases and Cancer: Methods and Protocols*, Methods in Molecular Biology, vol. 1731, https://doi.org/10.1007/978-1-4939-7595-2_25,

The ubiquitin-proteasome system (UPS) is a hierarchical and elaborate cellular system that impacts cell physiology by regulating the abundance of cellular proteins. Conjugation of the 76-amino acid protein, ubiquitin (Ub), onto a substrate protein directs the substrate for trafficking or degradation at the proteasome or lysosome. This process is enacted by several enzymes and enzyme complexes, including the E1, E2, and E3 Ub ligases and the deubiquitinase enzymes (DUBs). Ub monomers are covalently attached to a lysine residue within the substrate protein through the activity of the Ub ligases. Containing eight conjugation sites itself, Ub can bind to a substrate as a monomer, linear chain, or branched chain. The configuration of the ubiquitin chain marks substrate proteins for destruction, either at the proteasome or lysosome, or for intracellular trafficking [7]. For example, Ub chains linked at the lysine 48 residue (K48) are often directed to the proteasome for degradation, whereas K63-linked Ub chains sort to the endo-lysosomal pathway. Opposing the Ub ligases, DUBs remove or modify bound ubiquitin [8]. The dynamic balance between E3 ligase and DUB activity within a cell regulates key cellular activities including apoptosis, cell division, and cell signaling (Fig. 1). As such, both E3 ligases and DUBs are attractive targets for therapeutic intervention.

Emerging literature highlighting the role of DUBs in human disease and specifically cancer [9] continues to support the rationale behind their therapeutic targeting. The human genome encodes more than 90 distinct DUB enzymes grouped into five families. Four families function as cysteine isopeptidases, and members of the fifth family are metalloproteases [8]. Through DUB inhibition, certain proteins should favor degradation, allowing manipulation of cellular proteostasis, in a similar fashion to the proteasome inhibitors. As roughly 90 DUBs regulate most cellular proteins, it serves that DUBs are somewhat promiscuous in their

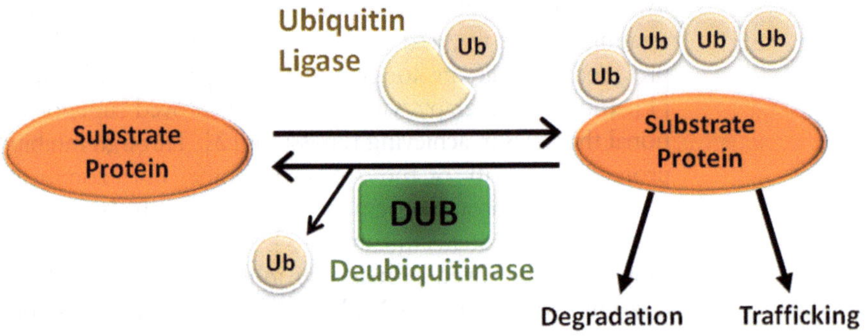

Fig. 1 Ubiquitin conjugation reversibly directs substrate protein trafficking and function. Substrate proteins are ubiquitinated by Ub ligase enzymes. The characteristics of the ubiquitin chain modification direct proteins to different cellular compartments, often for degradation. The process of ubiquitination is opposed by DUB enzymes. This dynamic balance determines protein abundance, affecting all vital cellular metabolic functions

activity but still function more specifically and discriminately than the proteasome [10]. While numerous DUB inhibitors are used in research and preclinical trials, none have advanced to clinical testing. Many of the published DUB inhibitors are poorly characterized [11]. Follow-up studies demonstrate that inhibitors lack specificity for published targets [10].

Activity-based assays are a useful tool to study DUB activity with the goal of drug discovery. Current commercially available high-throughput screening tools are less than ideal for multiple reasons: (1) these screens utilize a generic ubiquitin substrate with questionable generalizability to cell biology, (2) metalloprotease family DUBs are poorly represented, and (3) ideal buffer conditions can vary among enzymes, affecting their optimal activity. While we discuss a method for appropriate activity screening for DUB inhibitors, which is also adaptable for off-target DUB screening, this only begins the work of proper lead or tool compound development. Further characterization including biophysical testing, pharmacokinetic testing, and optimization using medicinal chemistry techniques is necessary, but beyond the scope of this work [11].

Here we present a protocol adapted from multiple published studies and methods regarding in vitro DUB assays [12–14]. This protocol provides a general framework to create a robust and adaptable assay for screening and optimization of novel compounds with proposed DUB inhibitory activity. The following protocol aims to (1) choose and/or create a biologically relevant substrate for DUB testing, (2) outline methods and troubleshooting to optimize in vitro DUB activity testing, and (3) describe methods for analysis with the goal of streamlining workflow.

2 Materials

1. DUB reaction buffer (generic): 50 mM Tris–HCl, pH 7.5, 150 mM sodium chloride, 0.25% Triton X-100, 25 mM potassium chloride, 5 mM magnesium chloride, and 0.1 mM tris(2-carboxyethyl)phosphine (TCEP).
2. DUB reaction buffer (cysteine isopeptidases): 50 mM Tris–HCl, pH 7.5, 150 mM sodium chloride, 0.25% Triton X-100, 25 mM potassium chloride, and 1 mM dithiothreitol (DTT).
3. DUB reaction buffer (metalloproteases): 50 mM Tris–HCl, pH 7.5, 150 mM sodium chloride, 0.25% Triton X-100, 25 mM potassium chloride, and 5 mM magnesium chloride.
4. K6, K11, K27, K29, K33, K48, K63, and linear di-ubiquitin chains.
5. 96-well plates.
6. Gel electrophoresis apparatus.

7. 12% SDS-PAGE gels.
8. Low molecular weight ladder.
9. 4× SDS or LDS protein sample buffer.
10. Silver stain kit.
11. Ubiquitin antibody that detects free ubiquitin chains and free ubiquitin monomers (i.e., VU-1 ubiquitin mouse monoclonal antibody from LifeSensors).
12. Dimethyl sulfoxide (DMSO).
13. Purified, recombinant DUB enzymes.
14. Denaturing buffer: 50 mM Tris–HCl, pH 7.5, 150 mM sodium chloride, 1% SDS, and 0.25% Triton X-100, supplemented with phosphatase and protease inhibitors (50 mM sodium fluoride, 2 mM sodium orthovanadate, 10 mM sodium pyrophosphate, 1 mM PMSF, and 2 μM leupeptin), including DUB-specific inhibitors (20 μM PR-619 and 5 mM *N*-ethylmaleimide).
15. Lysate dilution buffer: 50 mM Tris–HCl, pH 7.5, 150 mM sodium chloride, 0.25% Triton X-100, and 2 mM EDTA, supplemented with phosphatase and protease inhibitors (50 mM sodium fluoride, 2 mM sodium orthovanadate, 10 mM sodium pyrophosphate, 1 mM PMSF, and 2 μM leupeptin), including DUB-specific inhibitors (20 μM PR-619 and 5 mM *N*-ethylmaleimide).

3 Methods

Below we provide a protocol for the development of an in vitro DUB assay with the goal of drug discovery. As opposed to a high-throughput screen involving a generic ubiquitin-rhodamine substrate, these assays use a more biologically relevant substrate, specific to the tested DUB. The general concept presented here includes three major steps. First, characterize the proteolytic activity of a DUB for specific Ub linkages. Then, utilize the optimum Ub substrate to perform inhibitor efficacy screening and off-target screening. Finally, analyze the cleavage activity by silver staining or Western blotting in a medium-throughput assay (*see* **Note 1**).

3.1 In Vitro DUB Assay

Currently, there are >40 commercially available purified, recombinant DUB enzymes. In addition, the cDNA of all known DUBs encoded by the human genome is available. The linkage specificity and ideal enzyme concentrations for activities are known for many DUBs [10]. Prior to testing novel DUB inhibitors, it is important to first optimize reaction conditions, especially with a novel DUB. Furthermore, small differences in enzyme preparation and storage can affect results, making reaction optimization necessary in most cases. The optimization process can take several rounds of testing to determine ideal reaction conditions. While some DUBs are highly specific to a lysine linkage type at all concentrations, others become more promiscuous at higher concentrations. Furthermore, DUBs that show a preference to a Ub linkage type may also cleave other linkage types at a slower rate [10].

3.1.1 Determining Linkage Specificity of a Novel DUB (See **Note 2**, Fig. 2a)

1. Dilute the DUB or DUBs of interest to 20 μM (twice the final reaction concentrations) in DUB reaction buffer (*see* **Note 3**).
2. Also, dilute USP2 to 2 μM and/or AMSH to 20 μM in DUB reaction buffer (*see* **Note 3**).
3. Incubate at room temperature for 10 min (*see* **Note 4**).
4. Dilute an adequate volume of di-Ub chains of each linkage type (linear, K6-, K11-, K27-, K29-, K33-, K48-, and K63-linked di-ubiquitin).
5. Plate reactions in a 96-well plate.
6. Add 10 μL di-Ub mixture to 10 μL enzyme mixture to start the reactions.
7. Incubate at 37 °C.
8. Stop the reactions at appropriate time points (30 and 60 min) by removing 8 μL aliquots and immediately mixing with an equal amount of 4× protein sample buffer. As a negative control, DUB reaction buffer and di-Ub mixtures (4 μL of each) can be mixed directly into 4× sample buffer during reaction setup.
9. Resolve samples using SDS-PAGE gel electrophoresis. Recommend loading 10 μL of each sample on a 4–12% gradient Bis/Tris buffered polyacrylamide gel using a low molecular weight ladder.

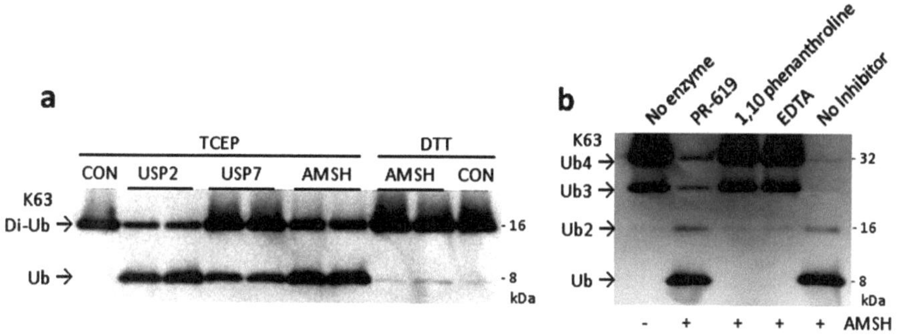

Fig. 2 DUBs break ubiquitin chains. (**a**) K63-linked di-Ub chains are cleaved by USP2, USP7, and AMSH in a DUB reaction buffer containing TCEP (0.1 mM) as the reducing agent. AMSH DUB activity is inhibited by higher concentrations of DTT (1.0 mM) in the buffer as a reducing agent. (**b**) AMSH DUB activity is inhibited by chelators of divalent cations (1,10-phenanthroline and EDTA) but retains DUB activity in the presence of cysteine isopeptidase inhibitor PR-619

10. Stain gels by silver staining according to the manufacturer's protocol or proceed to Western blotting (*see* **Note 5**).
11. Analyze results to determine need for further characterization of cleavage specificity.

In this assay, USP2 functions as a positive control and should cleave all linkage types at 2 μM. Cleavage activity in the negative control conditions (lacking DUB enzyme) indicates contamination of some reaction component or improper handling resulting in auto-deubiquitination of the di-Ub substrate. At higher DUB concentration, the enzyme may be more promiscuous compared to lower enzyme concentrations. Ideally, there is partial cleavage at the 30-min time point and complete cleavage at 60-min time points for compatible linkages. If the DUB cleaves all linkage types, a repeat assay at lower concentrations may be warranted. Alternatively, K48 and K63 linkages are the best-characterized linkages regarding biological activity. Further assay development with one of these linkage types may be appropriate.

3.1.2 Optimizing Reaction Conditions

1. Dilute the DUB of interest to 1, 2, 10, and 20 μM (twice the final reaction concentrations) in DUB reaction buffer.
2. Incubate at room temperature for 10 min.
3. Dilute di-Ub chains to 2 μM in DUB reaction buffer.
4. Add 10 μL di-Ub mixture to 10 μL enzyme mixture to start the reactions. Also, add 10 μL of di-Ub mixture to 10 μL of DUB reaction buffer as control.
5. Incubate at 37 °C for 30 and 60 min.
6. Stop the reactions at appropriate time points (30 and 60 min) by removing 8 μL aliquots and immediately mixing with an equal amount of 4× protein sample buffer. As a negative control, DUB reaction buffer and di-Ub mixtures (4 μL of each) can be mixed directly into 4× sample buffer during reaction setup.
7. Resolve samples using SDS-PAGE gel electrophoresis. Recommend loading 10 μL of each sample on a 4–12% gradient Bis/Tris buffered polyacrylamide gel using a low molecular weight ladder.
8. Stain gels by silver staining according to the manufacturer's protocol or proceed to Western blotting.

3.1.3 Screening DUB Inhibitors for Activity

1. Prepare 20× stocks of experimental inhibitors at desired concentrations (i.e., 0.2, 2, 20, and 200 μM) in DUB reaction buffer. Be sure to control for DMSO.
2. Prepare 5× stocks of control inhibitors, PR-619 (20 μM and 100 μM) and 1,10-phenanthroline (20 μM). Control for DMSO.

3. Dilute DUB of interest at ideal concentration, as determined in Subheading 3.2.1, in 10 μL DUB reaction buffer in a 96-well plate.
4. Add 1 μL of the 20× inhibitors to the DUB mixtures. Again, be sure to add DMSO to the control conditions to account for the vehicle for the inhibitors (*see* **Note 6**).
5. Incubate at room temperature for 20 min.
6. Dilute di-Ub chains to 2 μM in DUB reaction buffer.
7. Add 9 μL of di-Ub mixture to enzyme mixture with inhibitors.
8. Incubate at 37 °C for 60 min.
9. Stop the reactions at appropriate time points (30 and 60 min) by removing 8 μL aliquots and immediately mixing with an equal amount of 4× protein sample buffer. As a negative control, DUB reaction buffer and di-Ub mixtures (4 μL of each) can be mixed directly into 4× sample buffer during reaction setup.
10. Resolve samples using SDS-PAGE gel electrophoresis. Recommend loading 10 μL of each sample on a 4–12% gradient Bis/Tris buffered polyacrylamide gel using a low molecular weight ladder.
11. Stain gels by silver staining according to the manufacturer's protocol or proceed to Western blotting (Fig. 2b).

3.1.4 A Moderate-Throughput Off-Target Screen

1. Prepare DUB enzymes in triplicate in a 96-well plate. Dilute each enzyme to 2 μM in 10 μL of DUB reaction buffer. There are roughly 40 commercially available recombinant DUB enzymes that span all five families. JAMM family enzymes require a different buffer.
2. Dilute experimental inhibitor to 20× stock in DUB reaction buffer.
3. Dilute PR-619 to 100 μM (20×) and 1,10-phenanthroline to 20 μM (20×).
4. For each enzyme, add 1 μL DUB reaction buffer to the first well, 1 μL of the 20× experimental inhibitor to the second well, and 1 μL of the 20× known inhibitor to the third well (PR-619 for all cysteine isopeptidases and 1,10-phenanthroline for the metalloprotease DUBs).
5. Incubate at room temperature for 20 min.
6. Dilute di-Ub chains, specific to each enzyme, to 2 μM in DUB reaction buffer.
7. Add 9 μL of di-Ub mixture to enzyme mixture with inhibitors.
8. Incubate at 37 °C for 60 min.

9. Stop the reactions at appropriate time points (30 and 60 min) by removing 8 μL aliquots and immediately mixing with an equal amount of 4× protein sample buffer. As a negative control, DUB reaction buffer and di-Ub mixtures (4 μL of each) can be mixed directly into 4× sample buffer during reaction setup.
10. Resolve samples using SDS-PAGE gel electrophoresis. Recommend loading 10 μL of each sample on a 4–12% gradient Bis/Tris buffered polyacrylamide gel using a low molecular weight ladder.
11. Stain gels by silver staining according to the manufacturer's protocol or proceed to Western blotting.

3.2 Preparation of a Biologically Relevant Substrate

Many DUBs preferentially recognize and cleave certain ubiquitin linkages and have minimal activity against other linkage types. Others, such as USP2, cleave all ubiquitin linkages. When testing and developing novel DUB inhibitors, it follows that ubiquitin substrates should be appropriate for the DUB of interest. For example, AMSH is a DUB that cleaves only K63-linked polyubiquitin chains and has no known activity against a generic ubiquitin-rhodamine substrate. Appropriate substrates fall into two major categories. First, ubiquitin chains of varying length and linkage are commercially available for purchase. Native, untagged ubiquitin chains are detectable by Western blotting or silver staining. Others are available with a fluorescent probe that emits light after a cleavage event. Substrate preparation in this case mainly involves purchase and proper handling of the ubiquitin chains. The second option is to create a ubiquitinated substrate in a cellular system for use in the in vitro DUB assay. This allows for the demonstration of sufficiency of a certain DUB to deubiquitinate a target protein, which may be a novel association. The greater advantage to this approach lies in its obvious relevancy to cell biology, as the novel inhibitors are being tested against a known biological substrate of a given DUB. Below we describe our approach to creating a ubiquitinated substrate in a cell-based system.

1. Choose an appropriate mammalian model cell line for transfection. HEK 293 cells are useful due to their high transfection efficiency. The protein of interest will be ubiquitinated by the cell's native machinery. Depending on the protein of interest, variance in ubiquitination patterns may exist between cell lines.
2. Transfect cells with a mammalian expression vector encoding the protein of interest with a V5 tag.
3. Incubate for 24–48 h under standard conditions.

4. On the day of harvest, treat cells with MG-132 (20 μM) and leupeptin (50 μM) for 2 h to accumulate ubiquitinated proteins.
5. Wash cells with cold PBS using standard techniques.
6. Harvest in denaturing buffer.
7. Heat lysates to 95 °C for 5 min. Place back on ice for 5 min.
8. Sonicate lysates.
9. Lysates were then diluted 1:4 in lysate dilution buffer supplemented with the above mentioned phosphatase, protease, and DUB-specific inhibitors.
10. Lysates were clarified, and protein concentrations were determined.
11. Lysates were further diluted with dilution buffer to decrease the final SDS concentration to 0.1% or less.
12. Immunoprecipitation was performed by adding 1 μL of V5 antibody per 1 mg of lysate and rocking for 1 h at 4 °C. 12 μL of a 50% slurry of protein A/G resin was added per 1 mg of lysate and rocked for 1 h at 4 °C.
13. Lysates and resin were washed twice with lysate dilution buffer and then thrice with DUB reaction buffer (*see* **Note 3**).
14. Finally, resin was resuspended as a 30% slurry in reaction buffer and ready to proceed to in vitro DUB assay.
15. Add enzymes diluted in DUB reaction buffer and perform reactions as described above.
16. After stopping reactions with protein samples buffer and prior to analysis by Western blotting or silver staining, heat the samples to 95 °C to elute proteins from the beads. Load the supernatant into a gel apparatus and proceed as per above protocols for analysis.

4 Notes

1. There are commercially available di-Ub chains with fluorescent probes that can be used for higher-throughput assays to identify novel DUB inhibitors. Unfortunately, we observed that many of the inhibitors created problems with the assay, such as autofluorescence of the inhibitor. Also, the buffers suggested by the kits were not always optimal for the DUBs being tested. In some cases, fluorescent di-Ub probes are a useful tool.
2. As DUBs seem to recognize ubiquitin linkage types as opposed to specific substrate proteins, it is important to first characterize the spectrum of activity of a given DUB. Ub dimers, joined by each of the eight linkage possibilities, are commercially available

for purchase. Some DUBs preferentially cleave shorter ubiquitin chains. This preference coupled with relative ease of analysis makes di-Ub an attractive substrate for these assays.

3. In general, the cysteine isopeptidases require a reducing environment for DUB activity, whereas metalloproteases are inhibited by strong reductants. A generic buffer is presented that includes TCEP, which effectively reduces cysteine isopeptidases but does not reduce metals [15]. The subsequent incubation step at room temperature allows for reduction of the enzyme prior to initiation of the DUB assay. Alternatively, we provide buffers used successfully for reactions with only cysteine isopeptidases and another only for metalloprotease DUBs. Metalloprotease DUBs are zinc metalloproteases in the cell, but any divalent cation (Mg^{2+} in this protocol) is adequate. USP2 and AMSH controls are recommended for inclusion mainly to ensure proper buffer conditions. USP2 will cleave any Ub linkage type [10]. AMSH is K63 specific [10, 12] but is included at a metalloprotease control. Failure of USP2 or AMSH to cleave appropriate substrates likely indicates a problem with buffer composition that globally affects the assay.
4. Cysteine isopeptidases have higher activity levels in a reduced state. This benchtop incubation allows time for the reducing agents in the buffer to reduce the enzyme.
5. Western blotting is an alternative method of analysis. The ubiquitin antibody must detect ubiquitin chains of appropriate linkage types and also detect free ubiquitin.
6. The solvent that the inhibitors are dissolved in can greatly affect the enzyme kinetics. While important in all experiments, it is paramount to control for the DMSO, ethanol, or other solutions in which the inhibitors are dissolved.

References

1. Richardson PG, Barlogie B, Berenson J et al (2003) A phase 2 study of bortezomib in relapsed, refractory myeloma. N Engl J Med 348(26):2609–2617. https://doi.org/10.1056/NEJMoa030288
2. San Miguel JF, Schlag R, Khuageva NK et al (2008) Bortezomib plus melphalan and prednisone for initial treatment of multiple myeloma. N Engl J Med 359(9):906–917. https://doi.org/10.1056/NEJMoa0801479
3. Bonvini P, Zorzi E, Basso G et al (2007) Bortezomib-mediated 26S proteasome inhibition causes cell-cycle arrest and induces apoptosis in CD-30+ anaplastic large cell lymphoma. Leukemia 21(4):838–842. https://doi.org/10.1038/sj.leu.2404528
4. Jakubowiak AJ, Dytfeld D, Griffith KA et al (2012) A phase 1/2 study of carfilzomib in combination with lenalidomide and low-dose dexamethasone as a frontline treatment for multiple myeloma. Blood 120(9):1801–1809. https://doi.org/10.1182/blood-2012-04-422683
5. Siegel DS, Martin T, Wang M et al (2012) A phase 2 study of single-agent carfilzomib (PX-171-003-A1) in patients with relapsed and refractory multiple myeloma. Blood 120(14):2817–2825. https://doi.org/10.1182/blood-2012-05-425934
6. Kumar SK, Berdeja JG, Niesvizky R et al (2014) Safety and tolerability of ixazomib, an oral proteasome inhibitor, in combination with lenalidomide and dexamethasone in patients with previously untreated multiple

myeloma: an open-label phase 1/2 study. Lancet Oncol 15(13):1503–1512. https://doi.org/10.1016/S1470-2045(14)71125-8
7. Ciechanover A (2005) Proteolysis: from the lysosome to ubiquitin and the proteasome. Nat Rev Mol Cell Biol 6(1):79–87. https://doi.org/10.1038/nrm1552
8. Komander D, Clague MJ, Urbe S (2009) Breaking the chains: structure and function of the deubiquitinases. Nat Rev Mol Cell Biol 10(8):550–563. https://doi.org/10.1038/nrm2731
9. Weathington NM, Sznajder JI, Mallampalli RK (2013) The emerging role of the ubiquitin proteasome in pulmonary biology and disease. Am J Respir Crit Care Med 188(5):530–537. https://doi.org/10.1164/rccm.201304-0754PP
10. Ritorto MS, Ewan R, Perez-Oliva AB et al (2014) Screening of DUB activity and specificity by MALDI-TOF mass spectrometry. Nat Commun 5:4763. https://doi.org/10.1038/ncomms5763
11. Ndubaku C, Tsui V (2015) Inhibiting the deubiquitinating enzymes (DUBs). J Med Chem 58(4):1581–1595. https://doi.org/10.1021/jm501061a
12. McCullough J, Clague MJ, Urbe S (2004) AMSH is an endosome-associated ubiquitin isopeptidase. J Cell Biol 166(4):487–492. https://doi.org/10.1083/jcb.200401141
13. Hospenthal MK, Mevissen TE, Komander D (2015) Deubiquitinase-based analysis of ubiquitin chain architecture using ubiquitin chain restriction (UbiCRest). Nat Protoc 10(2):349–361. https://doi.org/10.1038/nprot.2015.018
14. Strayhorn WD, Wadzinski BE (2002) A novel in vitro assay for deubiquitination of I kappa B alpha. Arch Biochem Biophys 400(1):76–84. https://doi.org/10.1006/abbi.2002.2760
15. Getz EB, Xiao M, Chakrabarty T et al (1999) A comparison between the sulfhydryl reductants tris(2-carboxyethyl)phosphine and dithiothreitol for use in protein biochemistry. Anal Biochem 273(1):73–80. https://doi.org/10.1006/abio.1999.4203

Chapter 26

Generation of Highly Selective MMP Antibody Inhibitors

Dong Hyun Nam and Xin Ge

Abstract

Inhibiting individual MMPs of biomedical importance with high selectivity is critical for both fundamental research and therapy development. Here we describe the methods for discovery of inhibitory monoclonal antibodies from synthetic human antibody phage display libraries carrying convex paratopes encoded by long complementarity-determining region (CDR)-H3 segments. We demonstrate the application of this technique for isolation of highly specific and potent antibody inhibitors of human MMP-14.

Key words Inhibitory antibody, Long CDR, Synthetic library, Convex paratope

1 Introduction

Inhibition of MMPs using zinc-chelating compounds (e.g., hydroxamates) has been extensively studied as a therapeutic strategy to treat cancer [1]. Although preclinical results were encouraging, all these small-molecule inhibitors toward broad-spectrum MMPs failed in clinical trials due to severe side effects such as musculoskeletal pain and inflammation caused by the poor selectivity [2, 3]. It is now known that metalloproteinases play more complex and paradoxical roles in tumor progression beyond simple ECM degradation [4]. While many facets of proteolytic action are pro-tumorigenic, some metalloproteinases indeed exhibit tumor-suppressing effects in certain circumstances [5]. For example, MMP-8 favors host defense instead of stimulating tumor proliferation, suggesting its protective role in cancer processes [6]. In addition, metalloproteinases exert different roles at different steps of cancer progression, e.g., the opposing roles of MMP-9 at different microenvironments [7]. For these reasons, selectively blocking individual tumorigenesis-promoting metalloproteinase(s) at appropriate timeframe is highly desired for a successful therapy.

However, achieving target specificity and selectivity in small-molecule MMP inhibitors is remarkably challenging [8, 9]. Because the catalytic mechanism and catalytic domain fold are

Santiago Cal and Alvaro J. Obaya (eds.), *Proteases and Cancer: Methods and Protocols*, Methods in Molecular Biology, vol. 1731, https://doi.org/10.1007/978-1-4939-7595-2_26, © Springer Science+Business Media, LLC 2018

conserved among the MMP/ADAM/ADAMTS superfamily members, the available small-molecule inhibitors target multiple proteinases, resulting in off-target side effects [2, 3, 9, 10]. In this respect, antibody-based metalloproteinase inhibitors are emerging as both research tools and potential therapeutic agents [11–16] because of (a) high affinity and high specificity due to the large antigen-antibody interaction areas provided by multiple complementarity-determining regions (CDRs), (b) long half-life and the well-known mechanisms of antibody action, (c) low immunogenicity and low toxicity, and (d) multiple MMPs potentially targetable by antibodies [17].

Natural protease inhibitors exhibit a convex-shaped conformation that inserts into the enzyme active site and blocks the substrate access and/or catalytic function [18]. However, there is a low probability of generating antibodies with the convex antigen-binding sites (paratopes) from naive or immunized human or murine antibody libraries. The proteolytic pocket is often buried inside a major cleft or concave enzyme structure, and, as such, it is normally inaccessible by the cave-like, grooved, or flat antigen-binding surface in human and murine antibodies [19]. In contrast, dromedary antibodies are enriched in the long CDR-H3s encoding the extended convex-shaped paratopes, and, intriguingly, a large proportion of antibodies isolated from camels and llamas, compared with human and murine antibodies, bind the active-site pockets and inhibit enzymatic reactions [20–22]. However, the camelid antibodies would evoke an immune response in humans, and the availability of these animals is limited.

Here we describe the design and construction of human Fab libraries in which the long, convex-shaped, camelid-like paratopes are incorporated into the human antibody scaffold [23, 24] (Fig. 1). We demonstrate the application of these libraries to screen for inhibitors of MMP-14, a proinvasive and prometastatic human proteinase [25, 26], by phage panning. As results of screen, a panel of selective Fabs with a high inhibitory potency against MMP-14 was isolated. The methods described here should be generally applicable to other MMPs and proteases of biomedical importance.

2 Materials

2.1 Library Construction

2.1.1 Long CDR-H3 Assembly

1. Oligonucleotides (Table 1, Integrated DNA Technologies).
2. T4 DNA polymerase and dNTP mix.
3. T4 DNA ligase and buffer.
4. 10× annealing buffer: 10 mM Tris–HCl, pH 8.0, 500 mM NaCl, 10 mM EDTA.
5. TAE buffer: 40 mM Tris–acetate, 1.0 mM EDTA, pH 8.0.

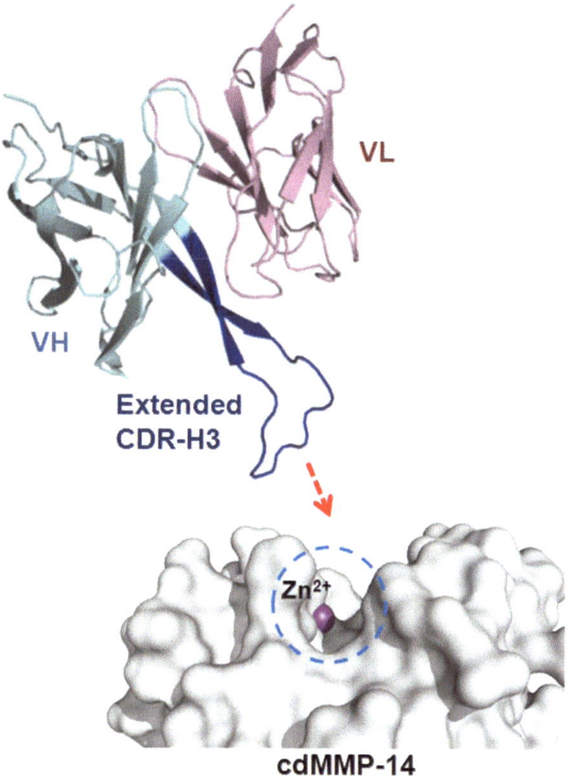

Fig. 1 Scheme that convex antibody paratope formed by an extended CDR-H3 mediates enzyme inhibition (reprinted from ref. 24)

Table 1
List of oligonucleotides for long CDR-H3 assembly

Name	Oligonucleotide sequences
VH1	Ggccgtttcactataagcgcagacacatccaaaaacacagcctacctgcagatgaacagc
VH2_23	P-ccgtgtattattgcgcgcgt(XYZ)$_{18}$(TAT)(GBN)atggactactggggtcaggg
VH2_25	P-ccgtgtattattgcgcgcgt(NNS)$_{20}$(TAT)(GBN)atggactactggggtcaggg
VH2_27	P-ccgtgtattattgcgcgcgt(NNS)$_{22}$(TAT)(GBN)atggactactggggtcaggg
VH3	P-acgcgcgcaataatacacggcagtgtcctcagctcttaagctgttcatctgcaggtaggc
VH4	Tggatgaccgaagcttgccgaggagacggtgaccagggttccctgaccccagtagtccat

Notes: (1) Overlapping regions are underlined with annealing temperatures of ~58 °C. (2) VH2 and VH3 are 5′-phosphorylated. (3) For CDR-H3 with 23 aa, XYZ codons were used, which contain unequal nucleotide ratios at each position of the codon triplet (*X* = 38% G, 19% A, 26% T, and 17% C; *Y* = 31% G, 34% A, 17% T, and 18% C; and *Z* = 24% G and 76% C). For CDR-H3 with 25 or 27 aa, NNS codon was used.

6. TAE/agarose gel: TAE buffer, 1.0% (w/v) agarose, 1:5000 (v/v) 10% ethidium bromide.
7. DNA Clean & Concentrator-5 kit (Zymo Research).

2.1.2 Preparation of Electrocompetent E. coli

1. *E. coli* XL-Blue.
2. *E. coli* Jude-I (DH10B F′[proAB lacI^Q lacZ ΔM15 Tn10(Tet^R)]) [27].
3. LB/Tet agar: LB (BD Difco), 1.5 g/L agar, 10 μg/mL tetracycline.
4. SOB/Tet: SOB (BD Difco), 10 μg/mL tetracycline.

2.1.3 In-Frame Selection of CDR-H3 Fragments

1. Plasmid pVH-bla [28].
2. Restriction enzymes AflII and HindIII with buffers.
3. Plasmid DNA miniprep kit.
4. DNA gel extraction kit (Zymo Research).
5. 0.2 mm gap electroporation cuvettes.
6. 2×YT/Amp/IPTG agar: 2×YT (BD Difco), 1.5 g/L agar, 50 μg/mL ampicillin, 0.5 mM isopropyl β-D-1-thiogalactopyranoside (IPTG).
7. 2×YT/Chlor: 2×YT, 34 μg/mL chloramphenicol.
8. 245 mm square bioassay dishes (Corning).
9. 80% glycerol, autoclaved.
10. Cell scrapper.

2.1.4 Cloning Functional CDR-H3 into Fab Phagemids

1. Plasmid pFab-pIII [29].
2. Fab phage F library [29].
3. Restriction enzyme BsmBI with buffer.
4. 2×YT/Amp: 2×YT, 100 μg/mL ampicillin.
5. 2×YT/Amp agar: 2×YT, 1.5 g/L agar, 100 μg/mL ampicillin.

2.2 Isolation of MMP-14-Specific Fab Clones by Phage Panning

2.2.1 Preparation of Fab Phage Libraries

1. 250 mL autoclavable polypropylene centrifuge bottles (*see* **Note 1**).
2. 2 L culture flasks (*see* **Note 1**).
3. M13KO7 helper phage (New England Biolabs).
4. 35 mg/mL kanamycin stock.
5. 5× PEG/NaCl: 20% PEG-8000 (w/v), 2.5 M NaCl.
6. Phage resuspension buffer: 50 mM Tris–HCl, pH 7.5, 150 mM NaCl, 5 mM $CaCl_2$, 0.1 mM $ZnCl_2$.
7. 0.22 μm sterile syringe filters.

2.2.2 Phage Panning on Immobilized MMP-14

1. Human MMP-14 catalytic domain [30, 31] (also *see* Chapter 7).
2. Human TIMP-2 N-terminal domain (n-TIMP2) [32].
3. Phosphate-buffered saline (PBS): 137 mM NaCl, 3 mM KCl, 8 mM Na_2HPO_4, 1.5 mM KH_2PO_4. Adjust pH to 7.2 with HCl and autoclave.
4. Streptavidin, 1 mg/mL (New England Biolabs).
5. Maxisorp 96-well immunoplates (Nunc).
6. Assay buffer: 50 mM Tris–HCl, pH 7.5, 150 mM NaCl, 5 mM $CaCl_2$, 0.1 mM $ZnCl_2$.
7. Blocking buffer: assay buffer, 0.5% (w/v) gelatin from porcine skin. Incubate on 45 °C in water bath with occasional shaking until completely dissolved.
8. Washing buffer: assay buffer, 0.05% (v/v) Tween 20.
9. 100 mM trimethylamine.

2.2.3 Monoclonal Phage ELISA

1. 2×YT/Amp/KO7: 2×YT, 100 μg/mL ampicillin, 10^{10} phage/mL of M13KO7.
2. Polystyrene 96-well round-bottom microplates.
3. Horseradish peroxidase/anti-M13 antibody conjugate (GE health).
4. TMB (3,3′,5,5′-tetramethylbenzidine) ELISA substrate solution (Pierce).

2.3 Antibody Characterizations

2.3.1 Fab Cloning, Expression, and Purification

1. Ni-NTA resin (Qiagen).
2. Restriction enzymes BglII and SalI-HF with buffers.
3. Ultrafiltration centrifugal units, 10 K MWCO (Millipore).
4. 15% SDS-PAGE gels.

2.3.2 Binding Affinity Measurements and Selectivity Tests

1. Catalytic domains of human MMP-2 [30, 31] and MMP-9 (*see* Chapter 7).
2. Goat anti-human IgG (Fab specific) peroxidase (Sigma-Adrich).

2.3.3 Inhibition Potency Measurement and Inhibition Mode Determination

1. Peptide M-2359: Mca-Lys-Pro-Leu-Gly-Leu-Dap(Dnp)-Ala-Arg-NH_2 (Bachem).
2. Black flat-bottom polystyrene NBS 96-well microplate (Corning).
3. 20% dimethyl sulfoxide (DMSO).

3 Methods

3.1 Library Construction

The construction of Fab library incorporated with long CDR-H3 segments consists of four steps (Fig. 2): **step 1**, oligonucleotide hybridization; **step 2**, synthesis of long CDR-H3 fragments; **step**

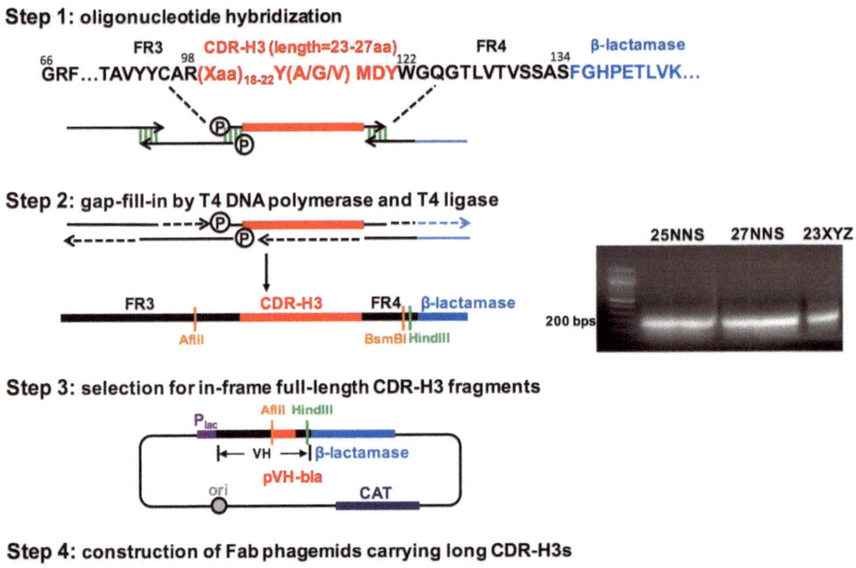

Fig. 2 Construction of synthetic antibody libraries with long CDR-H3s. (Step 1) Hybridization of degenerate oligonucleotides (Table 1) encoding long CDR-H3s with 23, 25, and 27 aa. (Step 2) CDR-H3 fragment assembly by T4 DNA polymerase and T4 DNA ligase. (Step 3) Assembled long CDR-H3 genes were subjected for full-length in-frame selection by fusing with β-lactamase (pVH-bla). (Step 4) Cloning the in-frame CDR-H3s into an existing Fab library to construct synthetic antibody library carrying long CDR-H3s with 23, 25, and 27 aa

3, selection of in-frame and full-length CDR-H3 fragments by cloning to the N-terminal of β-lactamase to remove truncated and reading frame shifted segments introduced by degenerated codons or mismatched assembly; and **step 4**, cloning of functional CDR-H3 fragments into Fab library phagemids.

3.1.1 Long CDR-H3 Assembly

1. Dissolve oligonucleotides (Table 1) with double-distilled water (DDW) to be 100 μM.
2. For oligo annealing, in PCR tubes add 84.5 μL DDW, 10 μL of 10× annealing buffer, 1.5 μL (150 pmol) VH1, 1.5 μL VH3, 1.5 μL VH4, and 1 μL (100 pmol) VH2_23 or VH2_25 or VH2_27 for different CDR-H3 length, respectively (*see* **Note 2**).
3. Place the tubes in a thermal cycler for annealing reaction: 95 °C 2 min; cooling from 95 to 25 °C over a period of 45 min; and holding at 4 °C. After reaction, briefly spin the tubes and store on ice or 4 °C until use.
4. For gap fill-in reaction, to 30 μL DDW add 50 μL annealed oligonucleotides, 5 μL 10 mM dNTP mixture, 10 μL T4 DNA ligase buffer, 2.5 μL (1000 units) T4 DNA ligase, and 2.5 μL (7.5 units) T4 DNA polymerase into PCR tubes.

5. Place the tubes in a thermal cycler for gap fill-in reaction: 37 °C 1 h; 75 °C 25 min to inactivate enzymes; holding at 4 °C until use.
6. Purify assembled DNA samples by electrophorese using 1% TAE/agarose gel with ethidium bromide for DNA visualization (typical results shown as Fig. 2 inset). Cut the target bands and recover the DNAs. These fragments are now ready for cloning into in-frame selection vector described in Subheading 3.1.3.

3.1.2 Preparation of Electrocompetent *E. coli*

1. Streak Jude-I or XL1-Blue stock on LB/Tet agar plates to grow fresh colonies overnight at 37 °C.
2. Seed a single colony in 5 mL SOB/Tet and grow overnight at 37 °C with shaking at 250 rpm.
3. Inoculate 2.5 mL overnight culture to 250 mL pre-warmed SOB/Tet and culture at 37 °C with shaking at 250 rpm until OD_{600} reaches to 0.8–1.0 (typically 2–3 h for Jude-I and 3–4 h for XL-1Blue).
4. Incubate the culture flasks on ice for 30 min.
5. Collect cells by centrifugation at 8500 × *g* at 4 °C for 5 min using two autoclaved prechilled 250 mL centrifuge bottles, and decant the supernatants.
6. Add 5 mL autoclaved cold DDW to each centrifuge bottle, and slowly shake the bottles in their standing position at 90 rpm 4 °C until cells are fully resuspended. Add 125 mL DDW to each bottle and slowly rotate to mix.
7. Centrifuge the cells at 8500 × *g* 4 °C for 5 min and decant supernatant.
8. Repeat **steps 5–7** twice to completely remove culture medium. Reduce DDW usages to 125 mL (62.5 mL each bottle) and 25 mL (12.5 mL each bottle) in the second and third washes.
9. Suspend cells in 1 mL DDW by shaking at 90 rpm 4 °C. Competent cells are ready for electroporation (Subheadings 3.1.3 and 3.1.4) and should be used in the same day to avoid loss of competency (*see* **Note 3**).

3.1.3 In-Frame Selection of CDR-H3 Fragments

1. Prepare 2×YT/agar with 50 μg/mL ampicillin and 0.5 mM IPTG (*see* **Note 4**).
2. Digest 15 μg plasmid pVH-bla and 1.5 μg assembled CDR-H3 fragments with AflII and HindIII, and gel purify the 4.8 kb and ~220 bp fragments, respectively.
3. Ligate 5 μg digested pVH-bla with 0.5 μg digested CDR-H3 fragments (at a molar ratio of vector to insert = 1:2) at room temperature for 6 h using T4 DNA ligase.

4. Desalt ligation product using DNA Clean & Concentrator-5 kit. Typically, 3 μg ligased DNA in 100 μL is obtained.
5. Mix 1.0 mL prepared electrocompetent cells with 3 μg desalted ligation product, and incubate on ice for 2 min.
6. Place ten 0.2 mm gap electroporation cuvettes on ice, and transfer 100 μL cell-DNA mixture to each cuvette (*see* **Note 5**).
7. Electroporate using MicroPulser (Bio-Rad) with voltage set at 2.5 kV (*see* **Note 6**).
8. Immediately add 1 mL SOB to cuvette, and mix with electroporated cells by gentle pipetting. Transfer the liquid to a 50 mL conical tube. Wash the cuvette with 1 mL SOB twice. Collect all electroporated cells.
9. Repeat electroporations for all cuvettes. Culture collected cells (~30 mL) at 37 °C for 1 h with shaking at 250 rpm.
10. Spread cultured cells on ten square dishes of 2×YT/Amp/IPTG agar. Allow the moisture completely adsorbed then incubate at 30 °C overnight. Save 30 μL transformed cell culture for library size determination by tittering (*see* **Note 7**).
11. In the following day, collect cells from the dishes with cell scrappers. Suspend library cells in 20% glycerol for storage at −80 °C.
12. When necessary, repeat **steps 2–11** until achieving desired library size.
13. To prepare pVH-bla library carrying in-frame long CDR-H3s, inoculate appropriate OD of library cells (>10-fold coverage of diversity) in LB/Amp and culture at 37 °C for 6 h. Extract plasmid DNA by miniprep.

3.1.4 Cloning Functional CDR-H3 into Fab Phagemids

1. Add >5 × 10^{10} phage particles of F library [29] to 200 mL exponentially growing *E. coli* XL1-Blue (OD_{600} = 0.4–0.5) in 2×YT/Tet (*see* **Note 8**).
2. Incubate 20 min at 37 °C without shaking.
3. Add ampicillin to be 100 μg/mL. Culture at 37 °C for 5–6 h with shaking at 250 rpm.
4. Extract F library plasmids pFab-pIII from 20 mL cell culture by miniprep (Fig. 3).
5. Digest 15 μg prepared F library pFab-pIII and 40 μg in-frame selected pVH-bla with AflII and BsmBI. Gel purify the 4.9 kb and 129–141 bp bands, respectively (*see* **Note 9**).
6. Ligate 5 μg purified pFab-pIII fragments with 0.5 μg prepared long CDR-H3 segments (at a molar ratio of vector to insert = 1:2) with T4 DNA ligase at room temperature for 6 h.

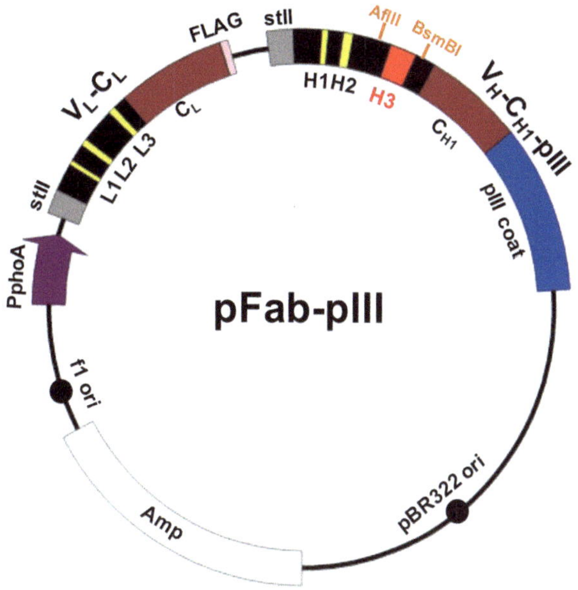

Fig. 3 Fab display phagemid pFab-pIII. A PhoA promoter drives bi-cistronic transcription encoding light chain (VL-CL) and variable and first constant domains of heavy chain (VH-CH1) fused with coat protein III (pIII). The stII signal peptides mediate secretion expression. Long CDR-H3 segments (red) are cloned between AflII and BsmBI cutting sites

7. Desalt ligated mixture using DNA Clean & Concentrator-5 kit.
8. Transform 3 μg ligated DNA to 1.0 mL freshly prepared XL1-Blue component cells by electroporation as details described in Subheading 3.1.3. Incubate the cells at 37 °C for 1 h.
9. Spread the culture on ten 245 mm square dishes of 2×YT/Amp agar and incubate at 30 °C overnight. Save 30 μL transformed cell culture for library size determination by tittering and quality check by DNA sequencing (*see* **Note 7**).
10. In the following day, scrape the cells from the dishes. Suspend library cells in 20% glycerol for storage at −80 °C.
11. If necessary, repeat **steps 5–10** until desired library size and quality are achieved.

3.2 Selection of Specific Fab Clones by Phage Panning

3.2.1 Preparation of Fab Phage Libraries

1. Inoculate 30 OD cells carrying constructed long CDR-H3 Fab library to 600 mL 2×YT/Amp (*see* **Note 10**).
2. Culture at 37 °C with shaking at 250 rpm to OD_{600} of 0.4–0.5 (approximately, 1.5–2.0 h) (*see* **Note 11**).
3. Add helper phages at a ratio of phages to bacterial cells = 10–20:1.

4. Incubate at 37 °C without shaking for 30 min for phage infection.
5. Add kanamycin to a final concentration of 35 μg/mL, and culture overnight at 30 °C with shaking (250 rpm) to produce Fab library phages.
6. Chill the culture on ice for 20 min. Clarify the media by centrifugation of *E. coli* cells at 4000 × *g* at 4 °C for 15 min, and transfer supernatant to a 2 L container (*see* **Note 12**).
7. Add cold PEG/NaCl solution as one-fifth volume of the supernatant. Incubate on ice for 1 h to precipitate phage particles.
8. Centrifuge at 10,000 × *g* 4 °C for 15 min to collect phages. White pellets should be seen. Discard supernatant and aspirate remaining liquid. Resuspend the phage pellets in 45 mL assay buffer (*see* **Note 13**).
9. Centrifuge the phage solution at 10,000 × *g* at 4 °C for 15 min to remove bacterial contaminants. Transfer the supernatant to a new tube.
10. Add cold PEG/NaCl solution (one-fifth volume of phage solution) to precipitate the phage. Incubate at 4 °C for 5 min. The solution should appear clouding.
11. Centrifuge at 10,000 × *g* at 4 °C for 15 min. Decant supernatant and aspirate remaining liquid (*see* **Note 14**).
12. Resuspend phage pellets with assay buffer in a volume that is 1/50 of the original culture volume. Filtrate the phage solution through 0.22 μm filters.
13. Estimate phage concentration spectrophotometrically (1 OD at 268 nm is equivalent to ~5 × 10^{12} phage/mL) [33]. This purified phage libraries can be used immediately for selection (Subheading 3.2.2), and the remaining phage can be stored at −80 °C in 15% glycerol. Use 20 μL purified phages for tittering measurement (*see* **Note 15**).

3.2.2 Selection of Fab Phage Clones on Immobilized cdMMP-14

In this protocol, cdMMP-14 is immobilized via biotinylation and streptavidin-coated plates. And nTIMP-2, a natural protein inhibitor of MMP-14, is exploited as the eluent. Because nTIMP-2 binds to the active site of native MMP-14 [18], this strategy results in enrichment of epitope-specific antibodies possessing inhibition function.

1. Coat immunoplate wells with 100 μL streptavidin solution (5 μg/mL in PBS buffer) for 2 h at room temperature or overnight at 4 °C. The number of wells required depends on library size (*see* **Note 16**).

2. Remove coating solution. Rinse with washing buffer twice. Block the wells with 250 μL blocking buffer (0.5% gelatin) for 2 h (*see* **Note 17**).
3. Remove blocking solution. Wash twice. Add 100 μL biotinylated cdMMP-14 (2 μg/mL in assay buffer) to each well and incubate for 20 min at room temperature.
4. Remove cdMMP-14 solution. Wash twice.
5. To deplete streptavidin binders, add 100 μL phage solution (containing 10^{12}–10^{13} Fab library phages in blocking buffer) to streptavidin-coated wells and incubate for 1 h at room temperature with shaking at 700 rpm.
6. After depletion, transfer phage supernatant to the wells coated with cdMMP-14. Incubate at room temperature for 1 h with shaking at 700 rpm.
7. Remove the phage solution and wash ten times with washing buffer and five times with assay buffer (*see* **Note 18**).
8. Add 100 μL 6 μM nTIMP-2 each well. Incubate for 1 h at room temperature for elution of phages carrying epitope-specific Fab clones.
9. To further elute all bound phages, add 100 μL 100 mM triethylamine per well and incubate for 5 min at room temperature (*see* **Note 19**).
10. Add 50 μL 1 M Tris–HCl (pH 8.0) per well for neutralization.
11. Incubate eluted phages with ten volumes of exponentially growing *E. coli* XL1-Blue (OD_{600} = 0.4–0.5 cultured in 2×YT/Tet) for 30 min at 37 °C without shaking for infection. Titrate input and output phages by serials dilutions.
12. Centrifuge cultured cells at 4500 × *g* at 4 °C for 15 min. Decant supernatant and resuspend with 1–2 mL 2×YT/Amp depending on the titers of output phages. Plate on LB/Amp agar, and incubate at 30 °C overnight.
13. The following day, scrape cells from the plates. Suspend cells in 20% glycerol for storage at −80 °C.
14. For the sequential rounds of panning, prepare phage antibody libraries as described in Subheading 3.2.1. Culture volume can be decreased to 50–100 mL depending on the titers of output phages.
15. Repeat the selection, **steps 1–13**, for total three or four rounds. Washing stringency can be increased to 20 times with washing buffer and five times with assay buffer. Selection pressure can also be given by reducing cdMMP-14 usage (to 1 μg/mL).

3.2.3 Monoclonal Phage ELISA

After multiple rounds of panning, individual Fab clones can be tested for cdMMP-14 binding by monoclonal phage ELISA.

1. Randomly pick colonies from agar plates using sterile pipette tips. Inoculate them to 96-well round-bottom microplates containing 200 μL 2×YT/Amp. Culture overnight at 30 °C with shaking at 250 rpm. These plates serve as the master plates (*see* **Note 20**).
2. In the next day, inoculate 96-well round-bottom microplates containing 200 μL 2×YT/Amp/KO7 with 2 μL overnight culture from the master plates for monoclonal phage production. Add glycerol to the master plates (20% final concentration) for storage at −80 °C.
3. Coat ELISA plates with either cdMMP-14 or blocking reagent only (negative control), as described in Subheading 3.2.2. Add 25 μL blocking buffer each well.
4. Centrifuge the phage culture plates at 4000 × *g* for 15 min. Transfer 25 μL supernatants to the prepared ELISA plates. Incubate at room temperature for 1 h.
5. Wash three times with washing buffer. Add 50 μL per well 1:5000 HRP-anti-M13 conjugate in blocking buffer. Incubate at room temperature for 30 min.
6. Wash plates four times with washing buffer and once with assay buffer. Add 50 μL per well of freshly prepared TMB solution. Allow signal development for 5–10 min.
7. Stop the reaction with 25 μL 2 M H_2SO_4. Read absorbance at 450 nm using a microplate reader.
8. Determine the specific bindings by comparing signals on cdMMP-14 over signals on blocking reagents (*see* **Note 21**).

3.3 Antibody Characterizations

3.3.1 Fab Cloning, Expression, and Purification

1. Inoculate the positive clones isolated in Subheading 3.2.3 from the master plates to 5 mL LB/Amp. Culture overnight at 37 °C with shaking at 250 rpm.
2. Extract the Fab display plasmids by miniprep. By applying standard molecular biology protocols, clone the VL-CL-VH fragments into the Fab expression plasmid [33] with BglII and SalI cutting sites.
3. Transform cloned Fab expression vectors into BL21(DE3) electrocompetent cells (Subheadings 3.1.2 and 3.1.3).
4. For Fab production, culture transformed cells in 500 mL 2×YT/Amp overnight at 30 °C.
5. Harvest cells by centrifugation and prepare periplasmic fraction by osmotic shock treatment [34].
6. Purify Fabs from periplasmic preparation [34] using Ni-NTA resin.
7. Verify the quality of purified Fabs using 15% SDS-PAGE gels.

3.3.2 Binding Affinity Measurements by ELISA

1. Coat 96-well microplates with biotinylated cdMMP-14, and block the plates with 0.5% gelatin as details described in Subheading 3.2.2.
2. Starting with 1 μM, twofold serially dilute purified Fabs with blocking buffer in cdMMP-14-coated wells. Incubate at room temperature for 1 h.
3. Discard Fab solutions and wash three times.
4. Incubate 50 μL 1/5000 goat anti-human IgG (Fab specific) HRP conjugate in blocking solution at room temperature for 1 h.
5. Decant the second antibody solution. Wash four times with washing buffer and one time with assay buffer.
6. Incubate with 50 μL/well TMB solution for 5–10 min. Add 25 μL 2 M H_2SO_4 solution to stop the reaction.
7. Measure absorbance at 450 nm using a microplate reader. Calculate affinity constant from a four-parameter, logistic, curve-fitting analysis to evaluate EC_{50} values of Fabs (a typical result shown in Fig. 4a).

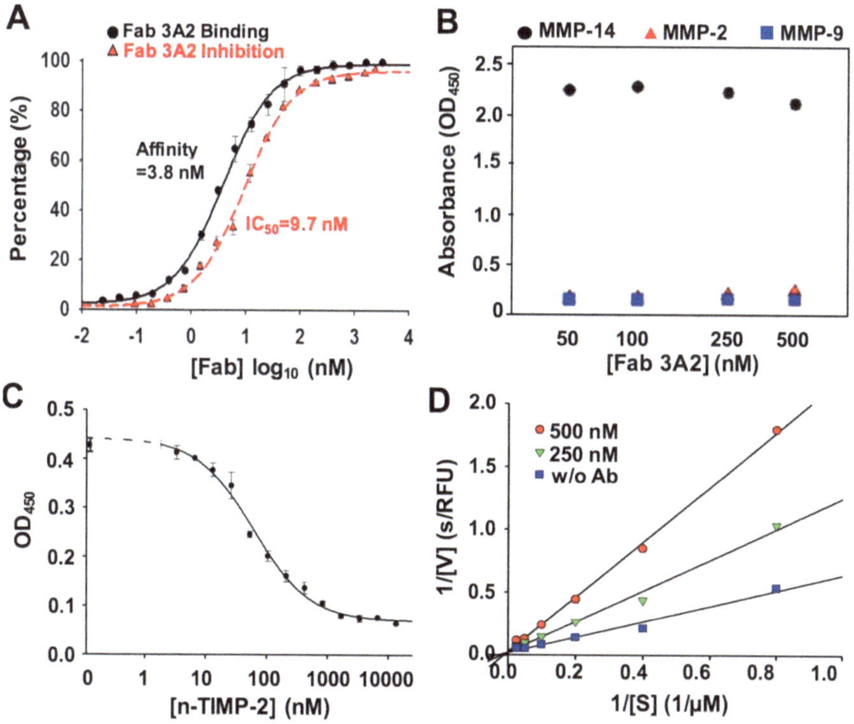

Fig. 4 Typical results of MMP inhibitory Fab characterizations (reprinted from ref. 24). (**a**) Binding affinity and inhibition potency measured by ELISA and FRET assays. (**b**) Selectivity tests. (**c**) Competitive ELISA with n-TIMP-2. (**d**) Determination of mode of inhibition

3.3.3 Selectivity Tests by Competitive ELISA

1. Coat 96-well microplates with biotinylated cdMMP-14, and block the plates with 0.5% gelatin as details described in Subheading 3.2.2.
2. Starting at 3 μM, twofold serially dilute purified cdMMP-2, cdMMP-9, and cdMMP-14 in the cdMMP-14-coated wells.
3. Incubate MMP solutions with Fabs of interest at their EC_{50} concentrations (measured in Subheading 3.3.2) at room temperature for 2 h.
4. Add antibody/antigen mixtures to 96-well microplate coated with biotinylated cdMMP-14. Incubate at room temperature for 15 min.
5. Develop the signals and measure the absorbance described in **steps 3–7** of Subheading 3.3.2. Typical results are shown in Fig. 4b.
6. Similarly, competitive ELISA with 4 nM to 10 μM nTIMP-2 can be performed. Typical results are shown in Fig. 4c.

3.3.4 Inhibition Potency Measurement by FRET Assays

1. Prepare 2 nM cdMMP-14 in assay buffer and 100 μM peptide M-2359 in 20% DMSO.
2. Starting at 10 μM, twofold serially dilute Fabs in 96-well black microplate.
3. Aliquot 25 μL 2 nM cdMMP-14 solution into each well containing 25 μL Fab solutions. Incubate the mixtures for 30 min to form antibody/antigen complex.
4. Add 1 μL peptide M-2359 solution to each well to start the reaction.
5. Monitor hydrolysis of the fluorogenic peptide with excitation at 328 nm and emission at 393 nm. Fluorescence is recorded continuously for 30 min, and the initial reaction rates are measured. Inhibition constants can be calculated by fitting the data to equation below, where V_i is the initial velocity in the presence of inhibitor, V_0 is the initial velocity in the absence of inhibitor, and $[I]$ is the inhibitor concentration. Typical results are shown in Fig. 4a.

$$\frac{V_i}{V_o}\% = \frac{1}{1+\frac{[I]}{IC_{50}}}\times 100.$$

6. Similarly, monitor hydrolysis reaction with 10 nM cdMMP-14, 0–40 μM M-2359, and fixed concentrations of Fab which show 35–70% inhibition. Determine kinetic parameters K_m and V_{max} by fitting to Lineweaver-Burk equation. Typical results are shown in Fig. 4d.

4 Notes

1. To avoid cross-contamination, keep a dedicated set of centrifuge bottles, culture flasks, and pipettes for phage experiments. Clean used bottles and flasks with 10% bleach solution. Discard used pipette tips directly to bleach solution.
2. Initial trails of annealing and gap fill-in reaction with equimolar of oligoes resulted in a smear band observed on DNA gels. Because oligoes VH1, VH3, and VH4 (60 mers) were not PAGE purified, truncated products were present due to DNA synthesis coupling efficiency. By increasing their usages to be 1.5 times of VH2 (PAGE-purified 94–106 mers) and reducing the reaction volume to 100 μL, clear assembled fragments were obtained.
3. To validate the competency, mix 100 μL (~20 OD) prepared electrocompetent cells with 300 ng plasmid DNA. Electroporate as details described in Subheading 3.1.3. 5×10^8 or more transformants indicate an acceptable competency for library construction.
4. The ampicillin and IPTG concentrations should be optimized [28].
5. To construct large libraries, enough amounts of cells, e.g., >200 OD, are needed. Each 0.2 mm gap electroporation cuvette can hold approximately 100 μL (~20 OD cells) and 300 ng ligated DNA.
6. The time of electroporation should read at 4.8–5.6 ms as indicator of a good transformation.
7. Serially dilute and culture on 2×YT/Amp/IPTG agar and 2×YT/chlor agar to determine library size and to observe selection effects. In the following day, count colony numbers on titration plates. Randomly pick a few colonies from 2×YT/Amp/IPTG agar and inoculate in 5 mL 2×YT/chlor for growth at 37 °C overnight. Extract plasmids for DNA sequencing to assess the quality of constructed library.
8. The design diversity of all other CDRs on the F library (approximately 2×10^8) should be covered >100-folds by enough number of phages.
9. Because the optimal temperature for BsmBI (55 °C) is different from AflII (37 °C), sequential digestion is needed.
10. For library preparation, the inoculum should be at least tenfold covering the library diversity, and the starting OD_{600} should be 0.05 or less.
11. Culturing at 37 °C improves phage infection efficiency likely by promoting F pilus expression. And overgrowth ($OD_{600} > 0.5$) will result in a lower infection rate.

12. Pelleted cells may appear sticky due to the toxicity of phage production and Fab expression to the *E. coli* host cells. It is recommended to use serological pipettes to collect the supernatant after centrifugation. Trace amounts of cells can be removed during phage purification steps.
13. To maintain MMPs in their native conformation, 0.1 mM Zn^{2+} and 5 mM Ca^{2+} present in assay buffer.
14. To remove the residue PEG/NaCl completely, we recommend to wash phage pellets by briefly rinsing with assay buffer and quickly decanting it. Because of excess number of phages prepared, the loss during wash does not affect panning results.
15. To decide the number of input phage for phage panning, it is necessary to estimate the phage concentration quickly using a spectrophotometer. Based on numerous tests, it is found that when OD_{268} is less than 0.5, the UV method agrees well with the titration results.
16. The phage concentration should not exceed 10^{13} phage/mL, and the total number of phage should exceed the library diversity by 1000-fold. It is also recommended to coat extra wells for polyclonal ELISA to track the progress of phage panning.
17. The blocking agent should be compatible with the antigen of interest. Common choice includes BSA, gelatin, skim milk, and ChemoBlocker. For biotinylated antigens, skim milk should not be used due to the presence of excessive biotin.
18. Washing in the first round of selection is relatively mild (generally ten times). As the copy numbers of positive clones increase after initial selection, in the sequential rounds of panning, more stringent washing conditions can be applied. To reduce nonspecific bindings, washing with a weak acidic buffer, e.g., pH 5.0 adjusted by citric acid, can also be considered [35].
19. Incubation longer than 10 min may reduce phage infectivity.
20. To avoid evaporation, 96-well culture plates can be placed in a closed box far away from the circulating fan. Place damp paper towel in the box.
21. In general, >5-fold signal increases are considered as positive.

References

1. Lee M, Fridman R, Mobashery S (2004) Extracellular proteases as targets for treatment of cancer metastasis. Chem Soc Rev 33(7): 401–409
2. Turk B (2006) Targeting proteases: Successes, failures and future prospects. Nat Rev Drug Discov 5(9):785–799
3. Zucker S, Cao J (2009) Selective matrix metalloproteinase (MMP) inhibitors in cancer therapy: Ready for prime time? Cancer Biol Ther 8(24):2371–2373
4. Kessenbrock K, Plaks V, Werb Z (2010) Matrix metalloproteinases: regulators of the tumor microenvironment. Cell 141(1):52–67

5. Overall CM, Kleifeld O (2006) Tumour microenvironment - opinion: Validating matrix metalloproteinases as drug targets and anti-targets for cancer therapy. Nat Rev Cancer 6(3):227–239
6. Decock J, Thirkettle S, Wagstaff L et al (2011) Matrix metalloproteinases: Protective roles in cancer. J Cell Mol Med 15(6):1254–1265
7. Egeblad M, Werb Z (2002) New functions for the matrix metalloproteinases in cancer progression. Nat Rev Cancer 2(3):161–174
8. Overall CM, López-Otín C (2002) Strategies for MMP inhibition in cancer: Innovations for the post-trial era. Nat Rev Cancer 2(9): 657–672
9. Cathcart J, Pulkoski-Gross A, Cao J (2015) Targeting matrix metalloproteinases in cancer: Bringing new life to old ideas. Genes Dis 2(1):26–34
10. Deu E, Verdoes M, Bogyo M (2012) New approaches for dissecting protease functions to improve probe development and drug discovery. Nat Struct Mol Biol 19(1):9–16
11. Devy L, Huang L, Naa L et al (2009) Selective inhibition of matrix metalloproteinase-14 blocks tumor growth, invasion, and angiogenesis. Cancer Res 69(4):1517–1526
12. Sela-Passwell N, Kikkeri R, Dym O et al (2011) Antibodies targeting the catalytic zinc complex of activated matrix metalloproteinases show therapeutic potential. Nat Med 18(1):143–147
13. Naito S, Takahashi T, Onoda J et al (2012) Development of a neutralizing antibody specific for the active form of matrix metalloproteinase-13. Biochemistry 51(44):8877–8884
14. Ager EI, Kozin SV, Kirkpatrick ND et al (2015) Blockade of MMP14 activity in murine breast carcinomas: implications for macrophages, vessels, and radiotherapy. J Natl Cancer Inst 107(4). https://doi.org/10.1093/jnci/djv017
15. Botkjaer KA, Kwok HF, Terp MG et al (2016) Development of a specific affinity-matured exosite inhibitor to MT1-MMP that efficiently inhibits tumor cell invasion in vitro and metastasis in vivo. Oncotarget 7(13):16773–16792
16. Sandborn WJ, Bhandari BR, Fogel R et al (2016) Randomised clinical trial: A phase 1, dose-ranging study of the anti-matrix metalloproteinase-9 monoclonal antibody GS-5745 versus placebo for ulcerative colitis. Aliment Pharmacol Ther 44(2):157–169
17. Drag M, Salvesen GS (2010) Emerging principles in protease-based drug discovery. Nat Rev Drug Discov 9(9):690–701
18. Fernandez-Catalan C, Bode W, Huber R et al (1998) Crystal structure of the complex formed by the membrane type 1-matrix metalloproteinase with the tissue inhibitor of metalloproteinases-2, the soluble progelatinase A receptor. EMBO J 17(17):5238–5248
19. Lauwereys M, Ghahroudi MA, Desmyter A et al (1998) Potent enzyme inhibitors derived from dromedary heavy chain antibodies. EMBO J 17(13):3512–3520
20. De Genst E, Silence K, Decanniere K et al (2006) Molecular basis for the preferential cleft recognition by dromedary heavy-chain antibodies. Proc Natl Acad Sci U S A 103(12): 4586–4591
21. Desmyter A, Transue TR, Ghahroudi MA et al (1996) Crystal structure of a camel single-domain V-H antibody fragment in complex with lysozyme. Nat Struct Biol 3(9):803–811
22. Schmitz KR, Bagchi A, Roovers RC et al (2013) Structural evaluation of EGFR inhibition mechanisms for nanobodies/VHH domains. Structure 21(7):1214–1224
23. Hoogenboom HR (2005) Selecting and screening recombinant antibody libraries. Nat Biotechnol 23(9):1105–1116
24. Nam DH, Rodriguez C, Remacle A et al (2016) Active-site Selective Protease inhibitors Discovered from Convex Paratope Synthetic Libraries. Proc Natl Acad Sci U S A 113(52): 14970–14975
25. Genís L, Gálvez BG, Gonzalo P et al (2006) MT1-MMP: Universal or particular player in angiogenesis? Cancer Metastasis Rev 25(1): 77–86
26. Morrison CJ, Butler GS, Rodríguez D et al (2009) Matrix metalloproteinase proteomics: Substrates, targets, and therapy. Curr Opin Cell Biol 21(5):645–653
27. Masip L, Klein-Marcuschamer D, Quan S et al (2008) Laboratory evolution of Escherichia coli thioredoxin for enhanced catalysis of protein oxidation in the periplasm reveals a phylogenetically conserved substrate specificity determinant. J Biol Chem 283(2):840–848
28. Ge X, Mazor Y, Hunicke-Smith SP et al (2010) Rapid Construction and Characterization of Synthetic Antibody Libraries Without DNA Amplification. Biotechnol Bioeng 106(3): 347–357
29. Persson H, Ye W, Wernimont A et al (2013) CDR-H3 diversity is not required for antigen recognition by synthetic antibodies. J Mol Biol 425(4):803–811
30. Koo HM, Kim JH, Hwang IK et al (2002) Refolding of the catalytic and hinge domains of human MT1-mMP expressed in Escherichia coli and its characterization. Mol Cells 13(1): 118–124

31. Nam DH, Ge X (2016) Direct production of functional matrix metalloproteinase--14 without refolding or activation and its application for in vitro inhibition assays. Biotechnol Bioeng 113(4):717–723
32. Lee KB, Nam DH, Nuhn JA et al (2017) Direct expression of active human tissue inhibitors of metalloproteinases by periplasmic secretion in Escherichia coli. Microb Cell Factories 16:73
33. Fellouse FA, Sidhu SS (2013) Making antibodies in bacteria. In: Kaser MR, Howard GC (eds) Making and Using Antibodies. CRC Press, Boca Raton, pp 151–172
34. Goldman ER, Hayhurst A, Lingerfelt BM et al (2003) 2,4,6-Trinitrotoluene detection using recombinant antibodies. J Environ Monit 5(3):380–383
35. Tur MK, Huhn M, Sasse S et al (2001) Selection of scFv phages on intact cells under low pH conditions leads to a significant loss of insert-free phages. BioTechniques 30: 404–413

Chapter 27

Strategies to Target Matrix Metalloproteinases as Therapeutic Approach in Cancer

Zoi Piperigkou, Dimitra Manou, Konstantina Karamanou, and Achilleas D. Theocharis

Abstract

Matrix metalloproteinases (MMPs) are a family of zinc-dependent endopeptidases that are capable of degrading numerous extracellular matrix (ECM) components thus participating in physiological and pathological processes. Apart from the remodeling of ECM, they affect cell-cell and cell-matrix interactions and are implicated in the development and progression of various diseases such as cancer. Numerous studies have demonstrated that MMPs evoke epithelial to mesenchymal transition (EMT) of cancer cells and affect their signaling, adhesion, migration and invasion to promote cancer cell aggressiveness. Various studies have suggested MMPs as suitable targets for treatment of malignancies, and several MMP inhibitors (MMPIs) have been developed. Although initial trials have failed to establish MMPIs as anticancer agents due to lack of specificity and side effects, new MMPIs have been developed with improved action that are currently being investigated. Furthermore, novel strategies that target MMPs for improving drug delivery and regulating their activity in tumors are presented. This review summarizes the implication of MMPs in cancer progression and discusses the advancements in their targeting.

Key words Therapeutic approach, MMP, Cancer, Clinical trial

1 Introduction

Cancer can be characterized as a complex disease and one of the most devastating public health problems worldwide [1]. Cancer progression requires the multistage process of metastasis, which can be distinguished into three main stages: withdrawal of cancer cells from the primary tumor, intravasation in the bloodstream and extravasation of tumor cells at distant sites. These processes require cell-cell and cell-matrix interactions as well as paracrine interactions between tumor and neighboring stromal cells [2, 3]. The initiating step for cancer cells to acquire migratory potential is the epithelial to mesenchymal transition (EMT), which refers to the reprogramming occurring to genetically and epigenetically modified cells [4–6]. During EMT, tumor cells lose cell junctions,

Santiago Cal and Alvaro J. Obaya (eds.), *Proteases and Cancer: Methods and Protocols*, Methods in Molecular Biology, vol. 1731, https://doi.org/10.1007/978-1-4939-7595-2_27, © Springer Science+Business Media, LLC 2018

undergo alterations in their morphology and obtain actin-rich extended protrusions. In addition, significant changes can be observed in gene expression of signaling and matrix components, including transcriptional activation of extracellular matrix (ECM)-degrading enzymes [7, 8]. Several biomarkers have been proposed as EMT indicators, such as the "E-cadherin switch" which is characterized by the downregulation of E-cadherin and other epithelial markers and upregulation of N-cadherin, vimentin, as well as other mesenchymal markers. Furthermore, EMT occurs in association with activation of several growth factor receptor cascades, alterations in the expression levels of miRNAs, and EMT-related transcription factors. Moreover, during EMT, the regulation of transcriptional machinery results in modified biosynthesis of a variety of intracellular proteins, cell surface receptors such as integrins, and matrix-degrading enzymes as matrix metalloproteinases (MMPs) [4, 5]. Importantly, E-cadherin has been proposed as a direct target for MMP-dependent shedding suggesting a direct role for MMPs in disassembly of cell junctions [9]. The establishment of distant metastases is facilitated by the reverse phenomenon of EMT, which is called MET (mesenchymal-to-epithelial transition) in which tumor cells regain their epithelial morphology, a process that helps them to survive and settle in the secondary site [10].

ECMs play a pivotal supportive and regulatory role as they act as physical barriers for the cells and enable the interplay between them, influencing many cellular properties, such as proliferation, survival, migration, and differentiation. ECMs are composed of distinct structural and functional macromolecules such as proteoglycans (PGs), glycosaminoglycans (GAGs), collagens, fibronectin, elastin, laminins, and several (glyco)proteins [11–14]. EMT and tumor microenvironment are interdependent, since tumor and surrounding cells (immune, stromal, and endothelial cells) interact with ECMs, rearrange their components, and facilitate tumor cells to acquire a mesenchymal phenotype [15]. Irregular ECM remodeling during tumorigenesis is in line with alterations observed in the expression and/or activation of ECM-degrading enzymes, such as MMPs, a disintegrin and metalloproteinases family (ADAMs), ADAMs with thrombospondin motifs (ADAMTs) and the components of plasminogen activation system [12, 16].

There is mounting evidence supporting the view that MMPs are among the principal mediators of ECM and tumor microenvironment, participating in the multistep processes of EMT and cancer progression; therefore, they have been considered as potential diagnostic and therapeutic biomarkers of several types of cancer [17]. MMPs are calcium-dependent zinc-containing endopeptidases and the main proteinases, which are responsible for the alterations taking place in the ECM, as they cleave the majority of ECM components [17–20]. The family of mammalian MMPs consists of

24 members that can be divided depending on their structural domain architecture, substrate recognition, and cellular localization. Concerning the latter feature, MMPs can be categorized into two groups: secreted and membrane-bound MMPs. According to their general structure and substrate specificity, MMPs can be divided into six groups: collagenases, gelatinases, membrane type, stromelysins, matrilysins, and other MMPs [21–24] (Fig. 1). MMPs are synthesized as inactive pro-forms and stepwise activation is required for the active enzymes [22]. Endogenous inhibitors called tissue inhibitors of MMPs (TIMPs) control MMP activities as their N-terminal site interacts with the catalytic site of MMPs and their C-terminal site facilitates the activation of pro-forms of MMP-2 and MMP-9 [21]. The interactions between TIMPs and MMPs can regulate the extent of proteolytic degradation of ECM components [21, 25]. In addition to the role of MMPs in ECM remodeling, MMPs can regulate crucial cellular processes such as proliferation, invasion, apoptosis, adhesion, tumor angiogenesis, immune surveillance, autophagy, differentiation and EMT [17, 26].

2 MMPs as Diverse Effectors in Cancer

The ability of cancer cells to degrade the basement membrane has been correlated with the metastatic potential of several cancers. There is mounting evidence supporting that MMPs are the principal regulators of matrix interactions with the surrounding cells, during carcinogenesis [16]. These matrix-degrading enzymes orchestrate various cellular processes involving cell-cell and cell-ECM interactions, which help cancer cells to achieve critical landmarks of cancer development, such as proliferation, migration, adhesion, invasion, angiogenesis and apoptosis [27, 28]. Overexpression of MMPs and TIMPs has been correlated with cancer cell aggressiveness and poor patient prognosis [29, 30]. Indeed, high expression levels of MMP-9 and MMP-2 in serum are correlated with poor prognosis for breast cancer patients [31]. MMPs regulate the bioavailability of several growth factors such as insulin-like growth factor (IGF) that are sequestered in the peritumor ECM, thus promoting tumor growth and cancer cell proliferation [32, 33]. Studies have indicated that many epidermal growth factor receptor (EGFR) ligands, such as heparin-binding epidermal growth factor-like growth factor (HB-EGF) and transforming growth factor α (TGF-α), are proteolytically shed by the cell surface from proteases like MMP-3, MMP-7, ADAM10, ADAM12, or ADAM17 [34, 35]. Moreover, syndecan-1 shedding is mainly caused by MMP-7 and MMP-9, and the subsequent soluble syndecan-1 can bind to growth factors such as HB-EGF and thus activate EGFR and downstream signaling pathways,

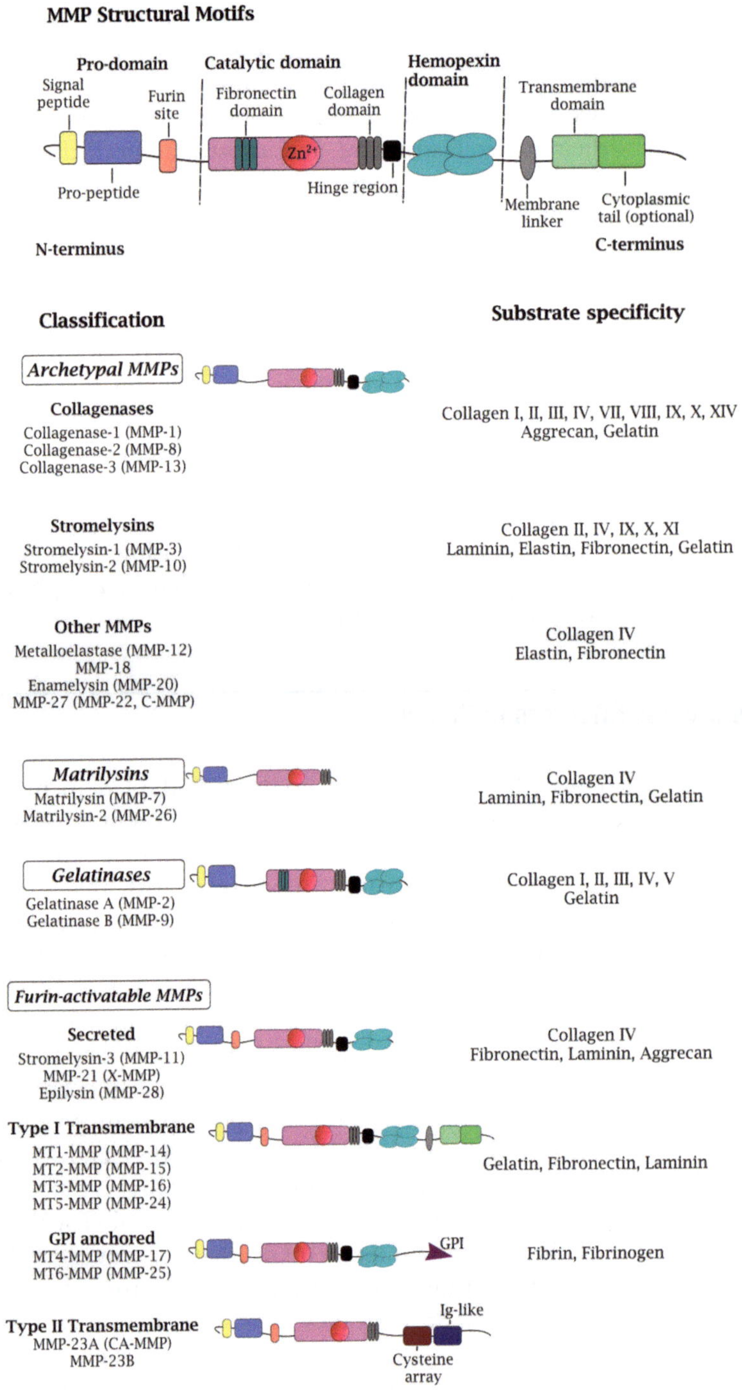

Fig. 1 Schematic representation of the generic structure of mammalian MMPs. Depending on their domain arrangement, the 24 MMP members are classified into four main categories (archetypal, matrilysins, gelatinases, and furin-activated MMPs). Their typical structure consists of a signal peptide, a pro-peptide, a catalytic domain, a hinge region and a hemopexin domain. Archetypal MMPs are subdivided into collagenases, stromelysins, and other MMPs, depending on their substrate specificity. Matrilysins lack of the hemopexin-like domain, whereas gelatinases have the characteristic fibronectin domain in their catalytic site. Furin-activated MMPs contain a furin-cleavage site following the pro-peptide and they are consisted of type I and II membrane-bound, secreted and GPI-anchored MMPs

promoting cancer progression [36, 37]. MMPs may also exert apoptotic or anti-apoptotic actions. For instance, MT1-MMP specifically interacts with TIMP-2 and activates Akt signaling cascade protecting cancer cells from apoptosis [38]. MMP-7 brings anti-apoptotic and chemoresistance signals to cancer cells by cleaving the ligand of the death receptor Fas [39, 40]. Moreover, MMPs exert significant influence in the growth of metastatic tumor cells and increase the motility of epithelial cells by regulating the dynamic cell-cell and cell-ECM interactions during these processes. It is worth noticing that ADAM10, MMP-1, and MMP-7 proteolytically shed the ectodomain of E-cadherin. The soluble E-cadherin inhibits the formation of cell aggregates, thus promoting EMT and increasing the migratory and invasive potential of breast cancer cells [41, 42].

Radisky et al. suggested that MMPs are implicated in EMT and tumor progression via three mechanisms: (a) increased MMP levels in the tumor microenvironment can directly promote EMT in epithelial cells, (b) tumor cells undergoing EMT can synthesize more MMPs in order to initiate the invasion and metastasis processes and (c) EMT can affect peritumoral cells that participate in tumor progression to further produce MMPs [22]. Specifically, the induction of EMT in many cancer cells resulted in activation of MMPs. For example, Shh-induced EMT resulted in MMP-9 activation in gastric cancer [43], with the same result found in EGFR [44]- and KLF8 [45]-induced EMT in squamous and breast cancer, respectively. Additionally, Wnt1-induced EMT is associated with MMP-3 activation and this inhibition resulted in repression of EMT characteristics [46], while in hepatocellular cancer cells, MT1-MMP and MMP-2 are upregulated by discoidin domain-containing receptor 2 (DDR2) through Erk2/Snail1 axis, leading to elevated invasion and metastasis [47]. Moreover, in pancreatic cancer, CD44 triggered EMT via activation of Snail which can regulate MT1-MMP expression [48]. Furthermore, suppression of estrogen receptor alpha (ERα) in MCF-7 breast cancer cells induced cell aggressiveness and EMT with a concomitant induction of the expression levels of many MMPs [49]. In contrast, a remarkable decrease in the expression of MMPs is observed in MDA-MB-231 breast cancer cells upon suppression of ERβ that is associated with reduction of the aggressiveness of breast cancer cells [50]. Moreover, in a mammary tumor model, transforming growth factor β (TGF-β) was found to promote the phosphorylation of the cap-binding protein eIF4E inducing EMT via the translation of Snail and MMP-3 mRNAs [51], whereas silencing of this translation initiation factor is associated with decreased EMT characteristics and MMP-9 and MMP-3 enzymatic activity [52]. Several studies have demonstrated the interplay of the small leucine-rich PG, lumican with MMPs in cancer progression [53–55]. Lumican modulates MT1-MMP activity in vitro and in vivo [53–55], evokes EMT/MET reprogramming affecting breast cancer cell aggressiveness and induces major changes in MMP expression levels, depending on the ER status of breast cancer cells [56]. MMP-dependent EMT activation has been found in many cancer cell types including the kidney, ovary, lens, lung, prostate, and breast [22, 26, 57, 58]. Important observation is the role of stromal-MMP-3 in breast cancer, where MMP-3-induced EMT was due to the expression of the alternative splice isoform of Rac1b leading to the production of reactive oxygen species (ROS) that in turn triggered the stimulation of NF-kB/Snail axis [57, 59]. Recent data also revealed the correlation between MMPs and EMT in oral squamous cancer cells. MT1-MMP-induced EMT upregulated Twist and ZEB and decreased the transcription of E-cadherin [60], while in another study the silencing of MMP-13 resulted in a less aggressive phenotype, with the opposite be found by its overexpression [61]. Vinnakota et al. found that M2-like macrophages can promote colon cancer cell invasion via MMPs [62], while Johansson et al. reported that cancer-associated fibroblasts (CAFs) can stimulate cetuximab resistance in head and neck squamous carcinoma cells via induction of MMPs [63]. CAFs via the secretion of MMP-9 can also induce EMT in prostate carcinoma cells [64], while CAF-originated MMP-13 can stimulate tumor angiogenesis through vascular endothelial growth factor (VEGF), thus resulting in increased invasion of melanoma and squamous cell carcinoma in vitro [65]. Vosseler et al. revealed the necessity of MMP production by both cancer and cancer-associated cells for the promotion of skin squamous cell carcinoma [66]. Taking under consideration the above data, MMPs are key mediators for EMT process and tumor progression; therefore, it is plausible to be considered as desirable biomarkers for pharmacological targeting in several types and stages of cancer. Because of these significant roles of MMPs in different steps of cancer progression, a growing number of MMP inhibitor programs have been initiated and evaluated in clinical trials for the selective targeting of cancer cells.

3 Regulation of MMPs

3.1 Transcriptional Regulation

The clarification of the molecular mechanisms through MMPs act may contribute to specific targeting of cancer cells with less recrudescence of patients [67]. A new approach for targeting MMPs is the activation of the transcription factor 3 (ATF3), which is known for the reduction of the migratory potential of glioblastoma cells through the direct regulation of the expression of MMPs. Overexpression of ATF3 is correlated with reduced expression and activation of MMP-2, MMP-7, and MMP-9 and decreased migration, while on the contrary knockdown of ATF3 is linked to increased migratory properties and low survival rates in several types of cancer [68–70]. MMP-14 (MT1-MMP) exhibits important anti-migratory properties in tumorigenic keratinocytes, through the downstream regulation of other MMP activities, as well as the activation of intracellular signaling pathways [71]. Since the transcription factor Snail is a great inducer of EMT in melanoma via suppression of E-cadherin gene expression, the association of MMP-14 with Snail-induced EMT in melanoma cells was clearly documented [55, 72, 73]. Cathcart et al. reported that the tumor suppressor protein p53 reduced the activity of MMP-14, while the silencing of the p53 expression deprived this effect in colon cancer cells. In addition to this, the pro-inflammatory cytokine interleukin 6 (IL-6) found to have synergistic effect in this novel regulatory mechanism of MMP-14. IL-6 enhanced p53 proteasomal degradation and simultaneously promoted the MMP-14-induced invasion and metastasis, resulting in increased invasive phenotype [74]. Most of the research work conducted regarding the transcriptional mechanism of action of MMPs is focused on the gelatinases, MMP-2 and MMP-9 [75]. On the other hand, several reports investigate the relationship between urokinase-type plasminogen activator (uPA) and MMP-9 in different types of malignancies. It is reported that uPA is highly expressed in several types of cancer, such as lung and ovarian. Increased levels of uPA along with plasminogen activator inhibitor 1 (PAI-1) can also be detected during metastasis and are indicators of low patient survival. The role of uPA, besides binding to the cell surface uPA receptor (uPAR) and, respectively, transforming plasminogen into plasmin, is also to activate the MMPs. The synergistic effect between uPA and MMP-9 was recently reported and proved to drive cancer cell aggressiveness and invasion [76–78]. At the same time, the expression of the epithelial marker E-cadherin was elevated, reversely to the expression of MMP-9, whereas the mesenchymal markers, vimentin and Snail, were decreased. Moreover, uPA and MMP-9 were suppressed with siRNA in breast cancer models, in order to evaluate the effects in tumor progression. The effective silencing of these two key molecules resulted in differentiated migratory, invasive and adhesive properties of breast cancer cells [79]. It is clear that inhibition of MMP-9 and its upstream regulatory pathways is crucial for cancer therapy. MMP-9 expression can be triggered by many key molecules, such as growth factors, like epidermal growth factor (EGF) or fibroblast growth factor 2 (FGF-2), and cytokines, like tumor necrosis factor α (TNF-α) and TPA (12-O-tetradecanoylphorbol-13-acetate), which is known for the activation of protein kinase C (PKC), which, respectively, is involved in the synthesis and secretion of MMP-9 [80–82]. During treatment with TPA, MMP-9 is expressed because of transcriptional alterations, such as the activation of NF-κB, which is a potent regulator of MMP-9 transcription [83, 84]. In a recent study, the molecular mechanism underlying the TPA-mediated functional properties and MMP-9 expression in low-invasive MCF-7 breast cancer cells was investigated. Specifically, an ethanol extract from *Peucedanum japonicum* Thunb. proved its inhibitory effect on the expression and activity of MMP-9 in combination with reduced nuclear translocation and transcriptional activation of NF-κB, mediated by TPA [85].

3.2 Proenzyme Activation

The structural basis for MMP activation is their synthesis as proenzymes or zymogens. During the transcriptional process, the synthesized peptide is removed from this form and consequently generates the proMMP. ProMMPs remain initially inactive because of the interaction of the cysteine residue of the PRCGXPD motif with the Zn^{2+} of the catalytic domain [86]. The activation of MMPs in extracellular level can be achieved with the contribution of other MMPs or other proteases. MMP-13 may be autoactivated by self-proteolysis and in turn can activate proMMP-9. MMP-9 is also capable of activating several MMPs such as proMMP-2 and proMMP-13. MMP-3 is responsible for rendering active several proMMPs, and specifically, Suzuki and his collaborators reported the transformation of proMMP-1 to the completely active MMP-1 form by MMP-3 [87, 88]. MMP-14 is also involved in the activation of MMP-8 and MMP-13 in vitro, as well as MMP-2, thus contributing in a proteolytic cascade where several MMPs can activate each other [89]. MMP-2 follows a revolutionary pattern of activation. It can be activated by MT-MMPs on a pericellular level, with the exception of MT4-MMP and MT2-MMP. Critical players in the activation of proMMP2 are MT1-MMP and TIMP2. They create a ternary complex from the binding positions of C-terminal sites, and consequently the "free" N-terminal inhibitory domain of TIMP2 binds pericellularly to the MT1-MMP. The next step is that an adjacent, uninhibited by TIMP2, MT1-MMP will cleave and activate the proMMP-2. After the interaction of proMMP-2 with the TIMP2, which is bound to MT1-MMP, proMMP-2 is ready to reintegrate to the cell surface [90]. Another scenario presented by Itoh and his research group is that TIMP2 renders MT1-MMP, after inhibition, as a receptor for proMMP-2, and this suggests that TIMP2 is a critical regulator of MT1-MMP [91]. Finally, intracellular activation is reported to occur because of the selective cleavage of endopeptidase furin, and several MMPs, like MMP-11, MMP-MMP-23 and MMP-28, favor this activation mode [92, 93].

4 Insights into Novel Therapeutic Approaches

It is well established that the enzymatic activity of MMPs in ECM remodeling plays a crucial role in cancer progression and upregulated MMP expression has been correlated with poor prognosis in several cancer types. Therefore, the development of novel agents that could effectively target MMPs is always in the efforts of pharmaceutical industry and cancer research. Significant points for targeting MMPs include their biosynthesis, secretion, activation and enzymatic activity. Several MMP inhibitors (MMPIs), natural or synthetic, designed to bind in the catalytic domain, made their way to clinical trials. Among the synthetic agents that target MMPs, the synthetic peptidomimetic and non-peptidomimetic inhibitors and the chemically modified tetracycline derivatives are included. Next-generation MMPIs are comprised of specific microRNAs, which block MMP transcription and monoclonal antibodies as catalytic domain inhibitors (Table 1).

4.1 Endogenous Inhibitors

The enzymatic activity of MMPs can be blocked by α-macroglobulin, a glycoprotein which can be found abundantly in human blood and fluids and has the role of a general proteinase inhibitor. TIMPs play a critical role in the ECM remodeling, as they regulate the activity of MMPs more specifically [23]. TIMPs are the natural blocking molecules of activated proteases; thus, they are nontoxic and non-immunogenic. These endogenous-secreted proteins inhibit all MMPs, while each TIMP targets more than one MMP. However, it is reported that TIMPs could trigger fundamental cellular processes in a MMP-independent manner. Modifications on the balanced interactions of MMPs and TIMPs may result in dysregulation of vascular diseases and in cancer progression [96, 97]. Although TIMP-1 is a broad-spectrum MMP inhibitor, studies have shown that its overexpression is associated with rapid cancer progression and poor patient prognosis [98–100]. TIMP-2 is secreted from cancer cells and together with MT1-MMP, it activates MMP-2, which are both crucial for cancer cell migration. Importantly, the N-terminal domain of TIMP2 (N-TIMP-2) exhibits high affinity for various MMPs [101]. A novel, combined, computational/directed evolution approach used to engineer protein-based inhibitors developed a mutant of N-TIMP-2 that was identified as the strongest MT1-MMP inhibitor investigated so far. This variant demonstrated improved affinity and specificity for MT1-MMP as compared to the wild-type N-TIMP-2, and it significantly inhibited the invasive potential in an in vitro breast cancer cell model [102]. In addition, reversion-inducing cysteine-rich protein with Kazal motifs (RECK) is a cell surface MMP inhibitor that regulates ECM integrity and

Table 1
MMP inhibitors in clinical trials

MMPIs	Type of drug/ source	Enzymes inhibited	Indication
Batimastat (BB-94)	Peptidomimetic (hydroxamate)	Broad spectrum (higher specificity: MMP-1, MMP-2, MMP-3, MMP-7, MMP-9)	Malignant ascites, malignant effusion (canceled in PIII) [28]
Marimastat (BB-2516)	Peptidomimetic (hydroxamate)	Broad spectrum (higher specificity: MMP-1, MMP-2, MMP-7, MMP-9, MMP-14)	Breast cancer, small cell lung cancer, non-small cell lung cancer (canceled in PIII) [28], vascular anomalies (completed PI) [94]
Trocade (Cipemastat/ Ro32-3555)	Peptidomimetic (hydroxamate)	MMP-1 with higher specificity and MMP-8, MMP-13	Rheumatoid arthritis (PIII) [95]
Ilomastat (GM-6001)	Peptidomimetic (hydroxamate)	Broad spectrum (higher specificity: MMP-1, MMP-2, MMP-8, MMP-9, MMP-26)	Corneal ulceration and diabetic retinopathy (PII–III) [95]
CGS27023A (MMI270)	Non-peptidomimetic (hydroxamate)	Broad spectrum (higher specificity: MMP-1, MMP-2, MMP-3, MMP-8, MMP-9)	Advanced solid cancer (canceled in PI) [95]
Prinomastat (AG 3340)	Non-peptidomimetic (hydroxamate)	Broad spectrum (higher specificity: MMP-2, MMP-3, MMP-7, MMP-9, MMP-13, MMP-14)	Non-small cell lung cancer and prostate cancer (canceled in PIII), glioblastoma multiforme (canceled in PII) [28, 94]
Tanomastat (BAY 12–9566)	Non-peptidomimetic (carboxylic acid)	MMP-2, MMP-3, MMP-9	Ovarian cancer, adenocarcinoma of the pancreas, non-small cell lung cancer, rheumatoid arthritis, rejection of organ transplant (canceled in PIII) [28]
Rebimastat (BMS-275291)	Non-peptidomimetic (thiol-based)	Broad spectrum (higher specificity: MMP-2, MMP-9 and MMP-1, MMP-8, MMP-14)	Hormone-resistant prostate cancer (PII), HIV-related Kaposi sarcoma (PI/II), advanced non-small cell lung cancer (PII/III, in combination with paclitaxel and carboplatin), breast cancer (canceled in PII) [94]

(continued)

Table 1
(continued)

MMPIs	Type of drug/ source	Enzymes inhibited	Indication
FP-025	Small molecule (non-hydroxamate based)	MMP-12	Healthy (PI) [94]
CTS1027	Small molecule (hydroxamate sulfone)	Broad Spectrum (higher specificity: MMP-2, MMP-13, no MMP-1)	Hepatitis C (PII) [94]
Antabuse (disulfiram)	Small molecule (sulfonamide)	MMP-2, MMP-9	Non-small cell lung cancer (PII/III, as add-on therapy to chemotherapy), metastatic pancreatic carcinoma (PI, with gemcitabine HCl, recruiting), glioblastoma (PI/II, PII, PII/III, recruiting, with copper), HIV infections (PI/II), stage IV melanoma (PI/II), prostate cancer (PI, recruiting, with copper) [94]
AZD1236	Small molecule (sulfonamide-based)	MMP-9, MMP-12	Chronic obstructive pulmonary disease (PII) [94]
S3304	Small molecule (sulfonamide derivative)	higher specificity: MMP-2, MMP-9	Adult solid tumors (PI), advanced non-small cell lung cancer (PI/II, unknown) [94]
Minocin (minocycline)	Chemically modified tetracycline	MMP-2, MMP-9	Central nervous system disease such as Alzheimer's disease (PII), amyotrophic lateral sclerosis (PIII), Huntington disease (PII/III), Parkinson's disease (PII), glioma (PI/II, in combination with bevacizumab and radiation), asthma (PII), aneurysm (PI/II, recruiting), prostate cancer (PIII, recruiting), mood disorders (PIV, PIII, recruiting) [94]

(continued)

Table 1
(continued)

MMPIs	Type of drug/ source	Enzymes inhibited	Indication
Periostat (doxycycline)	Chemically modified tetracycline	Broad spectrum (higher specificity: MMP-1, MMP-2, MMP-8, MMP-9)	Cystic fibrosis, type 2 diabetes, obesity and endometritis (PIV), nonischemic cardiomyopathy and aortic aneurysm (PII), primary systemic amyloidosis, tuberculosis, T-cell lymphoma, adenocarcinoma, resectable pancreatic cancer (recruiting, PII), non-Hodgkin lymphoma (canceled in PII), B-cell lymphoma (recruiting, ongoing), polycystic ovarian syndrome (PIII), syphilis (early PI) [94]
Metastat (COL-3)	Chemically modified tetracycline	Broad spectrum (higher specificity: MMP-1, MMP-2, MMP-8, MMP-9, MMP-13)	Refractory metastatic cancer and advanced solid tumors (PI), brain and central nervous system tumors (PI/II), AIDS-related Kaposi sarcoma (canceled in PII) [94]
Neovastat (AE-941)	Shark cartilage extract	Broad spectrum (higher specificity: MMP-1, MMP-2, MMP-7, MMP-9, MMP-13)	Relapsed or refractory multiple myeloma (PII), metastatic kidney cancer, and advanced colorectal/ breast cancer (PIII) [94]
Andecaliximab (GS-5745)	Monoclonal Ab	MMP-9	Ulcerative colitis (PII/III), rheumatoid arthritis, and chronic obstructive pulmonary disease (PI), Crohn's disease (PII), cystic fibrosis (PII, recruiting), rheumatoid arthritis (PII, as add-on therapy, recruiting), gastric adenocarcinoma (PI, PII, PIII, recruiting), advanced solid tumors (PI, recruiting) [94]

angiogenesis [103]. Tissue factor pathway inhibitor-2 (TFPI2) and procollagen C-terminal proteinase enhancer (PCPE) have structures similar to the inhibitory domain of TIMPs and exhibit significant MMP inhibitory activity [104, 105]. Interestingly, TFPI2 has been reported as a prognostic biomarker for hepatocellular carcinoma and oral squamous cell carcinoma [106, 107].

4.2 Early MMP Targeting Strategies

Several programs for development of MMPIs were initiated with the use of compounds that bind within the catalytic domain of MMPs. Batimastat is a broad-spectrum, competitive peptidomimetic MMPI that has been tested clinically. Even though it effectively inhibited MMP-1, MMP-2, MMP-3, MMP-7, MMP-9, and MMP-14 enzymatic activities and reduced tumor growth in breast and pancreatic cancer and melanoma, it failed in phase III (PIII) trials due to decreased oral bioavailability and poor solubility [108]. To overcome this disadvantage, the chemically similar analogue of batimastat, marimastat, was designed, which exhibited improved oral bioavailability with modest efficacy; however, it demonstrated significant musculoskeletal pain and inflammation in the patients; therefore, the development of this drug was also stopped [28]. CGS 27023A (Novartis) is a small-molecule inhibitor that targets MMP-2, MMP-8 and MMP-9 and has been developed from Novartis for advanced solid tumor therapy. It significantly inhibited angiogenesis, metastasis and tumor growth in in vivo breast and endometrial cancer models [109, 110]. Unfortunately, this drug was removed from the clinical trials in PI due to severe muscle pain in patients with non-small cell lung carcinoma [111]. Clinical trials with broad-spectrum MMPIs in late-stage cancer patients were terminated mainly due to their reduced efficacy and severe side effects. The efforts of designing next-generation MMPIs have been focused on the investigation and development of allosteric MMPIs with improved selectivity for one, specific MMP.

4.3 Next-Generation MMPIs in Clinical Trials

In order to improve the specificity and bioavailability of already established inhibitors, non-peptidomimetic MMPIs were also synthesized based on the 3D structure of specific MMP (Table 1). Two peptidomimetic MMPIs which entered clinical trials for inflammatory diseases are the collagenase-selective Trocade (cipemastat) and the broad-spectrum MMPI Ilomastat (GM-6001). Prinomastat (AG3340, Agouron), the optimized version of CGS 27023A, is a broad-spectrum non-peptidomimetic MMPI that has antiangiogenic and antimetastatic effects in in vivo models; however, its clinical study was canceled in PII due to the development of musculoskeletal syndrome [112]. Tanomastat (BAY 12–9566) is a non-peptidomimetic MMPI that specifically targets MMP-2, MMP-3 and MMP-9; however, there was no evidence that this drug could effectively decrease cancer progression [113]. NSC405020 is a novel small-molecule inhibitor that controls the biological activity of MT1-MMP, which retains its ability to activate MMP-2. Moreover, it selectively targets the hemopexin domain of MT1-MMP, thereby repressing its pro-tumorigenic activity in vivo [114]. Next-generation MMPIs also include tetracycline derivatives, which inhibit both enzymatic activity and transcription of MMPs. Periostat (CollaGenex Pharmaceuticals Inc.), a chemically modified tetracycline, doxycycline, is the only MMPI to be successfully launched and used for periodontal diseases. Additionally, many approved and ongoing studies in diseases such as musculoskeletal syndrome, type 2 diabetes, aortic aneurysm, and coronary artery disease include doxycycline in treatment schemes. Very encouraging is the conduction of several recruiting and ongoing studies testing doxycycline in combination with standard chemotherapy for use in cancer treatment [115]. Another chemically modified tetracycline is minocycline with a great range of applications in clinical trials (Table 1). Metastat (COL-3/CMT3) is another modified tetracycline derivative targeting many MMPs such as MMP-1, MMP-2, MMP-8, MMP-9, and MMP-13, but it presents many different side effects such as photosensitivity, phototoxicity, anemia, and sideroblastic anemia [116]. The selective MMPI AZD1326 (AstraZeneca) targeting MMP-9 and MMP-12 is currently tested in PII clinical trials for inflammation diseases, such as chronic obstructive pulmonary disease (COPD) and asthma. Another selective MMPI FP-025 (Foresee Pharmaceutical), against MMP-12, is considered as a high candidate for the treatment of the above diseases and for now is in PI clinical trials to clarify safety, tolerability, and pharmacokinetics in healthy patients [117, 118]. Other MMPIs focusing on malignancies and tested in clinical trials include Neovastat (Benefin/AE-941, Aeterna Zentaris), which is extracted from a natural source and it strongly inhibits MMP-2 activity [119, 120] and BMS-275291 (Bristol-Myers Squibb), a wide-spectrum MMPI [121]. A broad-spectrum MMP inhibitor is CTS1027 participating in clinical trials for hepatitis C (PII). A selective gelatinase inhibitor is disulfiram, assessing in clinical trials for the treatment of a variety of tumors and HIV infections. Moreover, S3304 is a sulfonamide derivate developed by Shionogi Pharmaceutical Co. Ltd. and seems to be well tolerated in patients with advanced and refractory solid tumors [116, 122].

4.4 Monoclonal Antibodies

More recently, the interest of the pharmaceutical industry was focused on the targeting of a specific MMP, because several broad-range MMPIs have failed in the clinical trials. In this context, at least three monoclonal antibodies (mAbs) against the catalytic domain of a single MMP have been developed to target several primary and metastatic cancers. DX-2400 is an antibody fragment (Fab) that selectively inhibits MT1-MMP enzymatic activity. DX-2400 significantly inhibited tumor growth, angiogenesis, invasion and metastasis in several preclinical models [123, 124]. Therapeutic promise has also been shown with full-length mAb REGA-3G12, which targets the catalytic domain of MMP-9 [125, 126]. This mAb selectively inhibits MMP-9 enzymatic activity, compared to MMP-2 [127]. GS-5745, a humanized full-length allosteric mAb against MMP-9, selectively inhibits its enzymatic activity. Recent study in a colorectal carcinoma model revealed that GS-5745 significantly attenuates tumor growth, invasion, and metastasis and it did not exhibit severe side effects (Table 1) [128]. Even though mAbs are characterized by limitations regarding high production costs, undesired effector functions, and selectivity restrictions due to the high homology of the catalytic sites of several MMPs, therapeutic approaches which are based on mAbs as allosteric inhibitors of MMPs, both when used as single agents and in combination with anticancer therapy, might exhibit improved efficacy.

4.5 MicroRNA-Mediated MMP Activity

Of particular interest in the understanding of cancer cell behavior is the field of microRNAs (miRNAs). They are endogenous non-coding RNA molecules, which have key roles in posttranscriptional regulation of several cellular processes [129]. Recent studies have associated various miRNAs with cell proliferation, resistance to apoptosis, differentiation, immunity and cancer initiation, progression and metastasis [130, 131]. Moreover, miRNAs are responsible for the regulation of ECM components and of their cellular receptors [132–134]. Recently, there has been considerable interest in the posttranscriptional regulation of MMPs, since they are directly regulated by miRNAs in various diseases, including osteoarthritis [135], glioblastoma and several malignancies [136]. Recent studies showed that miR-21 has been implicated in glioblastoma by regulating glioma cell proliferation, invasion and apoptosis. Moreover, this miRNA activates MMPs, through the downregulation of their inhibitors, contributing in glioma cells' aggressiveness. Specific inhibition of miR-21 with antisense oligonucleotides significantly upregulates RECK and TIMP-3 gene and protein levels, thus inhibiting MMP enzymatic activity in vitro and in vivo, serving as a novel anticancer therapy [137, 138]. Many miRNAs are found to regulate metastatic processes, including EMT, migration and invasion [139]. The induced overexpression of miR-146a in the highly metastatic brain-trophic metastatic MDA-MB-435-LvBr2 breast cancer cells significantly reduced the migratory and invasive potential of these cells through the induction of β-catenin and the following downregulation of MMP-1, uPA and uPAR [140]. A single miRNA is able to regulate the expression of different MMPs due to sequence homology in MMP structure. For instance, miR-143 downregulates gene and protein levels of MMP-2 and MMP-9 in pancreatic cancer cells [141]. MMP-13 is characterized as a direct target of miR-143 in osteosarcoma in vivo models [142]. Moreover, overexpression of miR-143 inhibits EGFR-dependent cell invasion, indirectly mediating MMP-9 expression in osteosarcoma [143]. These data demonstrate that a thorough understanding regarding the mechanisms of miRNA-mediated MMP expression will improve the clinical utility of miRNAs providing them as prognostic markers and personalized therapeutic targets in aggressive and metastatic malignancies.

4.6 Novel Targeting and Delivery Systems

In recent years, research has significantly developed in terms of delivery systems with an improved drug delivery potential for cancer therapy, such as the multifunctional liposomal nanocarriers. These are lipid bilayered vesicles that are utilized as novel drug delivery systems due to their efficiency, biocompatibility, solubility, low toxicity and ability to encapsulate a wide range of drugs via chemical conjugation [144]. An interesting example of liposome-based chemotherapeutic approaches targeting MMPs has been the doxorubicin-loaded polyethylene glycol (PEG) liposomes conjugated to a Fab fragment from MT1-MMP monoclonal antibody via a PEG spacer, which significantly decreased tumor growth in vivo, as compared with plain liposomes with doxorubicin [145]. In addition, liposome-based systems have been used as tools for active tumor site targeting. Such liposomal delivery systems of high selectivity include a monoclonal antibody with a MMP-2 cleavable peptide that recognizes the cancer cells. These MMP-sensitive liposomal probes are degraded in the presence of high MMP levels releasing the encapsulated therapeutic compound with cytotoxic effects for cancer cells [146]. A recent report demonstrated that the MCF-7 breast cancer cells secreting high levels of MMP-9 can be targeted by utilizing optimized liposomal formulations inducing the rapid release of the encapsulated contents from the liposomes in the tumor site [147].

Similar to liposome formulations, MMPs can be incorporated in nanostructures conjugated with cytotoxic compounds, for improving their efficacy in targeting cancer cells. Nanoparticles (NPs) are extremely small in size and possess a large surface area per unit of volume. Their novel physical characteristics of nanomaterials serve their drastically different chemical and biological properties compared to the same material in bulk form. Such unique chemical and biological properties of nanomaterials make them very attractive in medical applications including tumor-triggered targeting delivery systems [148–150]. An interesting example includes the effect of nano-heparin analogue of *Styela plicata* origin, on the aggressive MDA-MB-231 breast cancer cell line. Nano-styela heparin significantly inhibited cell proliferation, migration, and invasion in vitro and induced apoptosis in breast cancer cells and this was followed by a significant downregulation of MT1-MMP and uPA gene expression levels [151]. Biocompatible gold NPs (AuNPs) localized in the lysosomes significantly inhibited MMP activity by blocking Zn^{2+} on the active site of the enzyme, without cytotoxicity or inflammatory responses [152]. Multifunctional mesoporous silica NPs were loaded with β-cyclodextrin and an MMP substrate peptide in order to selectively target the MMP-rich tumor cells and subsequently induce the intracellular release of the cytotoxic drug [153].

5 Conclusion

MMPs are considered as key molecules in tumor development and have been correlated with the progression of various malignancies. They master ECM proteolysis and tissue remodeling facilitating tumor cell dissemination and metastasis. MMPs also trigger tumor cell aggressiveness by affecting numerous cell events such as proliferation, adhesion, migration, EMT and tumor stroma angiogenesis simultaneously. Plethora of information has been accumulated for the regulation of MMP expression, activity, and role in cancer and they have been pointed as therapeutic targets for disease treatment. Multiple MMPIs were developed and tested in clinical trials as anticancer drugs with unsatisfactory results in the past mostly due to the lack of specificity and severe side effects. Targeting MMPs still remains a viable and desirable therapeutic approach and new MMPIs have been developed with improved features and are currently in clinical trials. Furthermore, novel interventions for targeting MMPs are developed to improve delivery of chemotherapeutics enhancing their efficacy and reducing side effects. In addition, the epigenetic regulation of MMPs' expression by using miRNAs is proposed as a useful therapeutic tool for cancer treatment.

References

1. Jemal A, Siegel R, Xu J et al (2010) Cancer statistics, 2010. CA Cancer J Clin 60(5):277–300. https://doi.org/10.3322/caac.20073
2. Chambers AF, Groom AC, MacDonald IC (2002) Dissemination and growth of cancer cells in metastatic sites. Nat Rev Cancer 2(8):563–572. https://doi.org/10.1038/nrc865
3. Hanahan D, Weinberg RA (2011) Hallmarks of cancer: the next generation. Cell 144(5):646–674. https://doi.org/10.1016/j.cell.2011.02.013
4. Lamouille S, Xu J, Derynck R (2014) Molecular mechanisms of epithelial-mesenchymal transition. Nat Rev Mol Cell Biol 15(3):178–196. https://doi.org/10.1038/nrm3758
5. Zeisberg M, Neilson EG (2009) Biomarkers for epithelial-mesenchymal transitions. J Clin Invest 119(6):1429–1437. https://doi.org/10.1172/JCI36183
6. Kalluri R, Weinberg RA (2009) The basics of epithelial-mesenchymal transition. J Clin Invest 119(6):1420–1428. https://doi.org/10.1172/JCI39104
7. Thiery JP (2002) Epithelial-mesenchymal transitions in tumour progression. Nat Rev Cancer 2(6):442–454. https://doi.org/10.1038/nrc822
8. Thiery JP (2003) Epithelial-mesenchymal transitions in development and pathologies. Curr Opin Cell Biol 15(6):740–746
9. Rodríguez D, Morrison CJ, Overall CM (2010) Matrix metalloproteinases: what do they not do? New substrates and biological roles identified by murine models and proteomics. Biochim Biophys Acta 1803(1):39–54. https://doi.org/10.1016/j.bbamcr.2009.09.015
10. Yao D, Dai C, Peng S (2011) Mechanism of the mesenchymal-epithelial transition and its relationship with metastatic tumor formation. Mol Cancer Res 9(12):1608–1620. https://doi.org/10.1158/1541-7786.MCR-10-0568
11. Frantz C, Stewart KM, Weaver VM (2010) The extracellular matrix at a glance. J Cell Sci 123(Pt 24):4195–4200. https://doi.org/10.1242/jcs.023820
12. Theocharis AD, Skandalis SS, Gialeli C et al (2016) Extracellular matrix structure. Adv Drug Deliv Rev 97:4–27. https://doi.org/10.1016/j.addr.2015.11.001
13. Theocharis AD, Gialeli C, Hascall VC et al (2012) Extracellular matrix: a functional

scaffold. In: Karamanos NK (ed) Extracellular matrix: pathobiology and signaling. Walter de Gruyter GmbH & Co. KG, Berlin
14. Piperigkou Z, Mohr B, Karamanos N et al (2016) Shed proteoglycans in tumor stroma. Cell Tissue Res. https://doi.org/10.1007/s00441-016-2452-4
15. Lu P, Weaver VM, Werb Z (2012) The extracellular matrix: a dynamic niche in cancer progression. J Cell Biol 196(4):395–406. https://doi.org/10.1083/jcb.201102147
16. Kessenbrock K, Plaks V, Werb Z (2010) Matrix metalloproteinases: regulators of the tumor microenvironment. Cell 141(1):52–67. https://doi.org/10.1016/j.cell.2010.03.015
17. Gialeli C, Theocharis AD, Karamanos NK (2011) Roles of matrix metalloproteinases in cancer progression and their pharmacological targeting. FEBS J 278(1):16–27. https://doi.org/10.1111/j.1742-4658.2010.07919.x
18. Jackson BC, Nebert DW, Vasiliou V (2010) Update of human and mouse matrix metalloproteinase families. Hum Genomics 4(3):194–201
19. Brinckerhoff CE, Matrisian LM (2002) Matrix metalloproteinases: a tail of a frog that became a prince. Nat Rev Mol Cell Biol 3(3):207–214. https://doi.org/10.1038/nrm763
20. Sternlicht MD, Werb Z (2001) How matrix metalloproteinases regulate cell behavior. Annu Rev Cell Dev Biol 17:463–516. https://doi.org/10.1146/annurev.cellbio.17.1.463
21. Bourboulia D, Stetler-Stevenson WG (2010) Matrix metalloproteinases (MMPs) and tissue inhibitors of metalloproteinases (TIMPs): positive and negative regulators in tumor cell adhesion. Semin Cancer Biol 20(3):161–168. https://doi.org/10.1016/j.semcancer.2010.05.002
22. Radisky ES, Radisky DC (2010) Matrix metalloproteinase-induced epithelial-mesenchymal transition in breast cancer. J Mammary Gland Biol Neoplasia 15(2):201–212. https://doi.org/10.1007/s10911-010-9177-x
23. Visse R, Nagase H (2003) Matrix metalloproteinases and tissue inhibitors of metalloproteinases: structure, function, and biochemistry. Circ Res 92(8):827–839. https://doi.org/10.1161/01.RES.0000070112.80711.3D
24. Verma RP, Hansch C (2007) Matrix metalloproteinases (MMPs): chemical-biological functions and (Q)SARs. Bioorg Med Chem 15(6):2223–2268. https://doi.org/10.1016/j.bmc.2007.01.011
25. Bonnans C, Chou J, Werb Z (2014) Remodelling the extracellular matrix in development and disease. Nat Rev Mol Cell Biol 15(12):786–801. https://doi.org/10.1038/nrm3904
26. Brown GT, Murray GI (2015) Current mechanistic insights into the roles of matrix metalloproteinases in tumour invasion and metastasis. J Pathol 237(3):273–281. https://doi.org/10.1002/path.4586
27. Egeblad M, Werb Z (2002) New functions for the matrix metalloproteinases in cancer progression. Nat Rev Cancer 2(3):161–174. https://doi.org/10.1038/nrc745
28. Cathcart J, Pulkoski-Gross A, Cao J (2015) Targeting matrix metalloproteinases in cancer: bringing new life to old ideas. Genes Dis 2(1):26–34. https://doi.org/10.1016/j.gendis.2014.12.002
29. Szarvas T, vom Dorp F, Ergun S et al (2011) Matrix metalloproteinases and their clinical relevance in urinary bladder cancer. Nat Rev Urol 8(5):241–254. https://doi.org/10.1038/nrurol.2011.44
30. Hadler-Olsen E, Winberg JO, Uhlin-Hansen L (2013) Matrix metalloproteinases in cancer: their value as diagnostic and prognostic markers and therapeutic targets. Tumour Biol 34(4):2041–2051. https://doi.org/10.1007/s13277-013-0842-8
31. Ren F, Tang R, Zhang X et al (2015) Overexpression of MMP family members functions as prognostic biomarker for breast cancer patients: a systematic review and meta-analysis. PLoS One 10(8):e0135544. https://doi.org/10.1371/journal.pone.0135544
32. Overall CM, Lopez-Otin C (2002) Strategies for MMP inhibition in cancer: innovations for the post-trial era. Nat Rev Cancer 2(9):657–672. https://doi.org/10.1038/nrc884
33. Nakamura M, Miyamoto S, Maeda H et al (2005) Matrix metalloproteinase-7 degrades all insulin-like growth factor binding proteins and facilitates insulin-like growth factor bioavailability. Biochem Biophys Res Commun 333(3):1011–1016. https://doi.org/10.1016/j.bbrc.2005.06.010
34. Miller MA, Moss ML, Powell G et al (2015) Targeting autocrine HB-EGF signaling with specific ADAM12 inhibition using recombinant ADAM12 prodomain. Sci Rep 5:15150. https://doi.org/10.1038/srep15150
35. Witters L, Scherle P, Friedman S et al (2008) Synergistic inhibition with a dual epidermal growth factor receptor/HER-2/neu tyrosine kinase inhibitor and a disintegrin and metalloprotease inhibitor. Cancer Res 68(17):7083–7089. https://doi.org/10.1158/0008-5472.CAN-08-0739

36. Barbouri D, Afratis N, Gialeli C et al (2014) Syndecans as modulators and potential pharmacological targets in cancer progression. Front Oncol 4:4. https://doi.org/10.3389/fonc.2014.00004
37. Mythreye K, Blobe GC (2009) Proteoglycan signaling co-receptors: roles in cell adhesion, migration and invasion. Cell Signal 21(11):1548–1558. https://doi.org/10.1016/j.cellsig.2009.05.001
38. Valacca C, Tassone E, Mignatti P (2015) TIMP-2 interaction with MT1-MMP activates the AKT pathway and protects tumor cells from apoptosis. PLoS One 10(9):e0136797. https://doi.org/10.1371/journal.pone.0136797
39. Almendro V, Ametller E, Garcia-Recio S et al (2009) The role of MMP7 and its cross-talk with the FAS/FASL system during the acquisition of chemoresistance to oxaliplatin. PLoS One 4(3):e4728. https://doi.org/10.1371/journal.pone.0004728
40. Mitsiades N, Yu WH, Poulaki V et al (2001) Matrix metalloproteinase-7-mediated cleavage of Fas ligand protects tumor cells from chemotherapeutic drug cytotoxicity. Cancer Res 61(2):577–581
41. Noe V, Fingleton B, Jacobs K et al (2001) Release of an invasion promoter E-cadherin fragment by matrilysin and stromelysin-1. J Cell Sci 114(Pt 1):111–118
42. Maretzky T, Reiss K, Ludwig A et al (2005) ADAM10 mediates E-cadherin shedding and regulates epithelial cell-cell adhesion, migration, and beta-catenin translocation. Proc Natl Acad Sci U S A 102(26):9182–9187. https://doi.org/10.1073/pnas.0500918102
43. Yoo YA, Kang MH, Lee HJ et al (2011) Sonic hedgehog pathway promotes metastasis and lymphangiogenesis via activation of Akt, EMT, and MMP-9 pathway in gastric cancer. Cancer Res 71(22):7061–7070. https://doi.org/10.1158/0008-5472.CAN-11-1338
44. Zuo JH, Zhu W, Li MY et al (2011) Activation of EGFR promotes squamous carcinoma SCC10A cell migration and invasion via inducing EMT-like phenotype change and MMP-9-mediated degradation of E-cadherin. J Cell Biochem 112(9):2508–2517. https://doi.org/10.1002/jcb.23175
45. Wang X, Lu H, Urvalek AM et al (2011) KLF8 promotes human breast cancer cell invasion and metastasis by transcriptional activation of MMP9. Oncogene 30(16):1901–1911. https://doi.org/10.1038/onc.2010.563
46. Blavier L, Lazaryev A, Shi XH et al (2010) Stromelysin-1 (MMP-3) is a target and a regulator of Wnt1-induced epithelial-mesenchymal transition (EMT). Cancer Biol Ther 10(2):198–208
47. Xie B, Lin W, Ye J et al (2015) DDR2 facilitates hepatocellular carcinoma invasion and metastasis via activating ERK signaling and stabilizing SNAIL1. J Exp Clin Cancer Res 34:101.https://doi.org/10.1186/s13046-015-0218-6
48. Jiang W, Zhang Y, Kane KT et al (2015) CD44 regulates pancreatic cancer invasion through MT1-MMP. Mol Cancer Res 13(1):9–15. https://doi.org/10.1158/1541-7786.mcr-14-0076
49. Bouris P, Skandalis SS, Piperigkou Z et al (2015) Estrogen receptor alpha mediates epithelial to mesenchymal transition, expression of specific matrix effectors and functional properties of breast cancer cells. Matrix Biol 43:42–60. https://doi.org/10.1016/j.matbio.2015.02.008
50. Piperigkou Z, Bouris P, Onisto M et al (2016) Estrogen receptor beta modulates breast cancer cells functional properties, signaling and expression of matrix molecules. Matrix Biol 56:4–23. https://doi.org/10.1016/j.matbio.2016.05.003
51. Robichaud N, del Rincon SV, Huor B et al (2015) Phosphorylation of eIF4E promotes EMT and metastasis via translational control of SNAIL and MMP-3. Oncogene 34(16):2032–2042. https://doi.org/10.1038/onc.2014.146
52. Pettersson F, Del Rincon SV, Emond A et al (2015) Genetic and pharmacologic inhibition of eIF4E reduces breast cancer cell migration, invasion, and metastasis. Cancer Res 75(6):1102–1112. https://doi.org/10.1158/0008-5472.CAN-14-1996
53. Nikitovic D, Papoutsidakis A, Karamanos NK et al (2014) Lumican affects tumor cell functions, tumor-ECM interactions, angiogenesis and inflammatory response. Matrix Biol 35:206–214. https://doi.org/10.1016/j.matbio.2013.09.003
54. Brezillon S, Pietraszek K, Maquart FX et al (2013) Lumican effects in the control of tumour progression and their links with metalloproteinases and integrins. FEBS J 280(10):2369–2381. https://doi.org/10.1111/febs.12210
55. Stasiak M, Boncela J, Perreau C et al (2016) Lumican inhibits SNAIL-induced melanoma cell migration specifically by blocking MMP-14 activity. PLoS One 11(3):e0150226. https://doi.org/10.1371/journal.pone.0150226
56. Karamanou K, Franchi M, Piperigkou Z et al (2017) Lumican effectively regulates the estrogen receptors-associated functional

properties of breast cancer cells, expression of matrix effectors and epithelial-to-mesenchymal transition. Sci Rep 7:45138. https://doi.org/10.1038/srep45138

57. Nistico P, Bissell MJ, Radisky DC (2012) Epithelial-mesenchymal transition: general principles and pathological relevance with special emphasis on the role of matrix metalloproteinases. Cold Spring Harb Perspect Biol 4(2). https://doi.org/10.1101/cshperspect.a011908
58. Son H, Moon A (2010) Epithelial-mesenchymal transition and cell invasion. Toxicol Res 26(4):245–252. https://doi.org/10.5487/TR.2010.26.4.245
59. Cichon MA, Radisky DC (2014) ROS-induced epithelial-mesenchymal transition in mammary epithelial cells is mediated by NF-kB-dependent activation of Snail. Oncotarget 5(9):2827–2838. 10.18632/oncotarget.1940
60. Yang CC, Zhu LF, Xu XH et al (2013) Membrane type 1 matrix metalloproteinase induces an epithelial to mesenchymal transition and cancer stem cell-like properties in SCC9 cells. BMC Cancer 13:171. https://doi.org/10.1186/1471-2407-13-171
61. Huang SH, Law CH, Kuo PH et al (2016) MMP-13 is involved in oral cancer cell metastasis. Oncotarget 7(13):17144–17161. 10.18632/oncotarget.7942
62. Vinnakota K, Zhang Y, Selvanesan BC et al (2017) M2-like macrophages induce colon cancer cell invasion via matrix metalloproteinases. J Cell Physiol 232(12):3468–3480. https://doi.org/10.1002/jcp.25808
63. Johansson A-C, Ansell A, Jerhammar F et al (2012) Cancer-associated fibroblasts induce matrix metalloproteinase–mediated cetuximab resistance in head and neck squamous cell carcinoma cells. Mol Cancer Res 10(9):1158–1168. https://doi.org/10.1158/1541-7786.mcr-12-0030
64. Giannoni E, Bianchini F, Masieri L et al (2010) Reciprocal activation of prostate cancer cells and cancer-associated fibroblasts stimulates epithelial-mesenchymal transition and cancer stemness. Cancer Res 70(17):6945–6956. https://doi.org/10.1158/0008-5472.can-10-0785
65. Lederle W, Hartenstein B, Meides A et al (2010) MMP13 as a stromal mediator in controlling persistent angiogenesis in skin carcinoma. Carcinogenesis 31(7):1175–1184. https://doi.org/10.1093/carcin/bgp248
66. Vosseler S, Lederle W, Airola K et al (2009) Distinct progression-associated expression of tumor and stromal MMPs in HaCaT skin SCCs correlates with onset of invasion. Int J Cancer 125(10):2296–2306. https://doi.org/10.1002/ijc.24589
67. Devreotes P, Janetopoulos C (2003) Eukaryotic chemotaxis: distinctions between directional sensing and polarization. J Biol Chem 278(23):20445–20448. https://doi.org/10.1074/jbc.R300010200
68. Guenzle J, Wolf LJ, Garrelfs NW et al (2017) ATF3 reduces migration capacity by regulation of matrix metalloproteinases via NFkappaB and STAT3 inhibition in glioblastoma. Cell Death Discov 3:17006. https://doi.org/10.1038/cddiscovery.2017.6
69. Yuan X, Yu L, Li J et al (2013) ATF3 suppresses metastasis of bladder cancer by regulating gelsolin-mediated remodeling of the actin cytoskeleton. Cancer Res 73(12):3625–3637. https://doi.org/10.1158/0008-5472.CAN-12-3879
70. Xie JJ, Xie YM, Chen B et al (2014) ATF3 functions as a novel tumor suppressor with prognostic significance in esophageal squamous cell carcinoma. Oncotarget 5(18):8569–8582. 10.18632/oncotarget.2322
71. Baumann P, Zigrino P, Mauch C et al (2000) Membrane-type 1 matrix metalloproteinase-mediated progelatinase A activation in non-tumorigenic and tumorigenic human keratinocytes. Br J Cancer 83(10):1387–1393. https://doi.org/10.1054/bjoc.2000.1454
72. Dissanayake SK, Wade M, Johnson CE et al (2007) The Wnt5A/protein kinase C pathway mediates motility in melanoma cells via the inhibition of metastasis suppressors and initiation of an epithelial to mesenchymal transition. J Biol Chem 282(23):17259–17271. https://doi.org/10.1074/jbc.M700075200
73. Kuphal S, Palm HG, Poser I et al (2005) Snail-regulated genes in malignant melanoma. Melanoma Res 15(4):305–313
74. Cathcart JM, Banach A, Liu A et al (2016) Interleukin-6 increases matrix metalloproteinase-14 (MMP-14) levels via down-regulation of p53 to drive cancer progression. Oncotarget 7(38):61107–61120. 10.18632/oncotarget.11243
75. Jacob A, Prekeris R (2015) The regulation of MMP targeting to invadopodia during cancer metastasis. Front Cell Dev Biol 3:4. https://doi.org/10.3389/fcell.2015.00004
76. Basu A, Menicucci G, Maestas J et al (2009) Plasminogen activator inhibitor-1 (PAI-1) facilitates retinal angiogenesis in a model of oxygen-induced retinopathy. Invest Ophthalmol Vis Sci 50(10):4974–4981. https://doi.org/10.1167/iovs.09-3619

77. Rao JS, Gondi C, Chetty C et al (2005) Inhibition of invasion, angiogenesis, tumor growth, and metastasis by adenovirus-mediated transfer of antisense uPAR and MMP-9 in non-small cell lung cancer cells. Mol Cancer Ther 4(9):1399–1408. https://doi.org/10.1158/1535-7163.MCT-05-0082
78. Thummarati P, Wijitburaphat S, Prasopthum A et al (2012) High level of urokinase plasminogen activator contributes to cholangiocarcinoma invasion and metastasis. World J Gastroenterol 18(3):244–250. https://doi.org/10.3748/wjg.v18.i3.244
79. Moirangthem A, Bondhopadhyay B, Mukherjee M et al (2016) Simultaneous knockdown of uPA and MMP9 can reduce breast cancer progression by increasing cell-cell adhesion and modulating EMT genes. Sci Rep 6:21903. https://doi.org/10.1038/srep21903
80. Hozumi A, Nishimura Y, Nishiuma T et al (2001) Induction of MMP-9 in normal human bronchial epithelial cells by TNF-alpha via NF-kappa B-mediated pathway. Am J Physiol Lung Cell Mol Physiol 281(6):L1444–L1452
81. Lin CW, Hou WC, Shen SC et al (2008) Quercetin inhibition of tumor invasion via suppressing PKC delta/ERK/AP-1-dependent matrix metalloproteinase-9 activation in breast carcinoma cells. Carcinogenesis 29(9):1807–1815. https://doi.org/10.1093/carcin/bgn162
82. Weng CJ, Chau CF, Hsieh YS et al (2008) Lucidenic acid inhibits PMA-induced invasion of human hepatoma cells through inactivating MAPK/ERK signal transduction pathway and reducing binding activities of NF-kappaB and AP-1. Carcinogenesis 29(1):147–156. https://doi.org/10.1093/carcin/bgm261
83. Eberhardt W, Huwiler A, Beck KF et al (2000) Amplification of IL-1 beta-induced matrix metalloproteinase-9 expression by superoxide in rat glomerular mesangial cells is mediated by increased activities of NF-kappa B and activating protein-1 and involves activation of the mitogen-activated protein kinase pathways. J Immunol 165(10):5788–5797
84. Kim HR, Kim JM, Kim MS et al (2014) Saussurea lappa extract suppresses TPA-induced cell invasion via inhibition of NF-kappaB-dependent MMP-9 expression in MCF-7 breast cancer cells. BMC Complement Altern Med 14:170. https://doi.org/10.1186/1472-6882-14-170
85. Kim JM, Noh EM, Kim HR et al (2016) Suppression of TPA-induced cancer cell invasion by Peucedanum japonicum Thunb. extract through the inhibition of PKCalpha/NF-kappaB-dependent MMP-9 expression in MCF-7 cells. Int J Mol Med 37(1):108–114. https://doi.org/10.3892/ijmm.2015.2417
86. Benjamin MM, Khalil RA (2012) Matrix metalloproteinase inhibitors as investigative tools in the pathogenesis and management of vascular disease. EXS 103:209–279. https://doi.org/10.1007/978-3-0348-0364-9_7
87. Nagase H, Enghild JJ, Suzuki K et al (1990) Stepwise activation mechanisms of the precursor of matrix metalloproteinase 3 (stromelysin) by proteinases and (4-aminophenyl) mercuric acetate. Biochemistry 29(24):5783–5789
88. Nagase H, Ogata Y, Suzuki K et al (1991) Substrate specificities and activation mechanisms of matrix metalloproteinases. Biochem Soc Trans 19(3):715–718
89. Franco C, Patricia HR, Timo S et al (2017) Matrix metalloproteinases as regulators of periodontal inflammation. Int J Mol Sci 18(2). https://doi.org/10.3390/ijms18020440
90. Jiang B, Zhang Y, Liu J et al (2017) Ensnaring membrane type 1-matrix metalloproteinase (MT1-MMP) with tissue inhibitor of metalloproteinase (TIMP)-2 using the haemopexin domain of the protease as a carrier: a targeted approach in cancer inhibition. Oncotarget. 10.18632/oncotarget.15165
91. Itoh Y, Seiki M (2006) MT1-MMP: a potent modifier of pericellular microenvironment. J Cell Physiol 206:1):1–1):8. https://doi.org/10.1002/jcp.20431
92. Isaacson KJ, Martin Jensen M, Subrahmanyam NB et al (2017) Matrix-metalloproteinases as targets for controlled delivery in cancer: an analysis of upregulation and expression. J Control Release. https://doi.org/10.1016/j.jconrel.2017.01.034
93. Marchenko GN, Ratnikov BI, Rozanov DV et al (2001) Characterization of matrix metalloproteinase-26, a novel metalloproteinase widely expressed in cancer cells of epithelial origin. Biochem J 356(Pt 3):705–718
94. www.clinicaltrials.gov.
95. Tauro M, McGuire J, Lynch CC (2014) New approaches to selectively target cancer-associated matrix metalloproteinase activity. Cancer Metastasis Rev 33(4):1043–1057. https://doi.org/10.1007/s10555-014-9530-4
96. Raffetto JD, Khalil RA (2008) Matrix metalloproteinases and their inhibitors in vascular remodeling and vascular disease. Biochem Pharmacol 75(2):346–359. https://doi.org/10.1016/j.bcp.2007.07.004
97. Milia-Argeiti E, Huet E, Labropoulou VT et al (2012) Imbalance of MMP-2 and MMP-9 expression versus TIMP-1 and

TIMP-2 reflects increased invasiveness of human testicular germ cell tumours. Int J Androl 35(6):835–844. https://doi.org/10.1111/j.1365-2605.2012.01289.x
98. Aaberg-Jessen C, Christensen K, Offenberg H et al (2009) Low expression of tissue inhibitor of metalloproteinases-1 (TIMP-1) in glioblastoma predicts longer patient survival. J Neuro-Oncol 95(1):117–128. https://doi.org/10.1007/s11060-009-9910-8
99. Dechaphunkul A, Phukaoloun M, Kanjanapradit K et al (2012) Prognostic significance of tissue inhibitor of metalloproteinase-1 in breast cancer. Int J Breast Cancer 2012:290854. https://doi.org/10.1155/2012/290854
100. Jackson HW, Defamie V, Waterhouse P et al (2017) TIMPs: versatile extracellular regulators in cancer. Nat Rev Cancer 17(1):38–53. https://doi.org/10.1038/nrc.2016.115
101. Zurac S, Neagu M, Constantin C et al (2016) Variations in the expression of TIMP1, TIMP2 and TIMP3 in cutaneous melanoma with regression and their possible function as prognostic predictors. Oncol Lett 11(5):3354–3360. https://doi.org/10.3892/ol.2016.4391
102. Arkadash V, Yosef G, Shirian J et al (2017) Development of high affinity and high specificity inhibitors of matrix metalloproteinase 14 through computational design and directed evolution. J Biol Chem 292(8):3481–3495. https://doi.org/10.1074/jbc.M116.756718
103. Oh J, Takahashi R, Kondo S et al (2001) The membrane-anchored MMP inhibitor RECK is a key regulator of extracellular matrix integrity and angiogenesis. Cell 107(6):789–800
104. Herman MP, Sukhova GK, Kisiel W et al (2001) Tissue factor pathway inhibitor-2 is a novel inhibitor of matrix metalloproteinases with implications for atherosclerosis. J Clin Invest 107(9):1117–1126. https://doi.org/10.1172/JCI10403
105. Mott JD, Thomas CL, Rosenbach MT et al (2000) Post-translational proteolytic processing of procollagen C-terminal proteinase enhancer releases a metalloproteinase inhibitor. J Biol Chem 275(2):1384–1390
106. Lai YH, He RY, Chou JL et al (2014) Promoter hypermethylation and silencing of tissue factor pathway inhibitor-2 in oral squamous cell carcinoma. J Transl Med 12:237. https://doi.org/10.1186/s12967-014-0237-7
107. Sun FK, Sun Q, Fan YC et al (2016) Methylation of tissue factor pathway inhibitor 2 as a prognostic biomarker for hepatocellular carcinoma after hepatectomy. J Gastroenterol Hepatol 31(2):484–492. https://doi.org/10.1111/jgh.13154
108. Rasmussen HS, McCann PP (1997) Matrix metalloproteinase inhibition as a novel anticancer strategy: a review with special focus on batimastat and marimastat. Pharmacol Ther 75(1):69–75
109. Breyholz HJ, Wagner S, Levkau B et al (2007) A 18F-radiolabeled analogue of CGS 27023A as a potential agent for assessment of matrix-metalloproteinase activity in vivo. Q J Nucl Med Mol Imaging 51(1):24–32
110. Kopka K, Breyholz HJ, Wagner S et al (2004) Synthesis and preliminary biological evaluation of new radioiodinated MMP inhibitors for imaging MMP activity in vivo. Nucl Med Biol 31(2):257–267. https://doi.org/10.1016/j.nucmedbio.2003.08.003
111. Rao BG (2005) Recent developments in the design of specific matrix metalloproteinase inhibitors aided by structural and computational studies. Curr Pharm Des 11(3):295–322
112. Coussens LM, Fingleton B, Matrisian LM (2002) Matrix metalloproteinase inhibitors and cancer: trials and tribulations. Science 295(5564):2387–2392. https://doi.org/10.1126/science.1067100
113. Hirte H, Vergote IB, Jeffrey JR et al (2006) A phase III randomized trial of BAY 12-9566 (tanomastat) as maintenance therapy in patients with advanced ovarian cancer responsive to primary surgery and paclitaxel/platinum containing chemotherapy: a National Cancer Institute of Canada Clinical Trials Group Study. Gynecol Oncol 102(2):300–308. https://doi.org/10.1016/j.ygyno.2005.12.020
114. Remacle AG, Golubkov VS, Shiryaev SA et al (2012) Novel MT1-MMP small-molecule inhibitors based on insights into hemopexin domain function in tumor growth. Cancer Res 72(9):2339–2349. https://doi.org/10.1158/0008-5472.CAN-11-4149
115. Devy L, Dransfield DT (2011) New strategies for the next generation of matrix-metalloproteinase inhibitors: selectively targeting membrane-anchored mmps with therapeutic antibodies. Biochem Res Int 2011:191670. https://doi.org/10.1155/2011/191670
116. Hiroyuki O (2005) The pathogenic contribution of matrix metalloproteinases to lung cancer. Focus on lung cancer research. Nova Science Publishers, Inc., Hauppauge, NY
117. Amar S, Fields GB (2015) Potential clinical implications of recent matrix metalloproteinase inhibitor design strategies. Expert Rev Proteomics 12(5):445–447. https://doi.org/10.1586/14789450.2015.1069190
118. Chelluboina B, Nalamolu KR, Klopfenstein JD et al (2017) MMP-12, a promising thera-

peutic target for neurological diseases. Mol Neurobiol. https://doi.org/10.1007/s12035-017-0418-5
119. Gingras D, Batist G, Béliveau R (2001) Æ-941 (Neovastat®): a novel multifunctional antiangiogenic compound. Expert Rev Anticancer Ther 1(3):341–347. https://doi.org/10.1586/14737140.1.3.341
120. Gingras D, Boivin D, Deckers C et al (2003) Neovastat—a novel antiangiogenic drug for cancer therapy. Anti-Cancer Drugs 14(2):91–96. https://doi.org/10.1097/01.cad.0000054520.85618.3f
121. Poulaki V (2002) BMS-275291. bristol-myers squibb. Curr Opin Investig Drugs 3(3):500–504
122. Chiappori AA, Eckhardt SG, Bukowski R et al (2007) A phase I pharmacokinetic and pharmacodynamic study of s-3304, a novel matrix metalloproteinase inhibitor, in patients with advanced and refractory solid tumors. Clin Cancer Res 13(7):2091–2099. https://doi.org/10.1158/1078-0432.CCR-06-1586
123. Devy L, Huang L, Naa L et al (2009) Selective inhibition of matrix metalloproteinase-14 blocks tumor growth, invasion, and angiogenesis. Cancer Res 69(4):1517–1526. https://doi.org/10.1158/0008-5472.CAN-08-3255
124. Lemaitre V, D'Armiento J (2006) Matrix metalloproteinases in development and disease. Birth Defects Res C Embryo Today 78(1):1–10. https://doi.org/10.1002/bdrc.20065
125. Paemen L, Martens E, Masure S et al (1995) Monoclonal antibodies specific for natural human neutrophil gelatinase B used for affinity purification, quantitation by two-site ELISA and inhibition of enzymatic activity. Eur J Biochem 234(3):759–765
126. Martens E, Leyssen A, Van Aelst I et al (2007) A monoclonal antibody inhibits gelatinase B/MMP-9 by selective binding to part of the catalytic domain and not to the fibronectin or zinc binding domains. Biochim Biophys Acta 1770(2):178–186. https://doi.org/10.1016/j.bbagen.2006.10.012
127. Hu J, Van den Steen PE, Houde M et al (2004) Inhibitors of gelatinase B/matrix metalloproteinase-9 activity comparison of a peptidomimetic and polyhistidine with single-chain derivatives of a neutralizing monoclonal antibody. Biochem Pharmacol 67(5):1001–1009
128. Marshall DC, Lyman SK, McCauley S et al (2015) Selective allosteric inhibition of MMP9 is efficacious in preclinical models of ulcerative colitis and colorectal cancer. PLoS One 10(5):–e0127063. https://doi.org/10.1371/journal.pone.0127063
129. Ibrahim SA, Hassan H, Gotte M (2014) MicroRNA-dependent targeting of the extracellular matrix as a mechanism of regulating cell behavior. Biochim Biophys Acta 1840(8):2609–2620. https://doi.org/10.1016/j.bbagen.2014.01.022
130. Ma L, Teruya-Feldstein J, Weinberg RA (2007) Tumour invasion and metastasis initiated by microRNA-10b in breast cancer. Nature 449(7163):682–688. https://doi.org/10.1038/nature06174
131. Dai X, Chen A, Bai Z (2014) Integrative investigation on breast cancer in ER, PR and HER2-defined subgroups using mRNA and miRNA expression profiling. Sci Rep 4:6566. https://doi.org/10.1038/srep06566
132. Ibrahim SA, Hassan H, Gotte M (2014) MicroRNA regulation of proteoglycan function in cancer. FEBS J 281(22):5009–5022. https://doi.org/10.1111/febs.13026
133. Vigetti D, Viola M, Karousou E et al (2014) Epigenetics in extracellular matrix remodeling and hyaluronan metabolism. FEBS J 281(22):4980–4992. https://doi.org/10.1111/febs.12938
134. Ibrahim SA, Yip GW, Stock C et al (2012) Targeting of syndecan-1 by microRNA miR-10b promotes breast cancer cell motility and invasiveness via a Rho-GTPase- and E-cadherin-dependent mechanism. Int J Cancer 131(6):E884–E896. https://doi.org/10.1002/ijc.27629
135. Xu B, Li YY, Ma J et al (2016) Roles of microRNA and signaling pathway in osteoarthritis pathogenesis. J Zhejiang Univ Sci B 17(3):200–208. https://doi.org/10.1631/jzus.B1500267
136. Li L, Li H (2013) Role of microRNA-mediated MMP regulation in the treatment and diagnosis of malignant tumors. Cancer Biol Ther 14(9):796–805. https://doi.org/10.4161/cbt.25936
137. Gabriely G, Wurdinger T, Kesari S et al (2008) MicroRNA 21 promotes glioma invasion by targeting matrix metalloproteinase regulators. Mol Cell Biol 28(17):5369–5380. https://doi.org/10.1128/MCB.00479-08
138. Costa PM, Cardoso AL, Custodia C et al (2015) MiRNA-21 silencing mediated by tumor-targeted nanoparticles combined with sunitinib: a new multimodal gene therapy approach for glioblastoma. J Control Release 207:31–39. https://doi.org/10.1016/j.jconrel.2015.04.002
139. White NM, Fatoohi E, Metias M et al (2011) Metastamirs: a stepping stone towards improved cancer management. Nat Rev Clin Oncol 8(2):75–84. https://doi.org/10.1038/nrclinonc.2010.173

140. Hwang SJ, Seol HJ, Park YM et al (2012) MicroRNA-146a suppresses metastatic activity in brain metastasis. Mol Cells 34(3):329–334. https://doi.org/10.1007/s10059-012-0171-6
141. Hu Y, Ou Y, Wu K et al (2012) miR-143 inhibits the metastasis of pancreatic cancer and an associated signaling pathway. Tumour Biol 33(6):1863–1870. https://doi.org/10.1007/s13277-012-0446-8
142. Osaki M, Takeshita F, Sugimoto Y et al (2011) MicroRNA-143 regulates human osteosarcoma metastasis by regulating matrix metalloprotease-13 expression. Mol Ther 19(6):1123–1130. https://doi.org/10.1038/mt.2011.53
143. Wang Q, Cai J, Wang J et al (2014) MiR-143 inhibits EGFR-signaling-dependent osteosarcoma invasion. Tumour Biol 35(12):12743–12748. https://doi.org/10.1007/s13277-014-2600-y
144. Voinea M, Simionescu M (2002) Designing of 'intelligent' liposomes for efficient delivery of drugs. J Cell Mol Med 6(4):465–474
145. Hatakeyama H, Akita H, Ishida E et al (2007) Tumor targeting of doxorubicin by anti-MT1-MMP antibody-modified PEG liposomes. Int J Pharm 342(1–2):194–200. https://doi.org/10.1016/j.ijpharm.2007.04.037
146. Zhu L, Kate P, Torchilin VP (2012) Matrix metalloprotease 2-responsive multifunctional liposomal nanocarrier for enhanced tumor targeting. ACS Nano 6(4):3491–3498. https://doi.org/10.1021/nn300524f
147. Banerjee J, Hanson AJ, Gadam B et al (2009) Release of liposomal contents by cell-secreted matrix metalloproteinase-9. Bioconjug Chem 20(7):1332–1339. https://doi.org/10.1021/bc9000646
148. Nel A, Xia T, Madler L et al (2006) Toxic potential of materials at the nanolevel. Science 311(5761):622–627. https://doi.org/10.1126/science.1114397
149. Piperigkou Z, Karamanou K, Engin AB et al (2016) Emerging aspects of nanotoxicology in health and disease: from agriculture and food sector to cancer therapeutics. Food Chem Toxicol 91:42–57. https://doi.org/10.1016/j.fct.2016.03.003
150. Neagu M, Piperigkou Z, Karamanou K et al (2017) Protein bio-corona: critical issue in immune nanotoxicology. Arch Toxicol 91(3):1031–1048. https://doi.org/10.1007/s00204-016-1797-5
151. Piperigkou Z, Karamanou K, Afratis NA et al (2016) Biochemical and toxicological evaluation of nano-heparins in cell functional properties, proteasome activation and expression of key matrix molecules. Toxicol Lett 240(1):32–42. https://doi.org/10.1016/j.toxlet.2015.10.005
152. Hashimoto M, Sasaki JI, Yamaguchi S et al (2015) Gold nanoparticles inhibit matrix metalloproteases without cytotoxicity. J Dent Res 94(8):1085–1091. https://doi.org/10.1177/0022034515589282
153. Zhang J, Yuan ZF, Wang Y et al (2013) Multifunctional envelope-type mesoporous silica nanoparticles for tumor-triggered targeting drug delivery. J Am Chem Soc 135(13):5068–5073. https://doi.org/10.1021/ja312004m

INDEX

Santiago Cal and Alvaro J. Obaya (eds.), *Proteases and Cancer: Methods and Protocols*, Methods in Molecular Biology, vol. 1731, https://doi.org/10.1007/978-1-4939-7595-2, © Springer Science+Business Media, LLC 2018

MIX
Papier aus verantwortungsvollen Quellen
Paper from responsible sources
FSC® C105338

If you have any concerns about our products,
you can contact us on
ProductSafety@springernature.com

In case Publisher is established outside the EU,
the EU authorized representative is:
Springer Nature Customer Service Center GmbH
Europaplatz 3, 69115 Heidelberg, Germany

Printed by Libri Plureos GmbH
in Hamburg, Germany